Shinji Takahashi

An Atlas of Axial Transverse Tomography and its Clinical Application

With 576 Figures

Springer-Verlag Berlin · Heidelberg · New York 1969

SHINJI TAKAHASHI, M. D.
Professor of Radiology, Nagoya University School of Medicine,
Showaku, Nagoya, Japan

 Library of Congress Catalog Card Number 76—82421. Printed in Germany

Title-No. 1559

Preface

In spring this year it will be 23 years since I began to study rotation technique as applied to radiology. In applying this technique to roentgenography the name Rotation Radiography was adopted publicly in 1946. Since then this study has revealed that the technique is valuable not only in diagnosis but also in radiotherapy, and the name Conformation Radiotherapy was publicly announced in 1960.

Through these studies it became clear that it is possible to show the axial transverse cross section of the human body roentgenographically, which could be of great value medically, but it was realized that no detailed roentgenograms of the axial transverse cross section covering the whole of the normal human adult have been published so far. To prepare an atlas was therefore considered basic for the practical application of this method, since without it further developments of this type of roentgenography cannot be expected. Consequently it was decided first to prepare the atlas. In addition, the clinical application of this method to the diagnostic and therapeutic field was described with brief notes on the essential features of the method.

This work was planned a few years ago, but actual work commenced in September 1966. A further year was spent in the preparation of the manuscript, and its publication was made possible by the help of numerous coworkers. The preparation of the axial transverse tomograms has been our direct responsibility, but the revision of the anatomical diagrams drawn by us was made by courtesy of Dr. *Seiho Nishi*, Professor Emeritus of Anatomy, Tokyo University. The preparation of this book was made possible by the help of members of our Department staffs, especially of Drs. *T. Sasaki*, *S. Sakuma* and *A. Takeuchi*. In addition, Drs. *F. Hayashi*, *K. Ban*, *K. Hiramatsu*, *Y. Ayakawa*, *T. Fujita*, *T. Kato*, *S. Koga*, *Y. Tanaka* and others cooperated in the preparation of the respective figures, Mr. *K. Ito* in the conduct of the radiography, Mr. *R. Ando* in the preparation of the photographs, Mr. *H. Maekoshi* in the drawing of the anatomical figures and Miss *T. Nishikawa* in the arrangement and printing of the original manuscripts. Dr. *K. Morita* of the Czerny Krankenhaus, Heidelberg, kept in close contact with the publisher to expedite the printing. Dr. *T. Oyama* undertook the labors of translating one part of the manuscript from Japanese to English.

For the final decision of publication by Springer-Verlag, Professor *O. Olsson*, Lund, kindly gave recommendations and advice to me and the publisher.

I wish to take this opportunity to express my deep appreciation to all these persons.

Nagoya, May 1969 *Shinji Takahashi*

Contents

Introduction 1

Part 1. Axial Transverse Tomography of the Normal Adult 3

I. Conduct of Axial Transverse Tomography 5

1. Tomographic Apparatus 5

A. Roentgenography of Every Part of the Body 5

B. Quality of Image on the Tomogram 6

C. Low Magnification Rate of Image 8

D. Removal of Obstructive Shadows 8

2. Tomographic Technique 12

II. Interpretation of Axial Transverse Tomogram 13

Head 15

Neck 53

Chest 81

Upper Abdomen 139

Lower Abdomen 179

Arm 219

Leg 225

Part 2. Clinical Applications of Axial Transverse Tomography 233

Introduction 235

I. Application to Diagnosis 237

1. Features of Axial Transverse Tomography 237

2. Establishment of Diagnosis for Clinical Cases 241

II. Application to Pretherapeutic Procedure 289

1. Radiation Therapy 289

A. Planning for Irradiation 298

1. Determination of Region to be Treated 298

2. Selection of Irradiation Technique 299

B. Positioning of Patient 299

C. Confirmation of Correct Positioning 301

2. Surgical Operation 304

References 307

Author Index 315

Subject Index 319

Introduction

Knowledge of roentgenological anatomy is essential in roentgen diagnosis, as only when the normal state of the human body is known can abnormal, i.e. pathological findings be ascertained roentgenologically.

As for the axial transverse tomography, *de Abreau* (1), *Amisano* (4, 6), *Duhamel* et al. (19), *Frain* et al. (24—26, 28), *Gebauer* and *Wachsmann* (32), *Gebauer* (33), *Justztusz* (47), *de Maestri* (59), *Shimazaki* (117, 116), *Stevenson* (119,) *Takahashi* (121, 122, 126, 128), *Takahashi* et al. (123, 124, 129), *Vieten* (161), *Watson* (167) and especially *Vallebona* (147—158) have worked as pioneers in determining the fundamentals of this method of roentgenography or in applying this method to roentgen diagnosis.

In several European countries this roentgenographic method was developed from tomography, while in Japan it grew out of rotation radiography rather than the method of tomography.

The terms of this method thus differed individually, but in accordance with the recommendation of ICRU (1962) (p. 15, NBS Handbook 80) the term "axial transverse tomography" may perhaps be the most fitting.

This method is useful not only for diagnosis but also in undertaking treatment, especially in the field of radiotherapy, as it is necessary to know accurately and concretely the state of the lesion in the body, to set up an irradiation plan and to confirm whether or not the plan is being carried out properly. Such planning and confirmation are difficult to carry out by means of existing radiography methods alone. Axial transverse tomography can solve these problems, and thus it is believed that it should be used more widely in the fields of roentgen diagnosis and radiotherapy.

Monographs on axial transverse tomography, by *Bonte* et al. (169), *Farr* et al. (170), *Gebauer* et al. (171), *Gebauer* et al. (172), *Takahashi* (173—175), *Vallebona* et al. (176), *Vallebona* (177), total nine as far as I could collect, but these are mostly concerned with the diagnosis of chest diseases, though *Gebauer's* work contains good descriptions of almost all parts of the body.

In axial transverse tomography, despite the promise of wide clinical application, there is no monograph that explains systematically and clearly the roentgenological anatomy of every part of the body.

At present, when applying axial transverse tomography to all areas of the body for medical purposes, there is no other way but to refer to existing atlases illustrating anatomical cross sections of such regions prepared from cadavers. The books by *Doyen* et al. (178), *Hovelacque* et al. (179), *Nishi* et al. (180, 181), *Pernkopf* (182), *Roy-Camille* (183) and *Eycleshymer* (184) are listed in the bibliography. Distortion is sometimes seen in the figures due to their preparation post mortem. Further, some troubles arise because there is no way to refer the roentgen findings to the whole cadaver because the relevant roentgenogram is missing. In addition, an atlas containing cross-section figures of all parts of the human body in systematic order with thin layers of cross section is not usually obtainable even as an anatomical atlas.

These are the direct reasons for the publication of our monograph which takes as its subject the living standard adult.

To prepare the atlas of axial transverse tomograms, the level to be imaged should be determined as accurately as possible as, when the level in relation to the body axis at which the section is made moves even slightly, the appearance of the sectional figures will differ greatly. Again, unless the atlas of the axial transverse cross section is made systematically by one and the same author, there will be differences in the style of illustrating the axial transverse tomograms. One author will illustrate the figure of the axial transverse cross section right side left or left side right, and the other upside down or down side up, and this will cause confusion in the interpretation of tomograms based on such figures. It is hoped that the preparation of this atlas will contribute to the correction of such defects and drawbacks in existing books.

To avoid guesswork when giving anatomical interpretations of the cross sections, contrast medium was used as often as possible in order to obtain roentgen images of the various viscera and tissues. It was, of course, not possible to prepare roentgenograms of all body regions from the same individual. Needless to say, this was due to consideration of the roentgen dose to which the individual is exposed. The concentrated use of various contrast media was also avoided, as some of these media are not always harmless, and the administration of different contrast media can be a burden to the subject used. In other words, the study could fall into a study for its own sake. In view of the above, the subjects to be examined were made to vary in accordance with the several parts of the body and roentgen images of various organs of the same body region were prepared with or without the use of contrast medium and the diagrams of the anatomical figures were prepared by integration of these images.

Part 1

Axial Transverse Tomography of the Normal Adult

I. Conduct of Axial Transverse Tomography

A description will be made of the apparatus and of the tomographic procedure used in the preparation of this Atlas.

1. Tomographic Apparatus

Axial transverse tomography has been developed over the last twenty years. After the clinical value of this technique was proved by the pioneers, roentgenographic units for taking axial transverse tomograms have been commercially manufactured in Italy, France and Germany, and soon after in Japan. Most of this apparatus was of the type for taking tomograms of sitting or standing patients, e.g. axial transverse tomograph of erect type. In addition to this type, a unit for taking tomograms of lying patients, axial transverse tomograph of horizontal type, was suggested as superior to the erect type by *Janker* (45) and *Takahashi* (121, 128, 175), and a unit of this type has been manufactured since 1950 and is widely used in Japan.

Roentgenography here was carried out by an axial transverse tomograph of horizontal type. The patient is made to lie still on the tomography table while the roentgen tube and film are rotated around the patient from 0° to 360°. This apparatus was originally designed and manufactured to work with the range of rotation from 0° to 210°. Although a perfect image is obtained with the range of rotation of 360° (*Oliva* (83), *Bonte* et al. (169), *Frik* (29)), the range of rotation of 210° also provides good tomograms, suitable for clinical practice, when the following technique is applied as described below (*Takahashi* (124, 129)).

A. Roentgenography of Every Part of the Body

The tomographic table is made of wood and is 30 cm wide, 5.4 cm thick and 354 cm long. The rotation axis of the unit is approximately 12 cm above the surface of the tomography table. The position of the plane g to be cross sectioned, i.e. to be tomographed, is specific to the apparatus and is about 142.5 cm from the end of the table to which the tomography unit is attached. The plane g is the place where the lights converge from projectors located on both walls and on the bar of the support of the roentgen tube (T_1) for tomography. Hence, the part of the subject to be tomographed is easily adjusted to this plane g by means of the light projectors (Figs. 1 and 2).

The tomography table is approximately 2 times the length of the human body, so it is possible to place any part of the body on plane g with ease. With a unit of the erect type, it is usually difficult to take an axial transverse tomogram of every part of the body, though there is a paper on examination of the extremities made by means of this type of tomograph (*Lacroix* (51)).

In axial transverse tomography a normal roentgenogram of the body part to be tomographed is also taken with the patient in the same posture. On this normal roentgenogram the axial transverse level of the body at which the tomography is made should be clearly indicated. The location of the plane g crosses the focus of the roentgen tube T_2 fixed to the ceiling, while the cassette holder B is placed horizontally below the table. On the front cover of the cassette, either right across or halfway across, a lead line is placed to meet or coincide with the plane g. Directly before or after the axial transverse tomography, a normal roentgenogram of the part of the body being tomographed is taken with roentgen tube T_2 and film B.

When the subject to be examined lies supine on the bare table, the X-ray absorption rates of the soft tissues of the body are approximately equal to those of the tomography table and cause the contours of the dorsal regions of the body to be indistinct, due to lack of contrast between them. Hence, a cotton mat 3 cm thick is placed on the tomography table. This procedure makes it possible to produce a roentgen image of the entire contour of the cross section of the body by axial transverse tomography.

B. Quality of Image on the Tomogram

In general, the nearer contour of the body imaged on the axial transverse tomogram is too dense and renders interpretation between that part and the ground density of the tomogram difficult. Hence, a moving filter (*Matsuda* (72, 73)) was attached to the radiation mouth of the tube housing. This made the density of the contour and the ground density reasonable and made interpretation easy (Fig. 3).

Next, a wedge grid whose grid ratio is high at one side and low at the opposite side was placed with the high grid ratio close to the body and the grid itself perpendicular to the central X-rays and covering the entire area of the film (*Matsuda* (75)). This helped to remove the fog induced by scattered rays increasing at the parts of the film close to the body, and generally to improve the contrast of the tomograms.

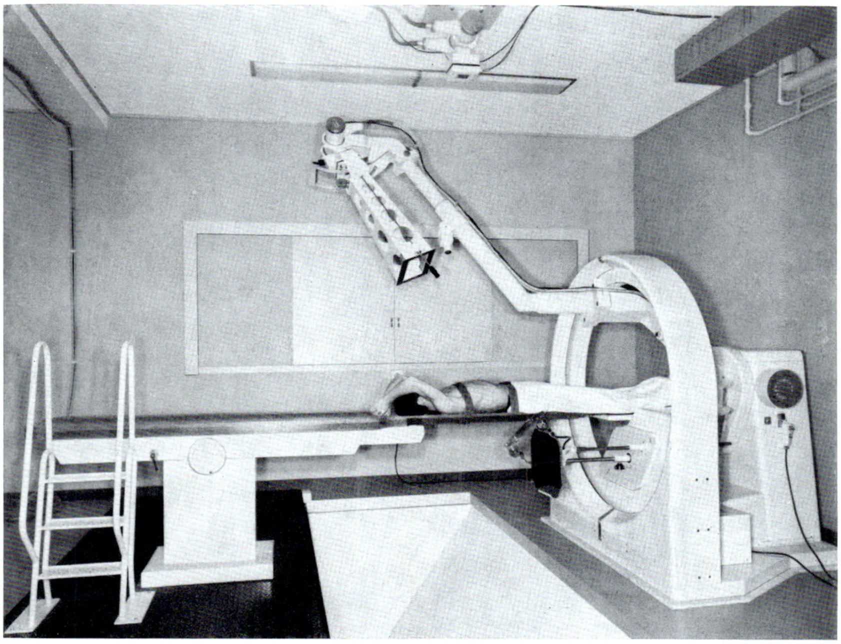

Fig. 1. Axial transverse tomograph of horizontal type (Toshiba) in action

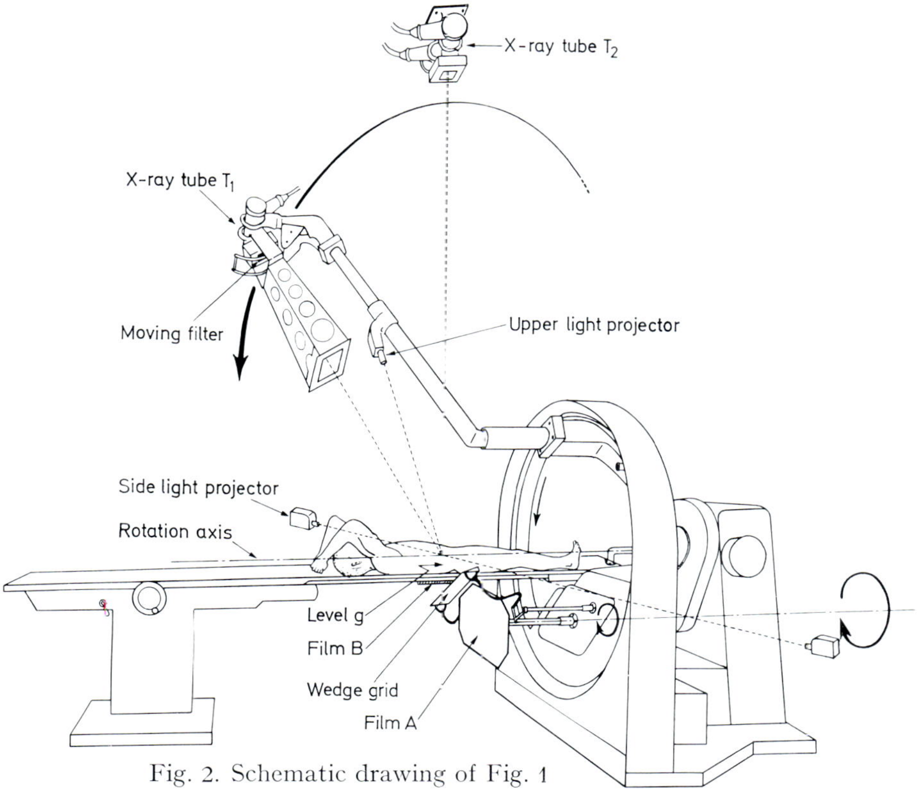

Fig. 2. Schematic drawing of Fig. 1

As these axial transverse tomograms are taken by high voltage technique (125 kVp), the contrast of bony tissues is poor as compared with that taken by low voltage technique. However, as soft tissue and bony tissue are reasonably distinct, the taking of tomograms by high voltage technique does not hinder the establishment of correct diagnoses. Moreover, high voltage technique has the advantage of removing the obstructive shadow, harmonising density and reducing the dose to which the patient is exposed during tomography (*Matsuda* (70), *Takahashi* (138)). As the angle of inclination of the central X-ray to the film is rather small, i.e. 20° in this tomography, the thickness of the layer is thin. As compared with the 30° usual in other countries, contrast of images is lower but obstructive shadows are markedly decreased (*Takahashi* (123)).

In this apparatus the play of the rotation axis during rotation is negligible. The adjustment of the alignment of the focus of the tube, rotation centers of the X-ray unit and the film was checked (*Matsuda* (74)).

The focus of the X-ray tube is small, 1 mm in size, while the capacity of the tube is fairly large with the maximal voltage of 150 kVp. 67 mA for 15 seconds.

As a result the penumbra of the roentgenograms is small, while the sharpness of the image is very good. Even with such a small bone as the lingual bone, the images were so sharp as to render differentiation of the substantia compacta from the substantia spongiosa possible.

C. Low Magnification Rate of Image

In this apparatus the distance between the tube focus and rotation axis is 212.5 cm, while that between the rotation center of the apparatus and that of the film is 62.5 cm, with a magnification rate of 1.24 times.

For roentgenography of the chest and abdomen a film of 14 × 17 inch size was used. The rectangular cassette is cut away at its 4 corners. The cassette is placed as near as possible to the rotation center of the apparatus. As the magnification rate of the image is small, the entire contours of the axial transverse cross section of the normal standard Japanese body can be contained within the film with exception of the upper part of the chest. This is convenient for diagnosis as well as for the planning of therapy.

D. Removal of Obstructive Shadows

Obstructive shadows are a problem for the establishment of correct diagnosis, especially in tomography of the chest (*Takahashi* et al. (130), *Takahashi* (134)).

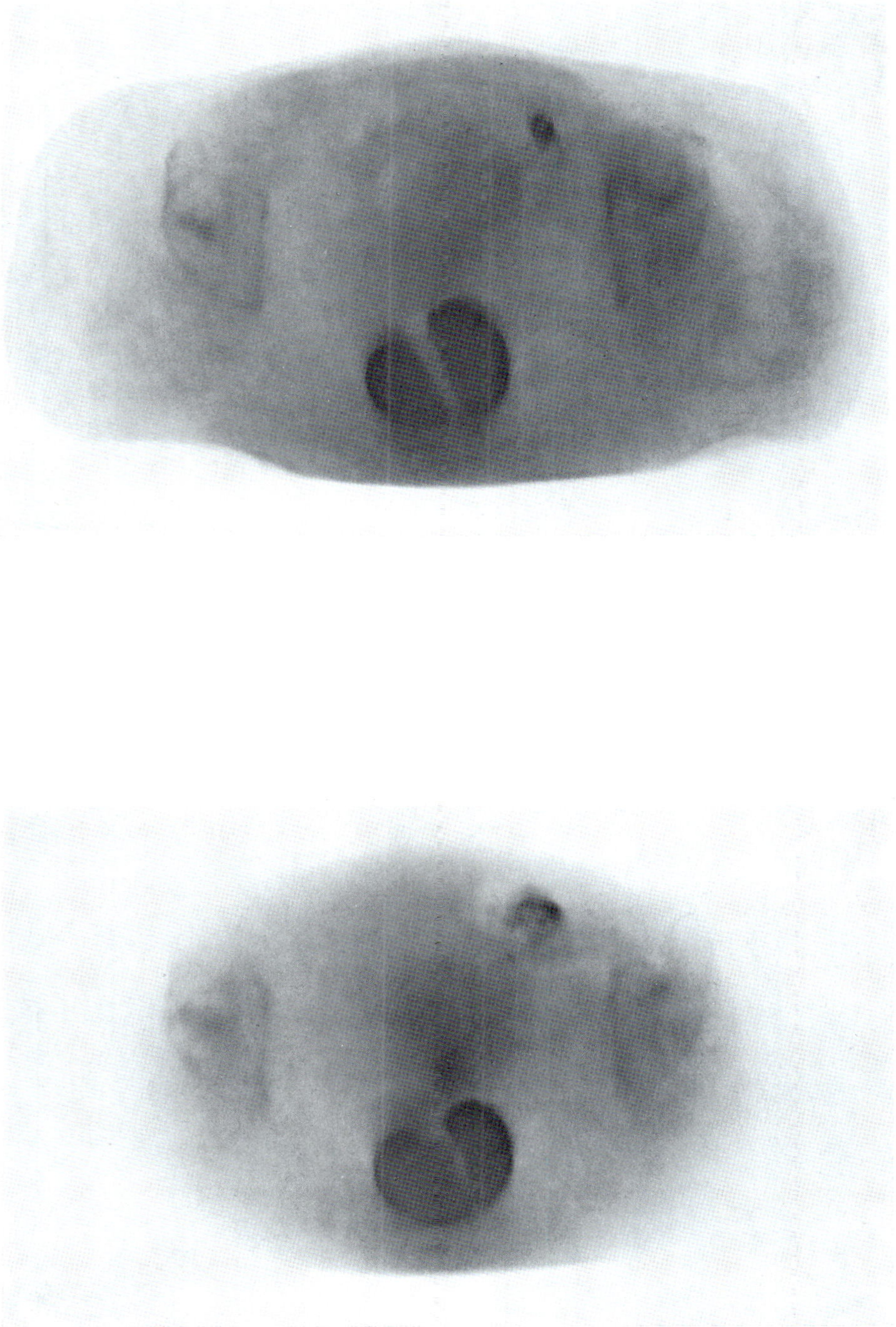

A

B

Fig. 3 A and B. Axial transverse tomograms of the pelvis at the same level in the same person. A with moving filter. B without moving filter. Entire contour of the body is seen perfectly on A, but imperfectly on B

Obstructive shadows that look like rib shadows in the lung field, or linear shadows imaged sagittally along the thoracic spine to the posterior lung field will induce the wrong diagnosis.

In order to reduce the frequency of occurrence of these shadows a) the inclination angle of the tube (inclination of the central X-ray to the film) is reduced to 20°; b) the central X-ray is inclined from the head to the feet i.e. craniocaudal direction of the central X-ray (*Takeuchi* (143, 144)); c) if possible, the range of rotation is made complete, i.e. rotate from 0° to 360°; and d) exposure is made with the high voltage technique. Clinically, the range of rotation from 0° to 220° is considered suitable and satisfactory, as the size of the room is usually limited and the obstructive shadow does not usually interfere with correct diagnosis, if the axial transverse tomography is carried out with the central X-ray directed craniocaudally to the supine patient. In the preparation of this Atlas, however, the tube was rotated from 0° to 360°, because increasing the range of rotation to 360° happens sometimes to eliminate the obstructive shadows found with 0° to 220° (Fig. 4). Obstructive shadows become practically negligible and it is thus possible to prepare standard illustrations of axial transverse cross sections of the body. In regions other than the chest these obstructive shadows do not usually appear and it is thus not necessary to rotate the tube from 0° to 360°. However, in order to maintain the standardized exposure conditions, the inclination angle of the tube and range of rotation were not changed throughout.

Fig. 4A—C. Overlap of obstructive shadow of ribs into the lung field. Axial transverse tomograms of the chest at the same level in the same person. A rotation angle of 360°: negligible obstructive shadow (↗). B rotation angle of 220°, with the craniocaudal direction of central X-ray: slight obstructive shadow (↗). C rotation angle of 220°, with the caudalocranial direction of central X-ray: excessive obstructive shadow (↗)

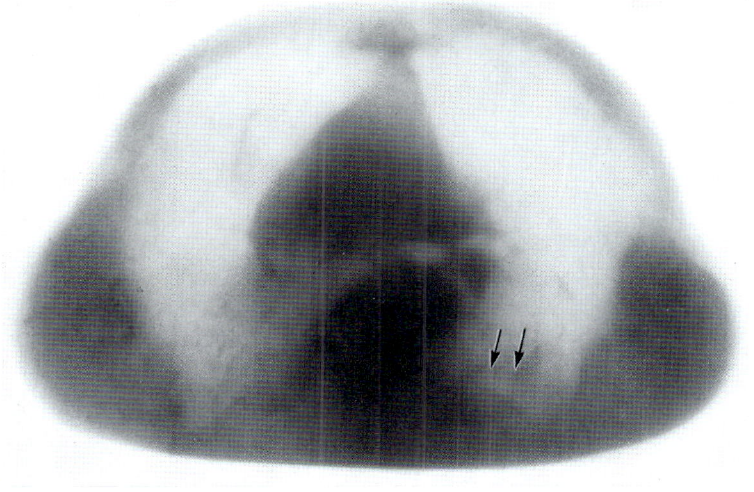
A

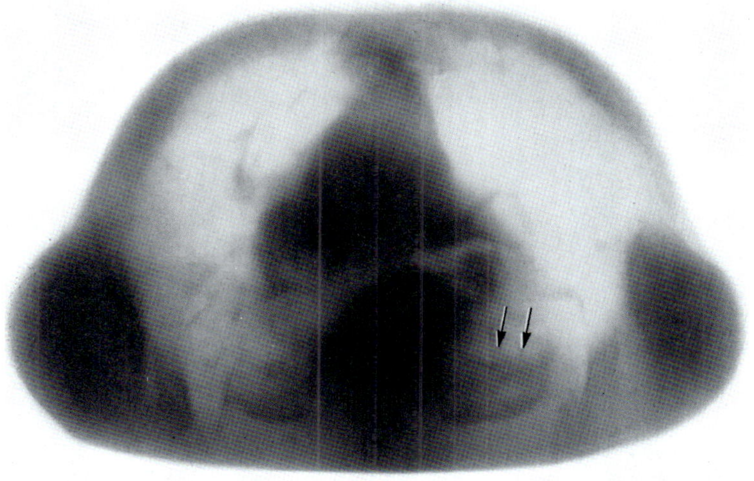
B

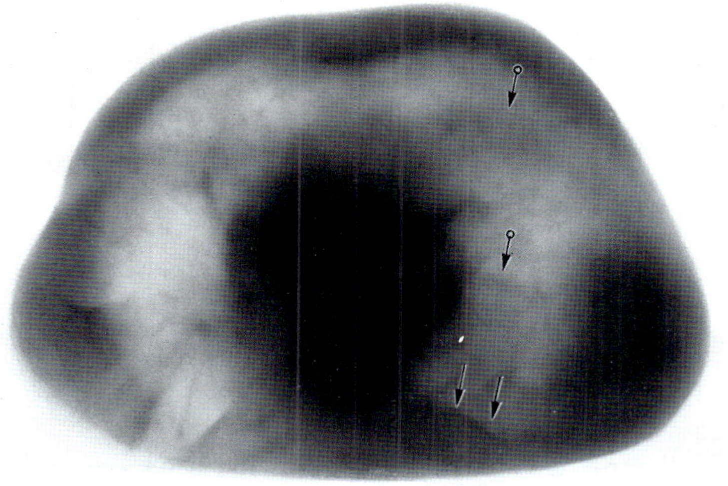
C

2. Tomographic Technique

The subject is made to lie on the mat of the roentgenography table on his back, and the transverse section of the part of the body to be tomographed is adjusted to the lights from the projectors. A normal roentgenogram is taken with the X-ray tube (T_2) secured to the ceiling, with the body kept still and the subject holding his breath. The roentgenographic conditions for various body regions are shown in Table 1. All persons used as subjects in the illustration of this Atlas are cancer patients who have passed the reproductive age. The parts selected to be tomographed are normal. For example, in tomography of the chest a patient suffering from the cancer of uterus is employed, with no abnormal findings in the chest, either clinically or roentgenologically. The patients were told of the nature of this Atlas and agreed to take part in the preparation of illustrations. In order to show the tissues and organs of the sections as clearly as possible on the tomogram, contrast medium is employed. In preparing the illustrations of the upper abdomen or the neck, air is insufflated into the retro-peritoneal or mediastinal space before the tomography is carried out. Without such a procedure the findings on the tomograms will be very poor.

Radiation hazards for technicians are negligible as the control room is separate from the tomography room. Exposure of patients per transverse tomography is shown in Table 1. In order to reduce the patient dose, the X-ray beams are prevented from protruding beyond the film by the diaphragm of the radiation mouth. Further, the amount of normal roentgenography was kept to the minimum, although it would have been desirable to take one a.p. roentgenogram with every axial transverse tomography.

Table 1. *Exposure conditions and air dose at the rotation center of the unit for one axial transverse tomography*

	kV	mA	sec	Intensifying screens	Air dose (mR)
Head	110	5	15	MS	150
Neck	95	5	15	MS	100
Chest	120	3	15	MS	110
Abdomen	125	10	15	MS	340
Arm	60—65	5	15	MS	35— 43
Leg	70—90	5	15	MS	50—100

Focus film distance: 262.8 cm. Wedge grid and moving filter used. MS: medium speed screen

II. Interpretation of Axial Transverse Tomogram

Up to the present research work on the individual parts of the body in the normal adult has appeared in several papers: axial transverse encephalotomography was studied by *di Chiro* (17), *Takahashi* et al. (131), the head by *Takahashi* et al. (132), the neck by *Takahashi* (133), the chest by *Duhamel* (26), *Gardella* (31), *Gebauer* (34), *Matsuda* (63), *Ono* (87), *Retzepis* (95), the gall bladder by *Imaoka* (44), the stomach and duodenum by *Matsuda* et al. (65), and *Sasaki* (110), the upper abdomen by the pneumoretroperitoneal technique by *de Albertis* (2), *Macarini* et al. (58), *Matsuda* et al. (66) or *Sasaki* (111) and by the pneumoperitoneal technique by *Sato* (113). The axial transverse tomography of the pelvis was reported by *Kubota* et al. (50).

In this Atlas, series of axial transverse tomograms taken for each level of every part of the human body will be illustrated, the illustrations extending across 2 pages for each level.

First, in order to know at what level and how the tomogram is taken, see the top of the right page, where at top left is shown a normal roentgenogram in the anteroposterior view of the subject taken at time of the transverse tomography; the horizontal line drawn through the roentgenogram represents the level at which the tomography is made. At the top right is a diagram, drawn from normal photographs taken in lateral view at time of tomography, which shows the level relative to the body at which the transverse tomography is carried out.

On the left page a tomogram is shown at the top. In the lower part of this page is a tomogram identical with that at the top but developed with less density and retouched, as it is sometimes difficult to reproduce all the details of the original tomogram. However, it should be emphasized here that *in this retouched illustration of the tomogram only the findings actually seen on the original tomogram are drawn*. In other words, there are no imaginary findings on the figure. The anatomical terms are attached to these roentgen findings to facilitate interpretation.

At the bottom of the right page is a diagram showing as faithfully as possible the topographical relation with the axial transverse tomogram. However, as muscles, tendons, nerves etc. do not produce roentgen images, reference was made to existing anatomical atlases (178—184) and these features were inserted, though compared with these anatomical section figures the muscles have been inserted as simply as possible, due to special stress on the practical utility of this Atlas and the desire to avoid as much as possible the insertion by mere conjecture of findings that did not actually appear. Illustrations and diagrams of the tomogram are reduced accurately to one third the size of the original tomogram.

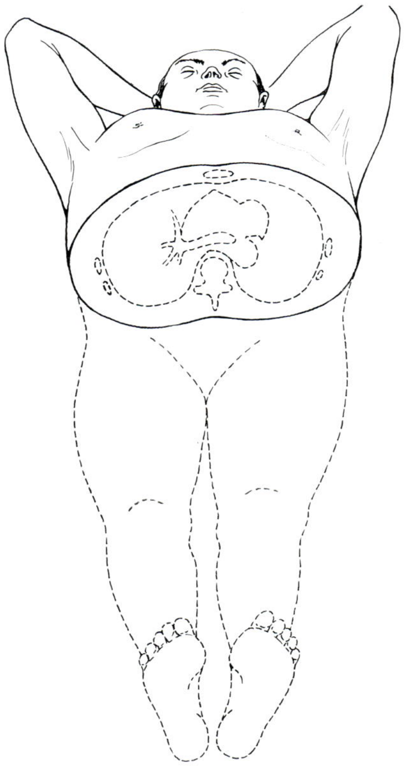

Fig. 5. Schematic drawing of our manner of viewing the axial transverse tomogram. An axial transverse cross section of the upper part of the body is inspected

As indicated in the figures, the transverse section figures were prepared as such for this Atlas (Fig. 5). After cutting the body in the supine position at the required levels of body axis, the lower part is removed and the sectional surface of the upper part observed from the horizontal direction.

This arrangement of the illustrations has been our practice since we developed rotation radiography in 1946 (*Takahashi* (174, 175)) for the following clinical reasons: when an interpretation of the axial transverse tomogram is made, the normal roentgenogram with the horizontal line is placed adjacent to the axial transverse tomogram in the viewing box and examined. For convenience of interpretation, the right of the axial transverse cross section view of the body is better placed to the left of the figure, so as to be similar to the normal roentgenogram taken posteroanteriorly.

This manner of viewing the illustration, that is, with the back of the body at the bottom of the illustration, is convenient for planning the positioning of the patient in radiation therapy.

On the following pages, the axial transverse tomograms are arranged in the order of the head, the neck, the chest, the upper abdomen, the female and male lower abdomen, and the arm and the leg.

Appendices are attached to each group of parts of the body in order to add the information which is difficult to include in the relevant illustrations.

Head

Eight axial transverse tomograms, including encephalotomogram, taken parallel to the orbitomeatal line

and

Ten axial transverse tomograms, including encephalotomogram, taken parallel to the acanthiomeatal line.

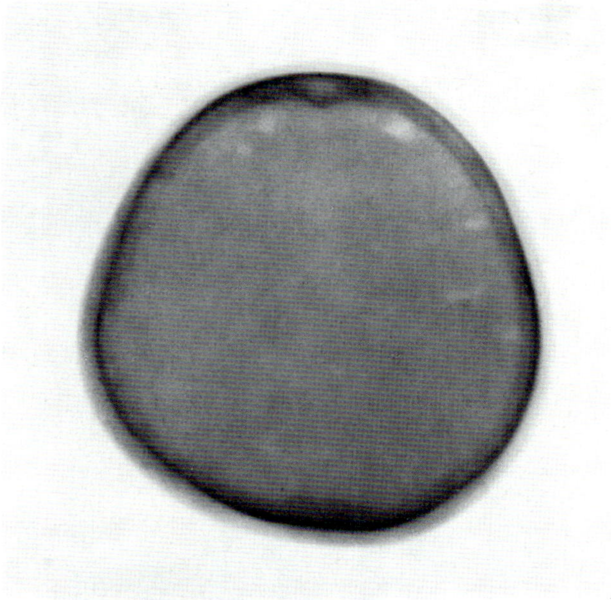

Fig. 6. Axial transverse tomogram

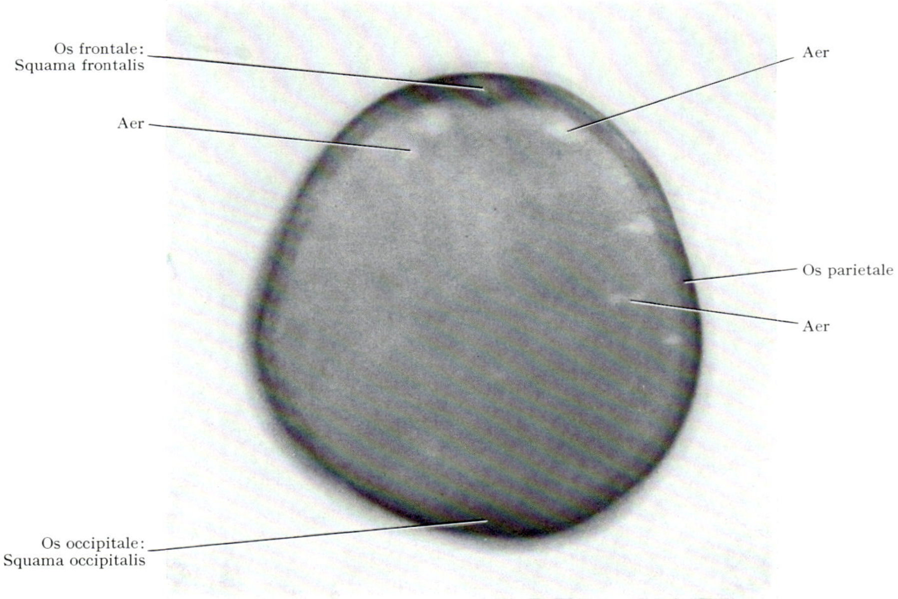

Fig. 7. Interpretation

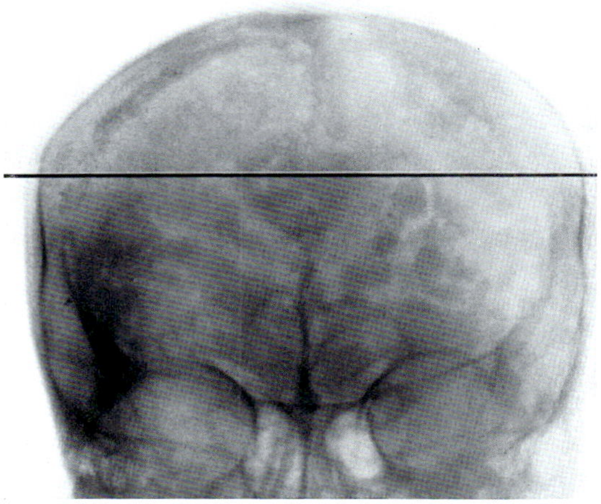

Fig. 8. Normal roentgenogram. Horizontal line showing the level tomographed

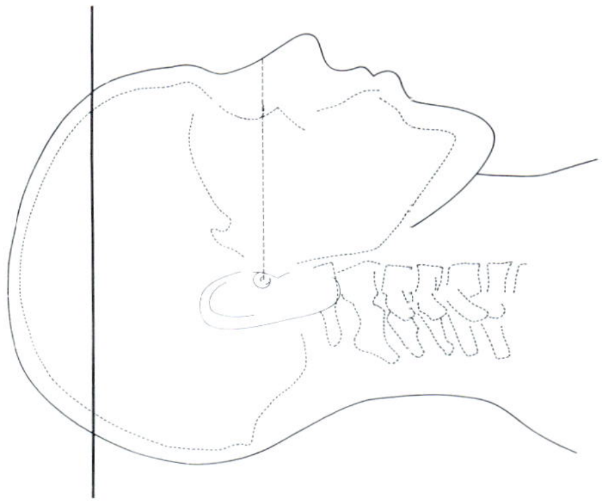

Fig. 9. Schema of tomographed level (solid line) 8 cm above the orbitomeatal line (dashed line)

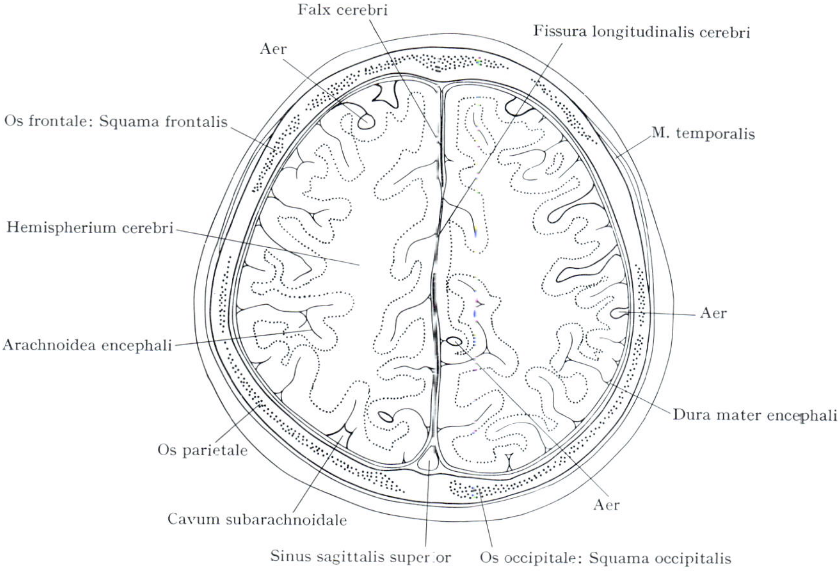

Fig. 10. Anatomical chart

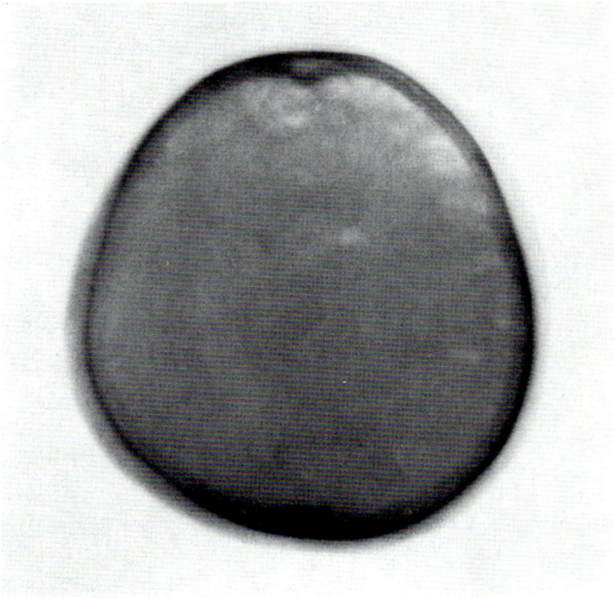

Fig. 11. Axial transverse tomogram

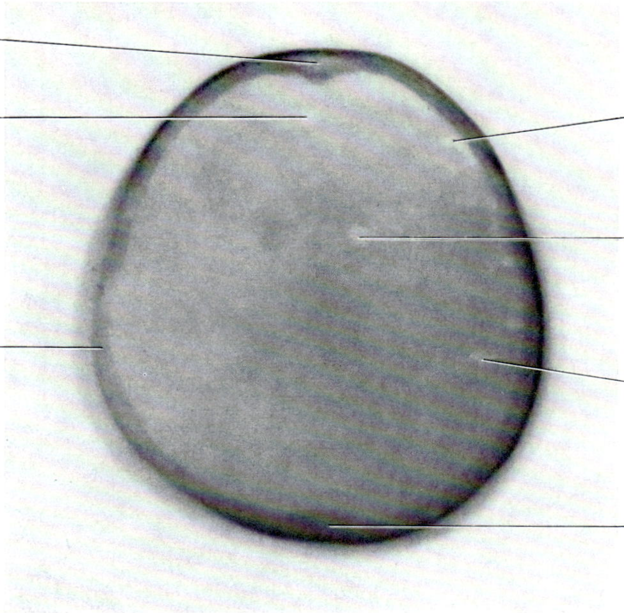

Fig. 12. Interpretation

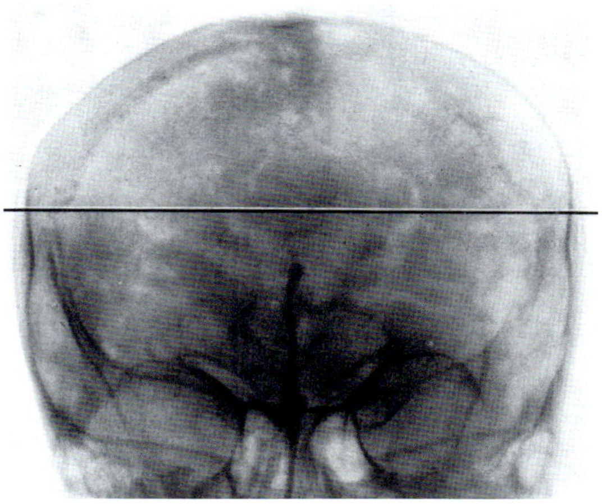

Fig. 13. Normal roentgenogram. Horizontal line showing the level tomographed

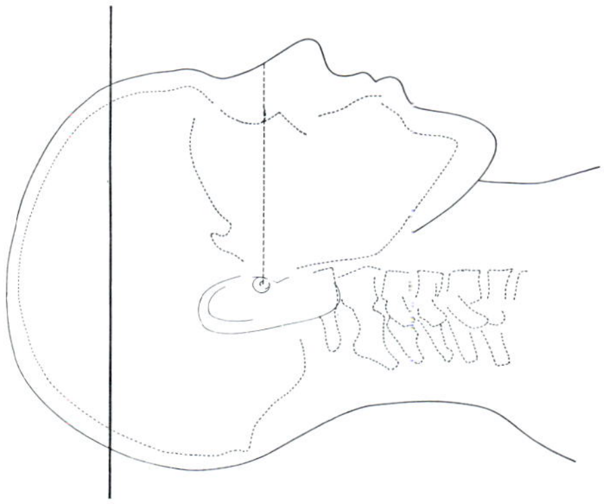

Fig. 14. Schema of tomographed level (solid line) 7 cm above the orbitomeatal line (dashed line)

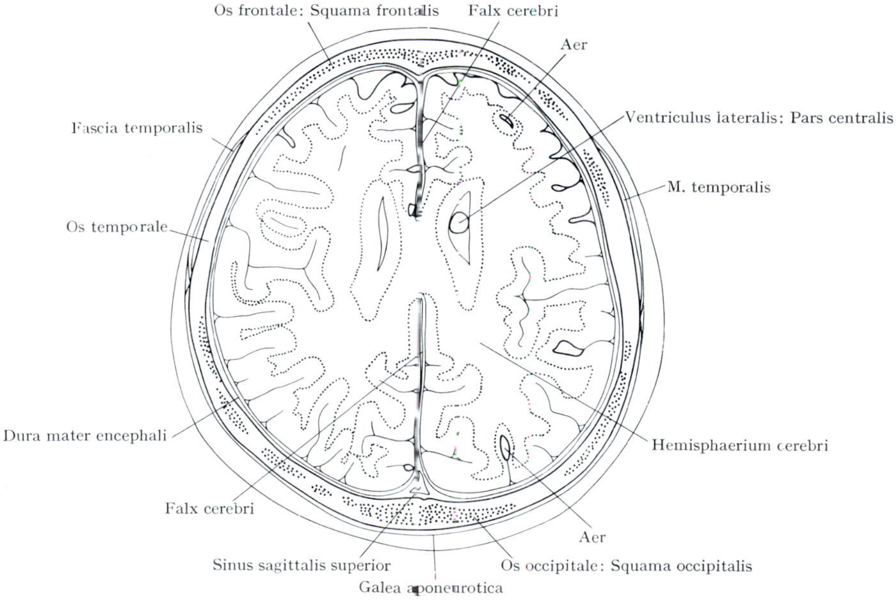

Fig. 15. Anatomical chart

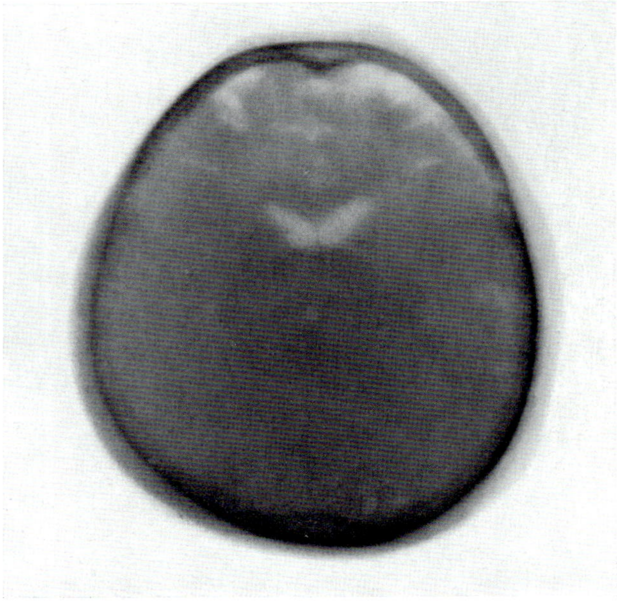

Fig. 16. Axial transverse tomogram

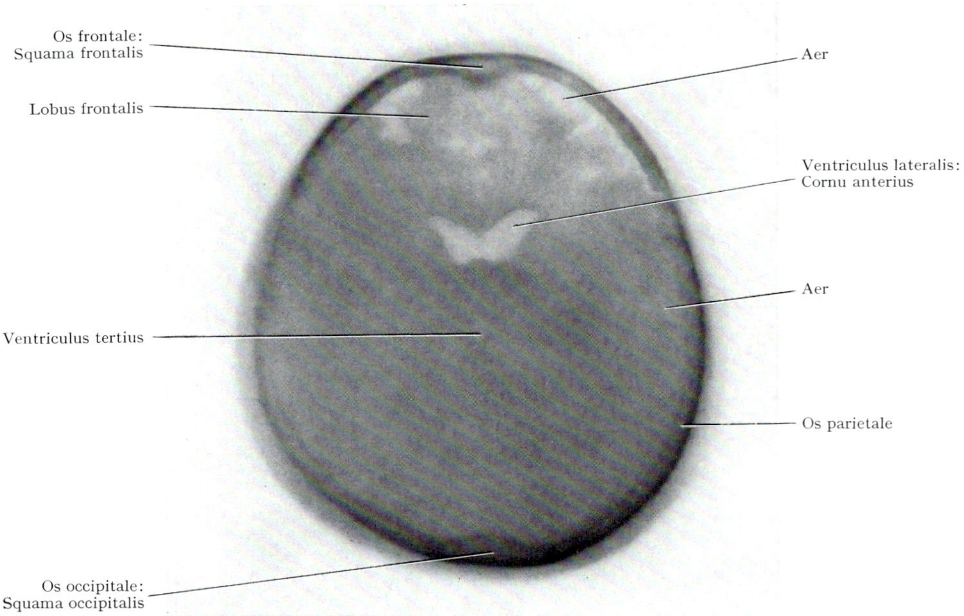

Fig. 17. Interpretation

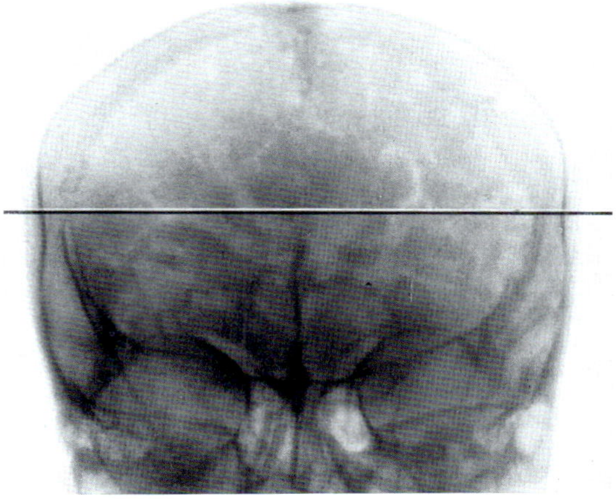

Fig. 18. Normal roentgenogram. Horizontal line showing the level tomographed

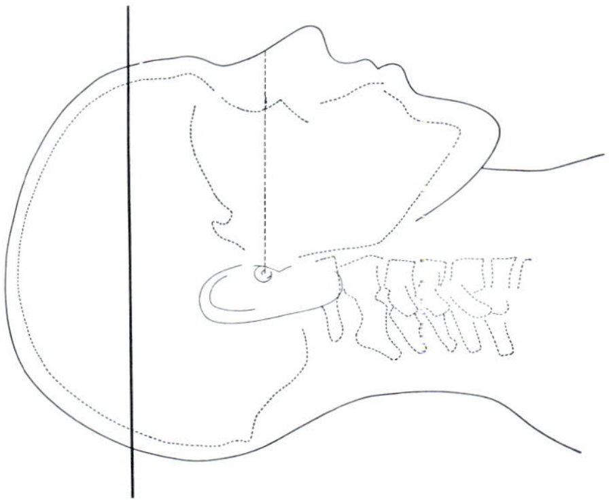

Fig. 19. Schema of tomographed level (solid line) 6 cm above the orbitomeatal line (dashed line)

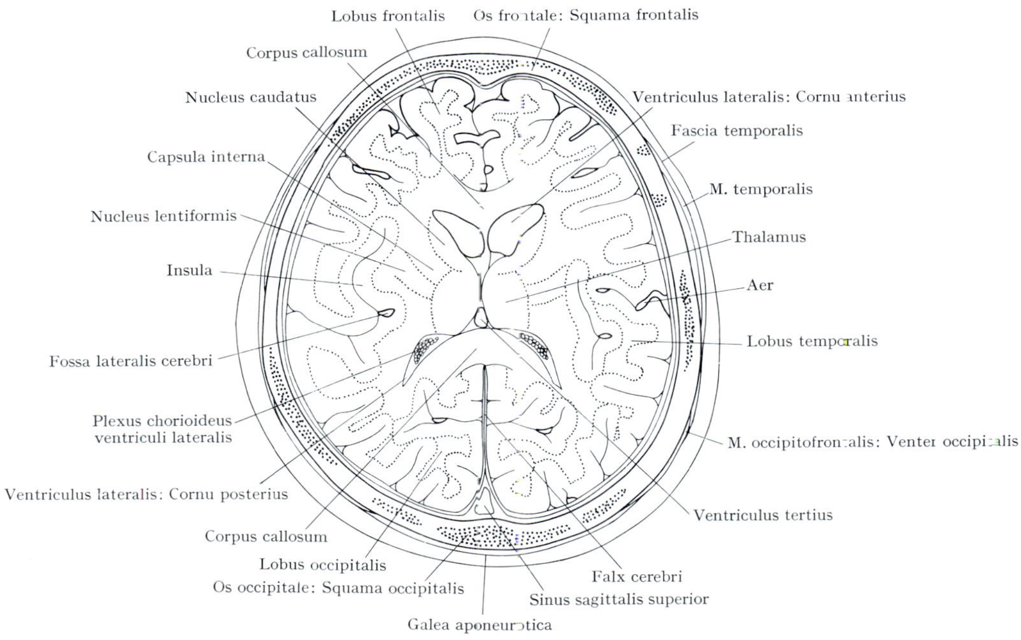

Fig. 20. Anatomical chart

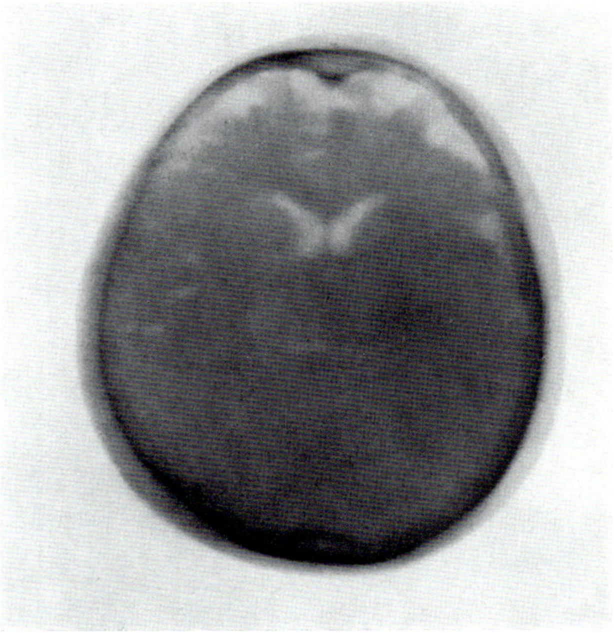

Fig. 21. Axial transverse tomogram

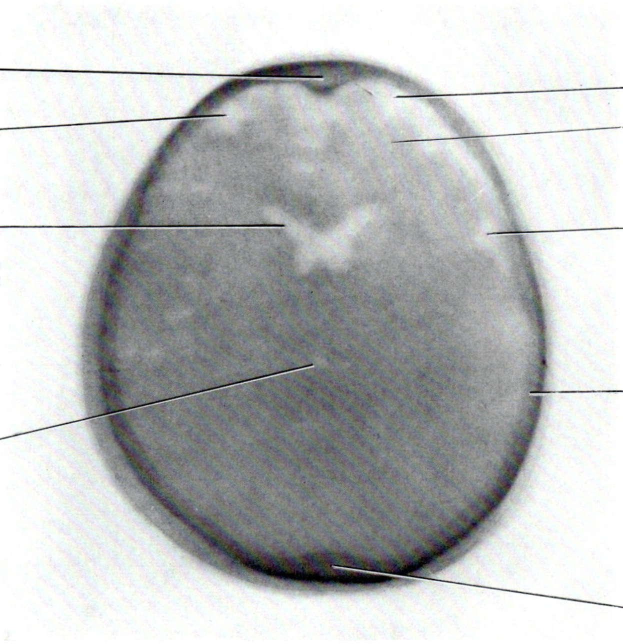

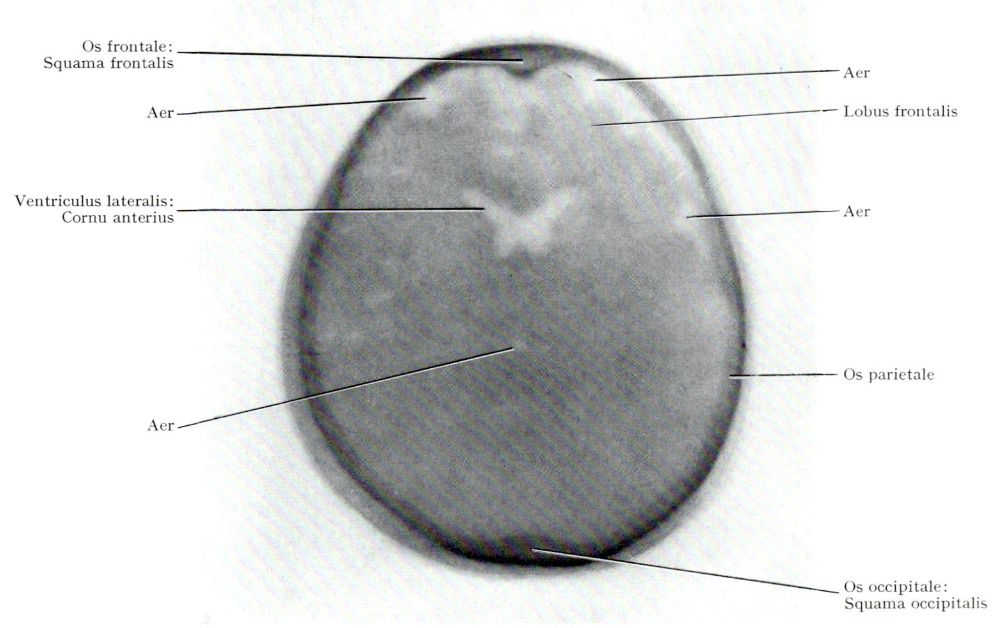

Fig. 22. Interpretation

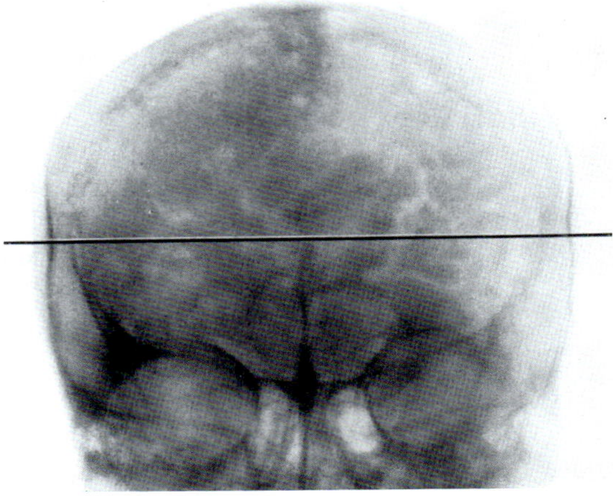

Fig. 23. Normal roentgenogram. Horizontal line showing the level tomographed

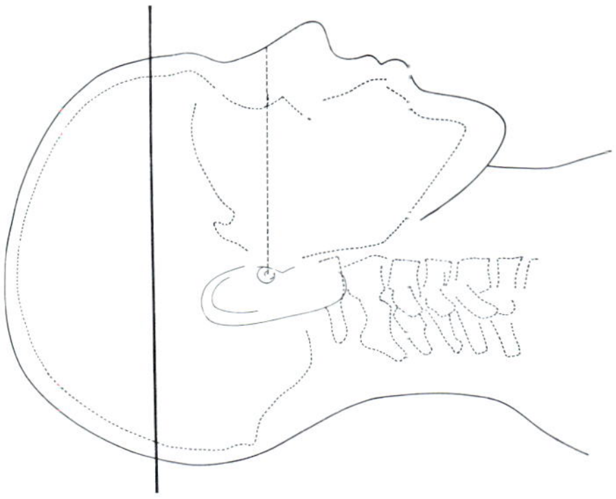

Fig. 24. Schema of tomographed level (solid line) 5 cm above the orbitomeatal line (dashed line)

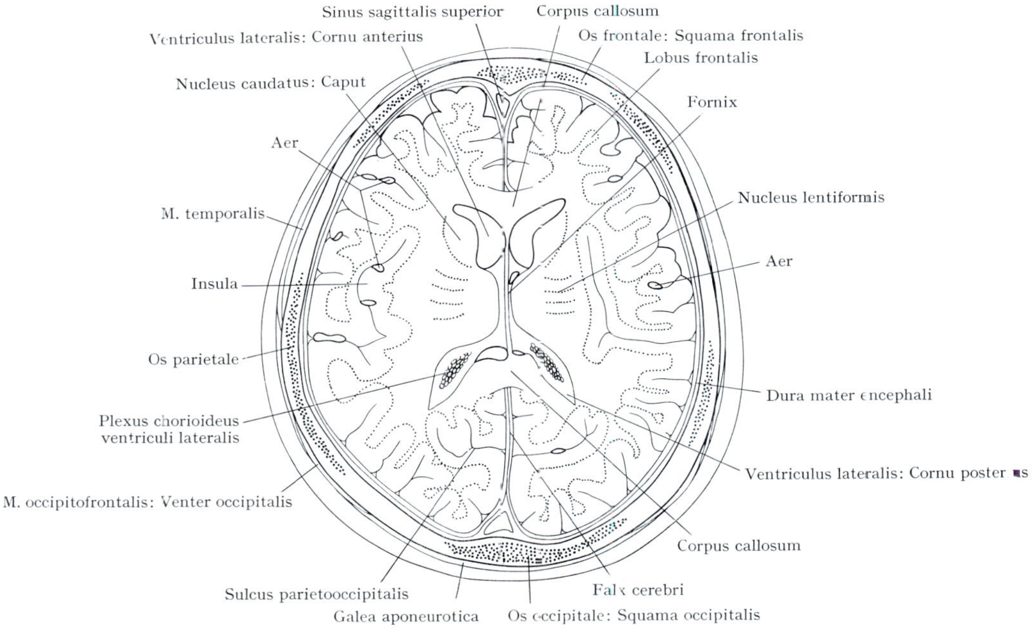

Fig. 25. Anatomical chart

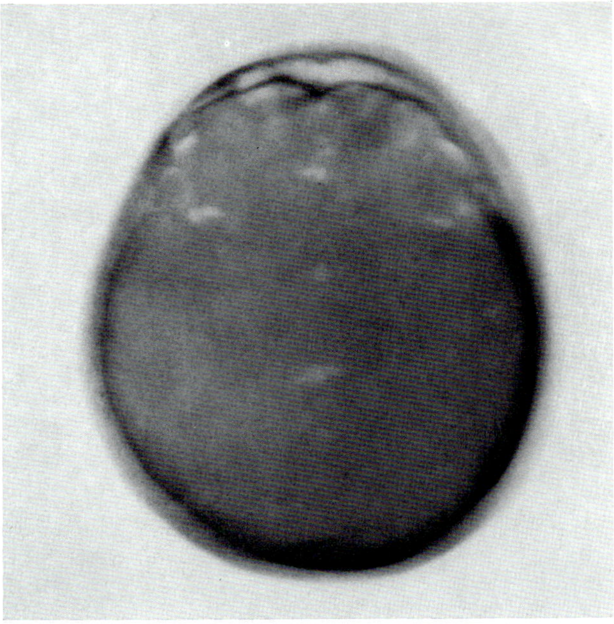

Fig. 26. Axial transverse tomogram

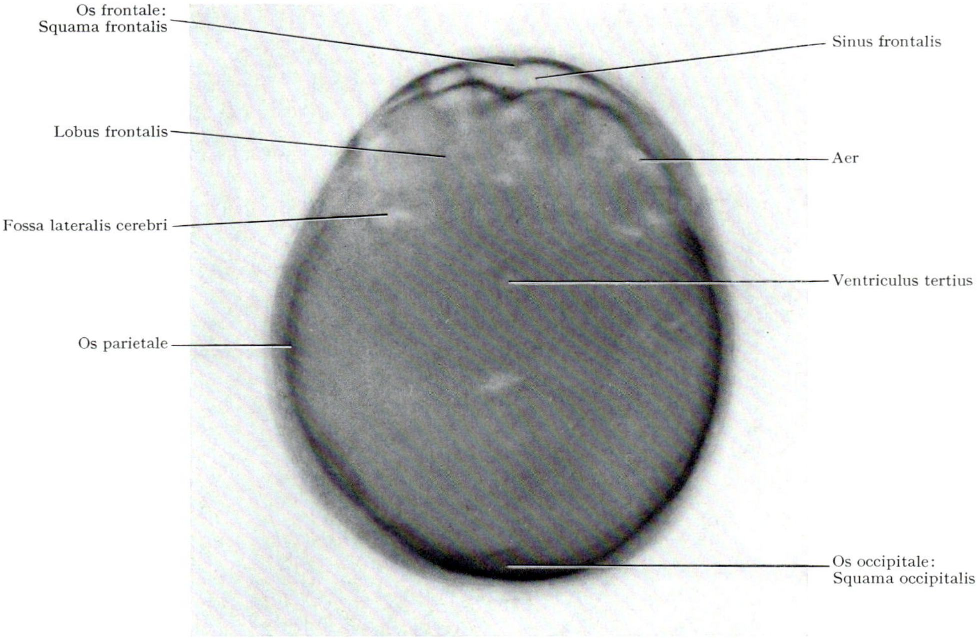

Fig. 27. Interpretation

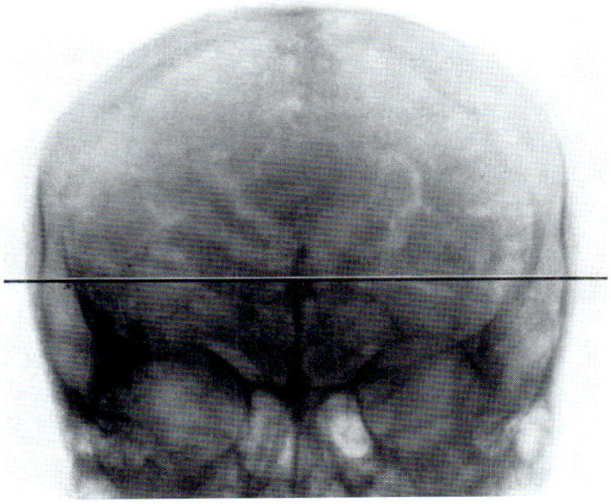

Fig. 28. Normal roentgenogram. Horizontal line showing the level tomographed

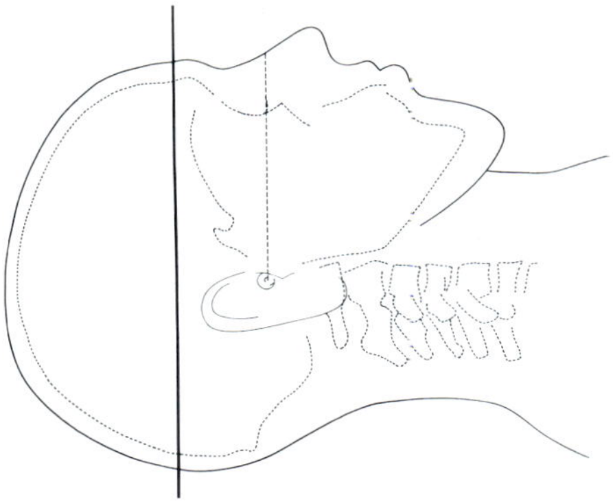

Fig. 29. Schema of tomographed level (solid line) 4 cm above the orbitomeatal line (dashed line)

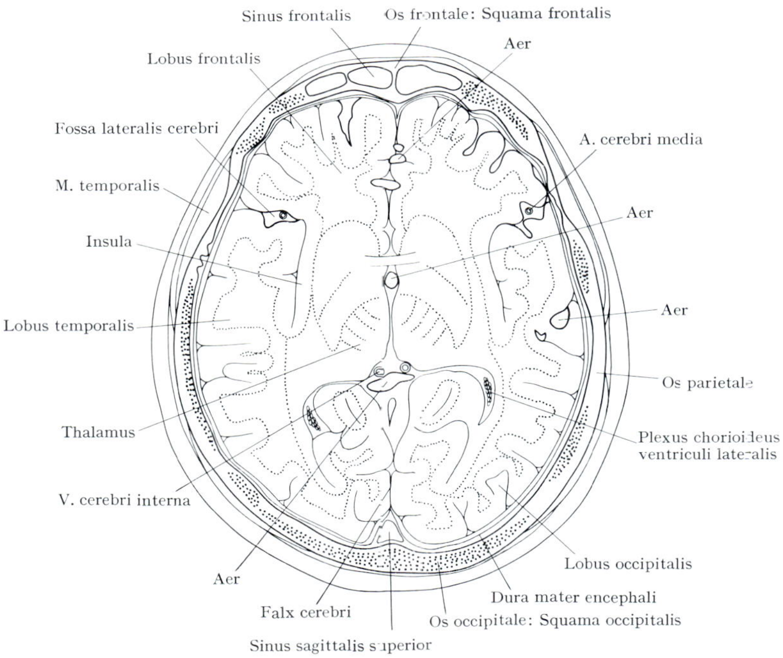

Fig. 30. Anatomical chart

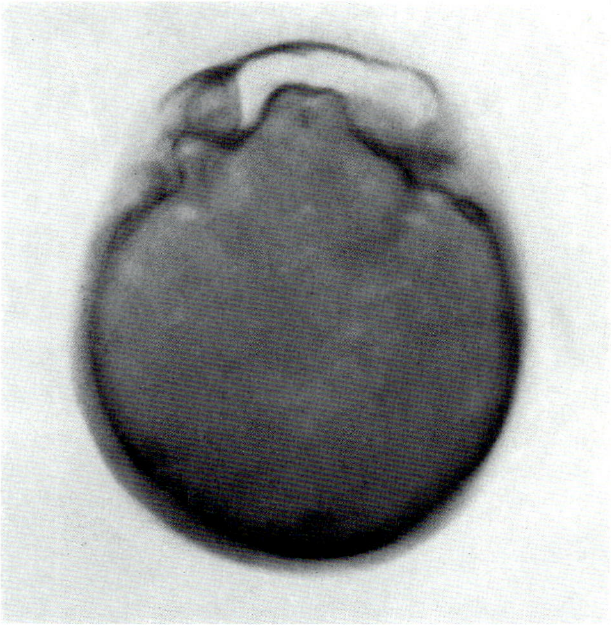

Fig. 31. Axial transverse tomogram

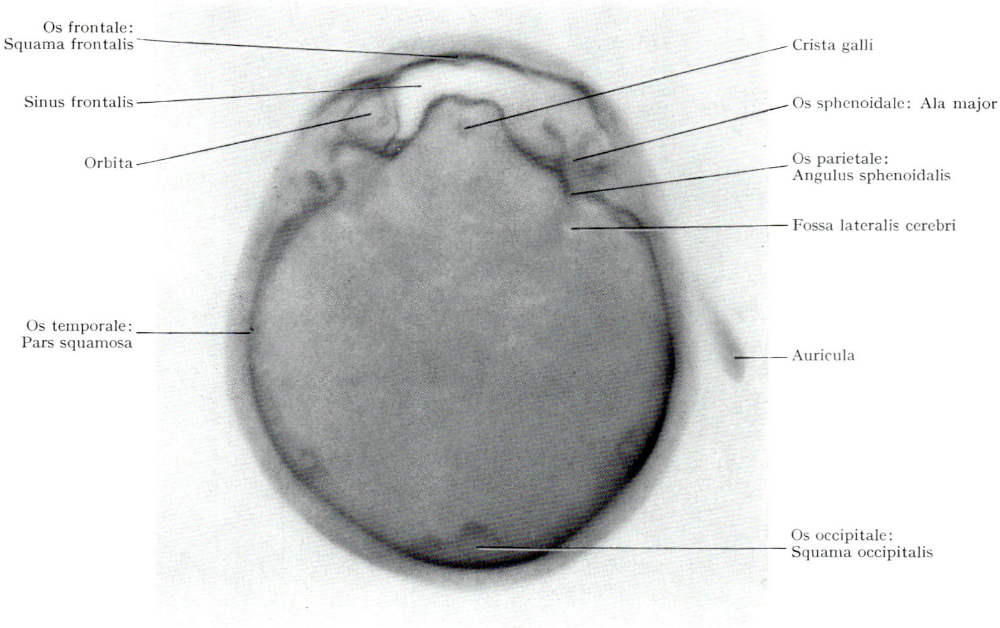

Fig. 32. Interpretation

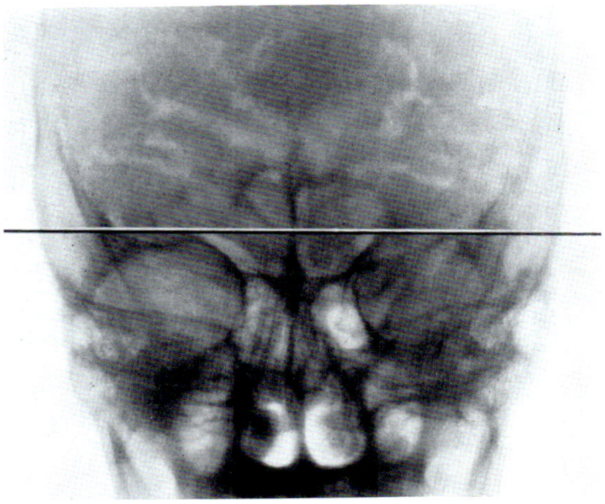

Fig. 33. Normal roentgenogram. Horizontal line showing the level tomographed

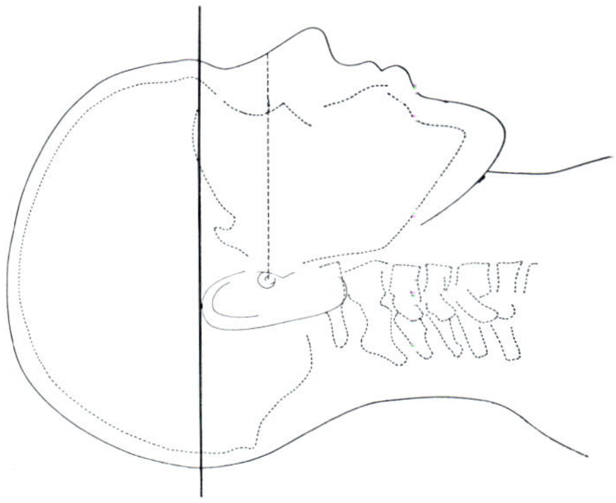

Fig. 34. Schema of tomographed level (solid line) 3 cm above the orbitomeatal line (dashed line)

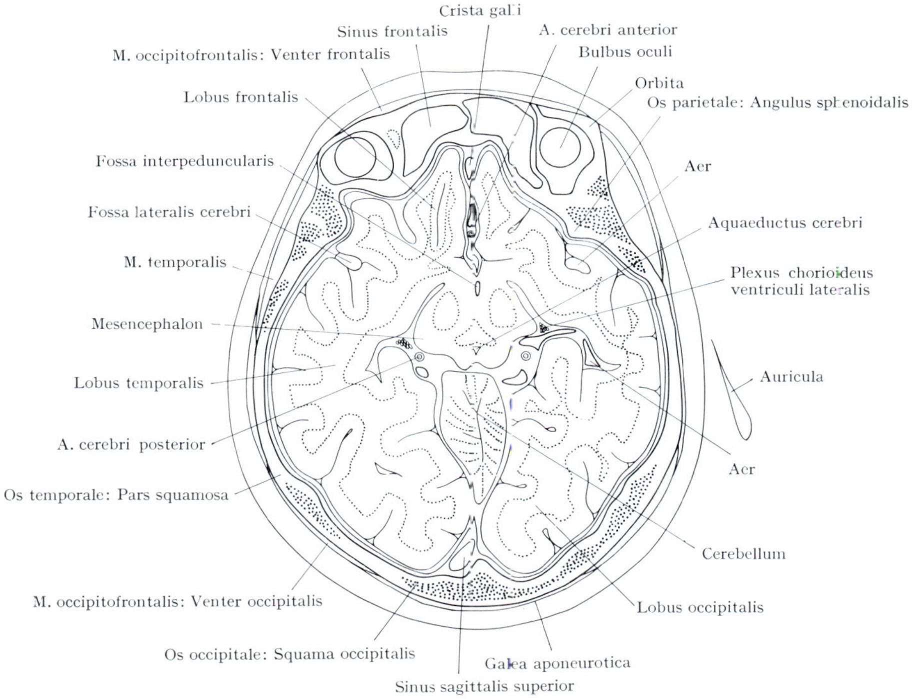

Fig. 35. Anatomical chart

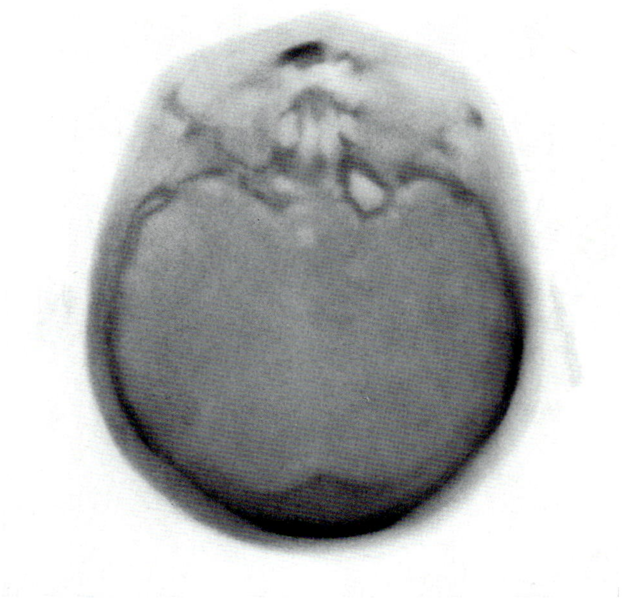

Fig. 36. Axial transverse tomogram

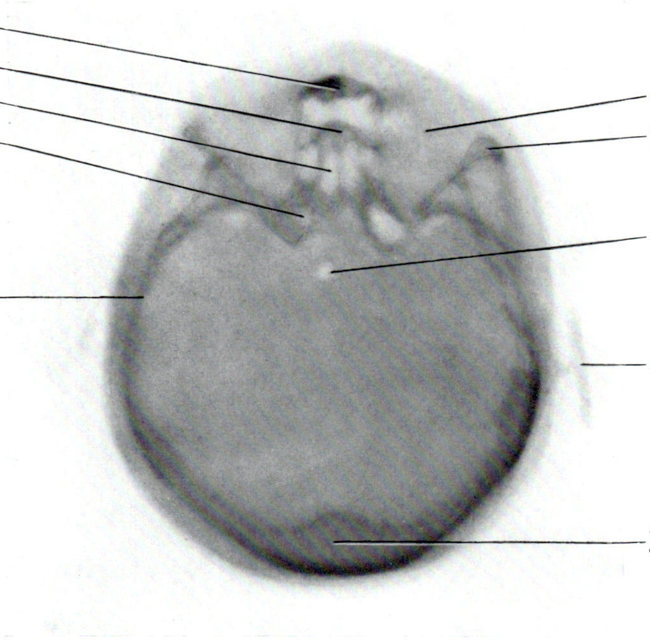

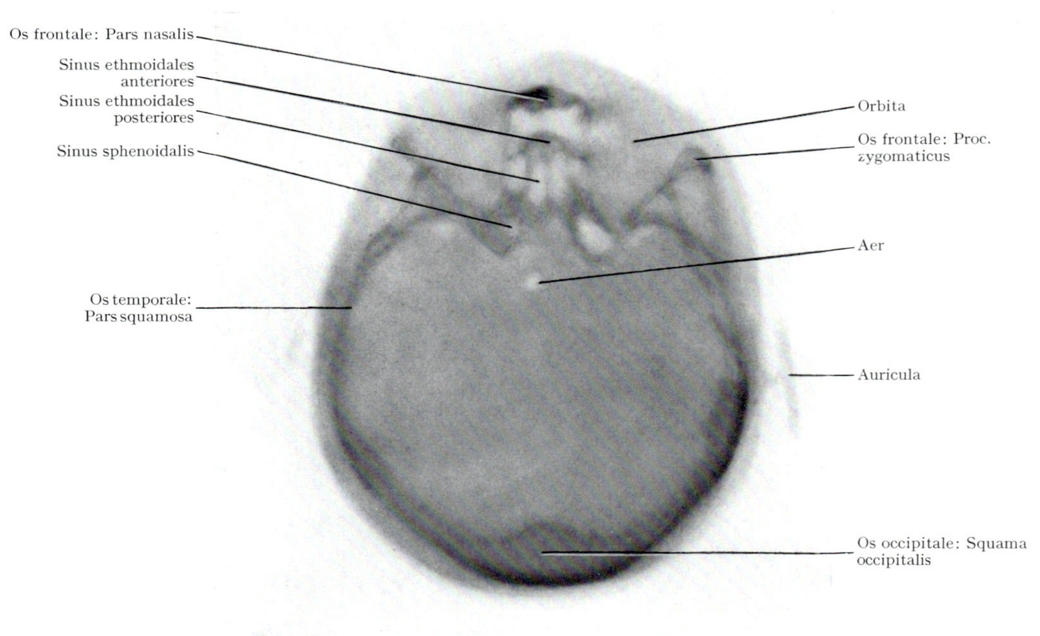

Fig. 37. Interpretation

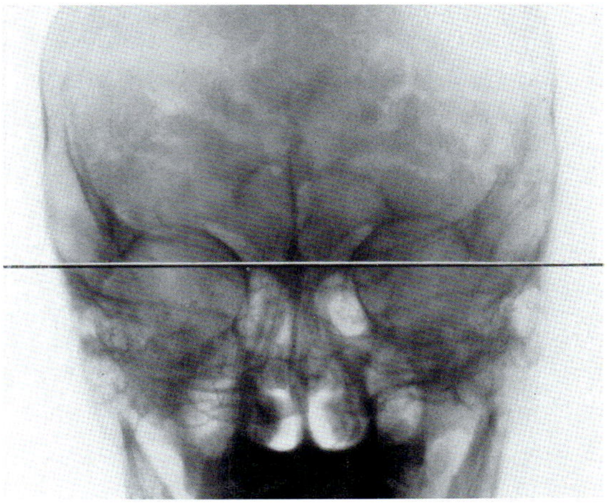

Fig. 38. Normal roentgenogram. Horizontal line showing the level tomographed

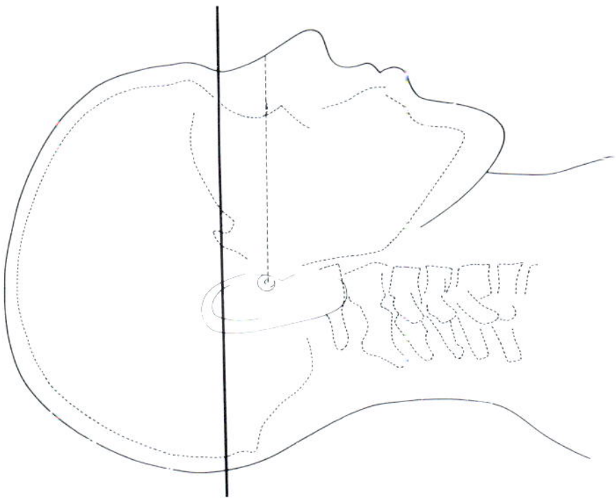

Fig. 39. Schema of tomographed level (solid line) 2 cm above the orbitomeatal line (dashed line)

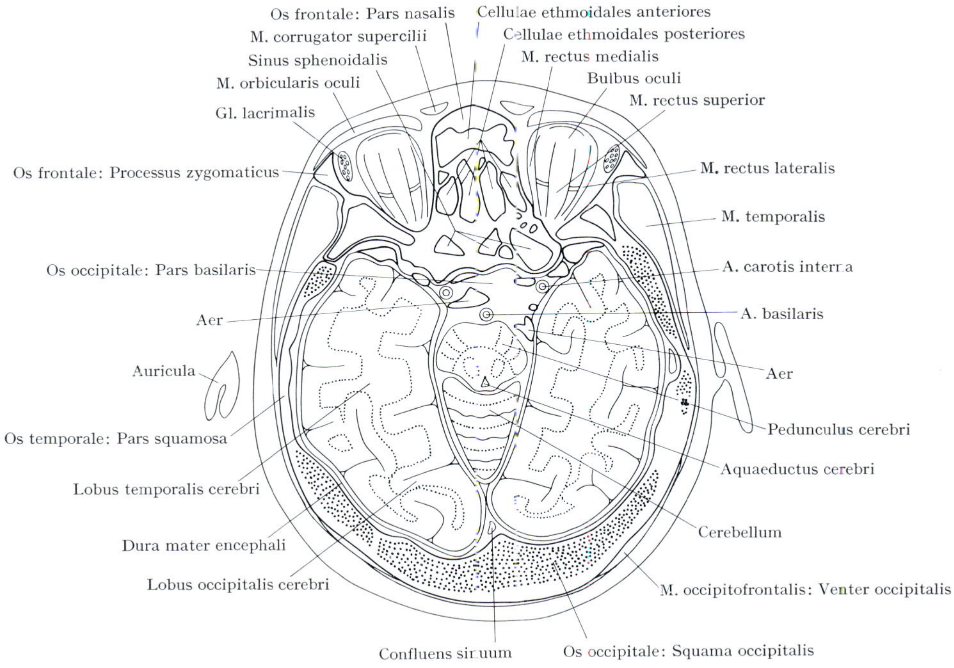

Fig. 40. Anatomical chart

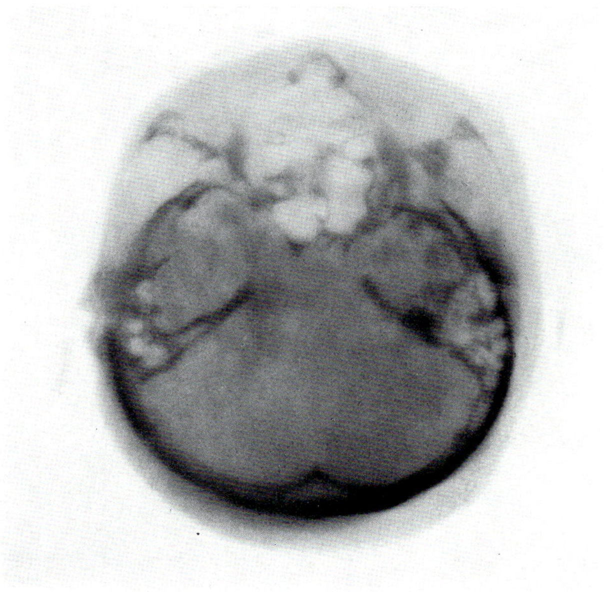

Fig. 41. Axial transverse tomogram

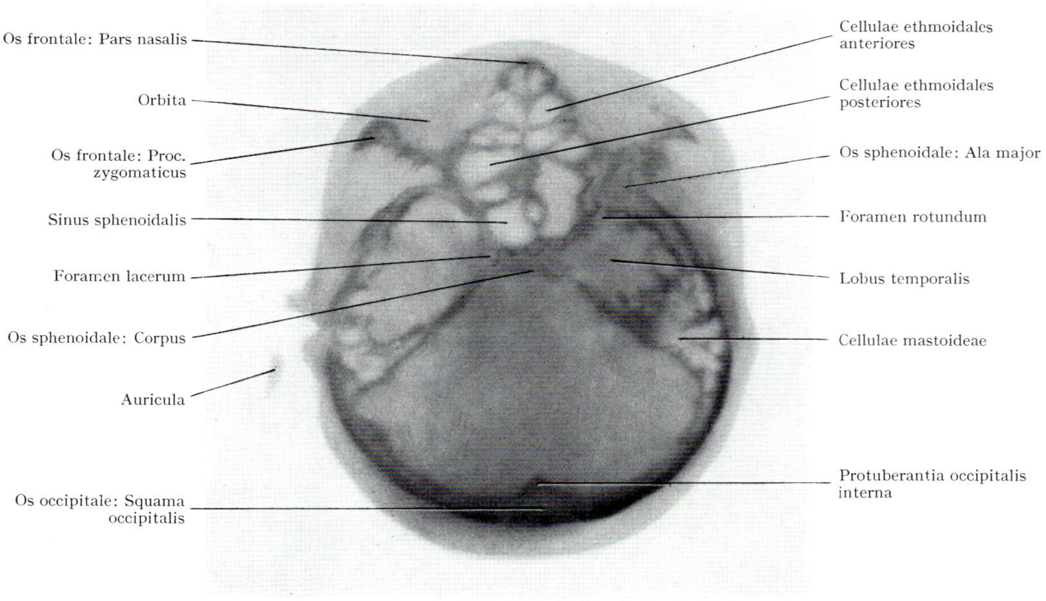

Fig. 42. Interpretation

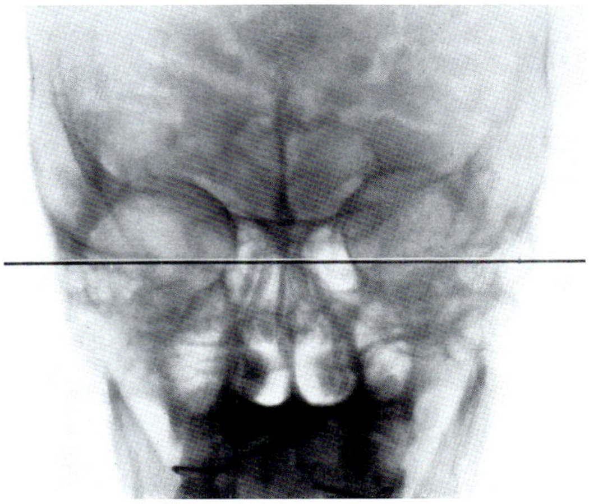

Fig. 43. Normal roentgenogram. Horizontal line showing the level tomographed

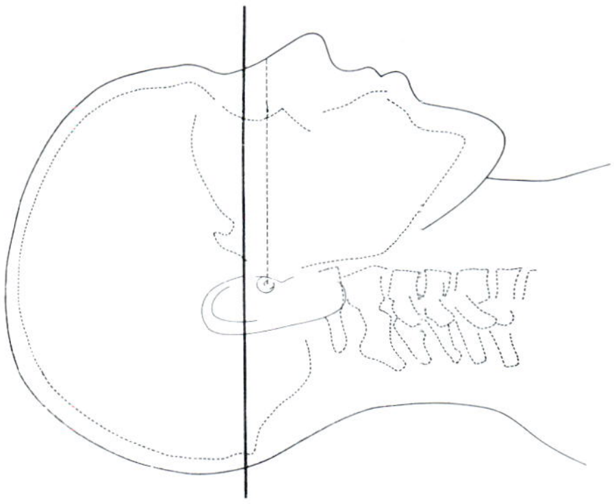

Fig. 44. Schema of tomographed level (solid line) 1 cm above the orbitomeatal line (dashed line)

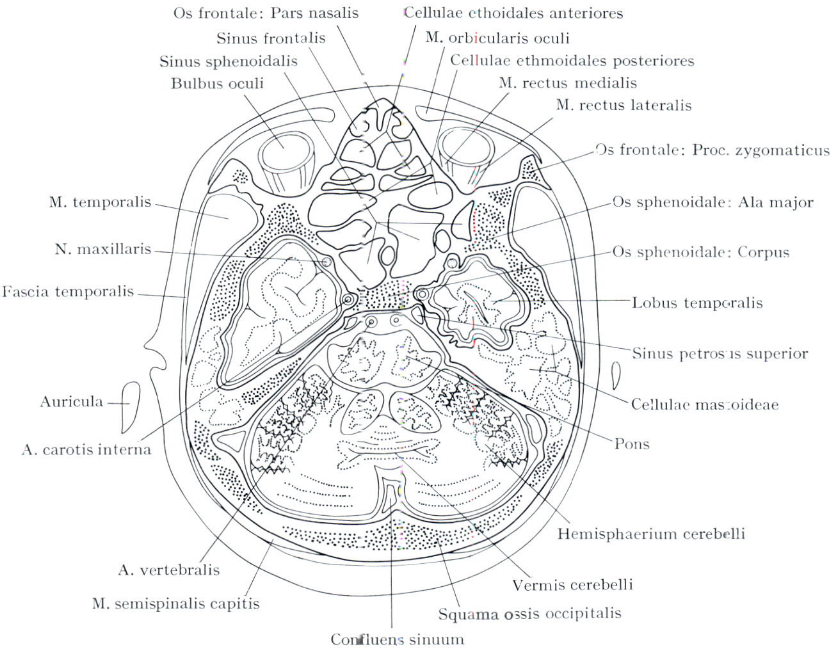

Fig. 45. Anatomical chart

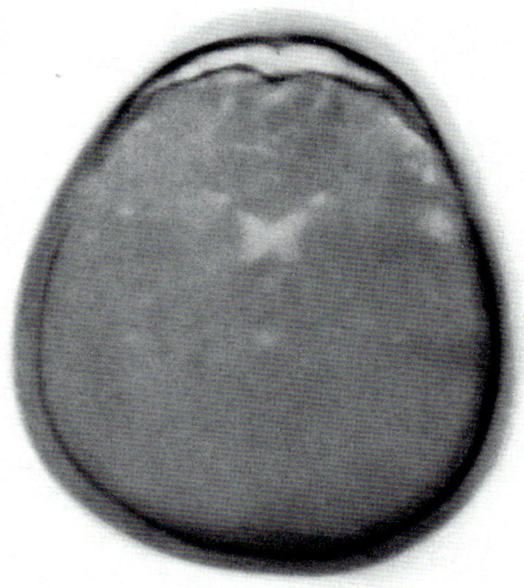

Fig. 46. Axial transverse tomogram

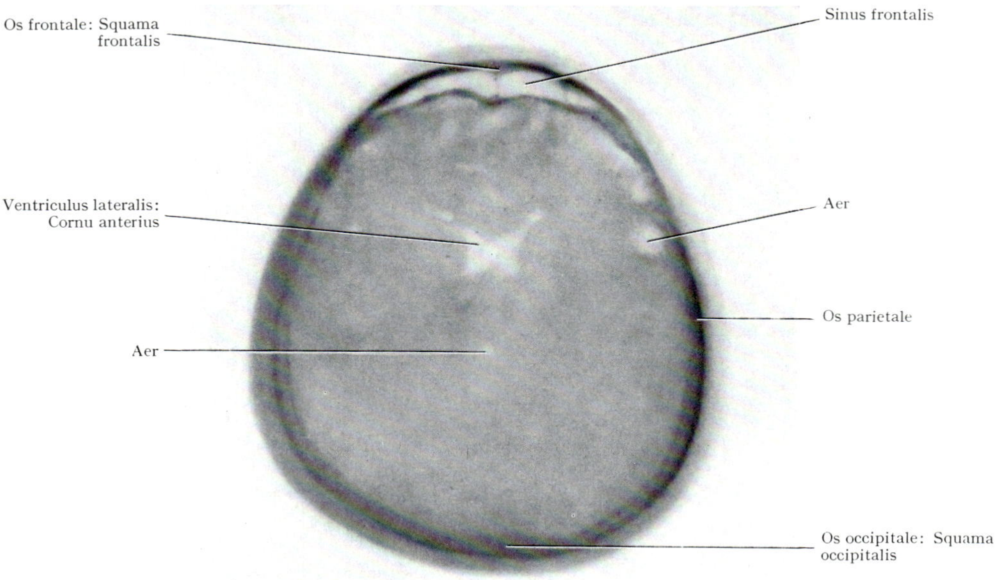

Fig. 47. Interpretation

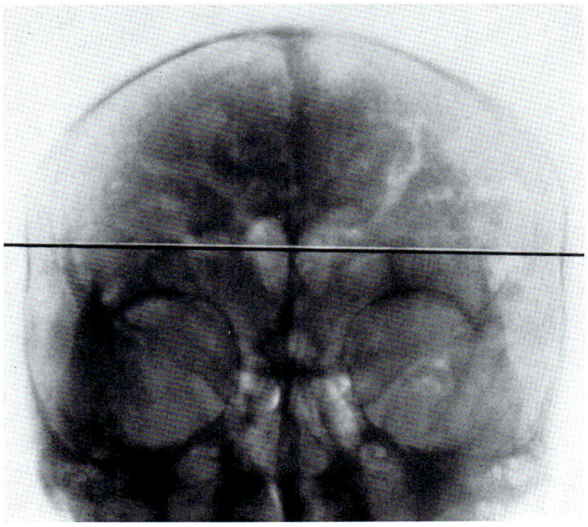

Fig. 48. Normal roentgenogram. Horizontal line showing the level tomographed

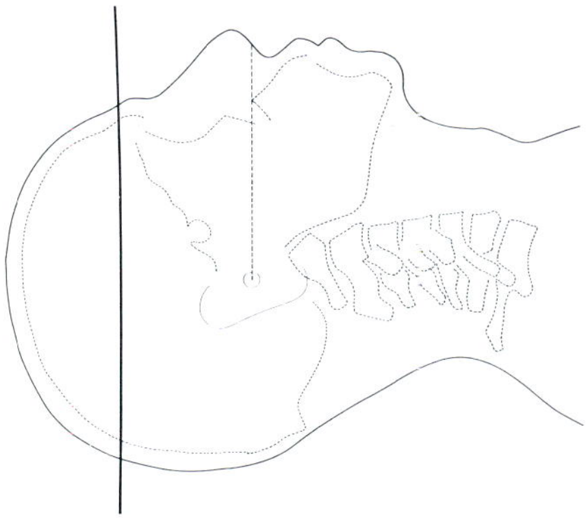

Fig. 49. Schema of tomographed level (solid line) 6 cm above the acanthiomeatal line (dashed line)

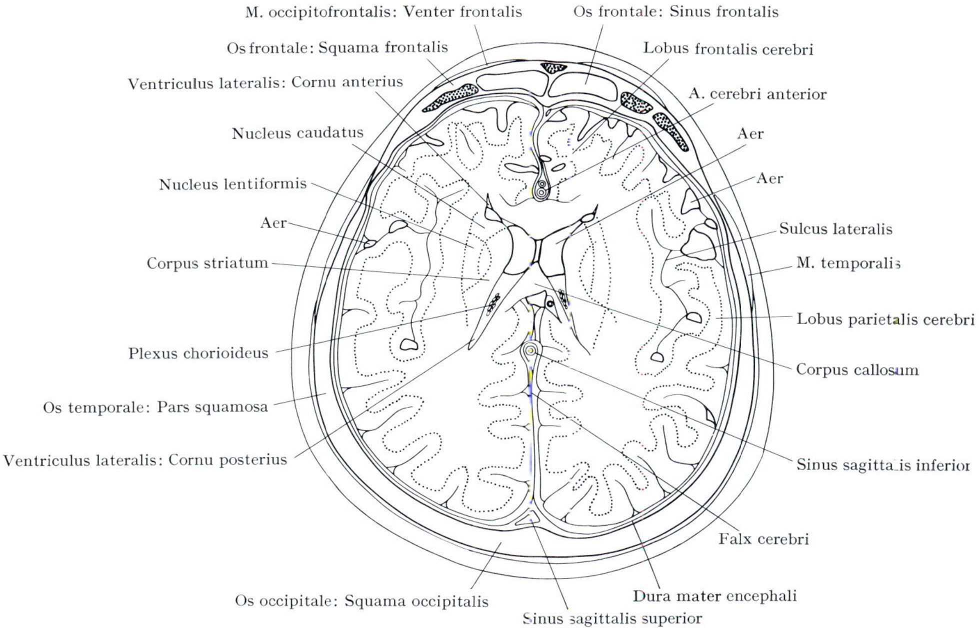

Fig. 50. Anatomical chart

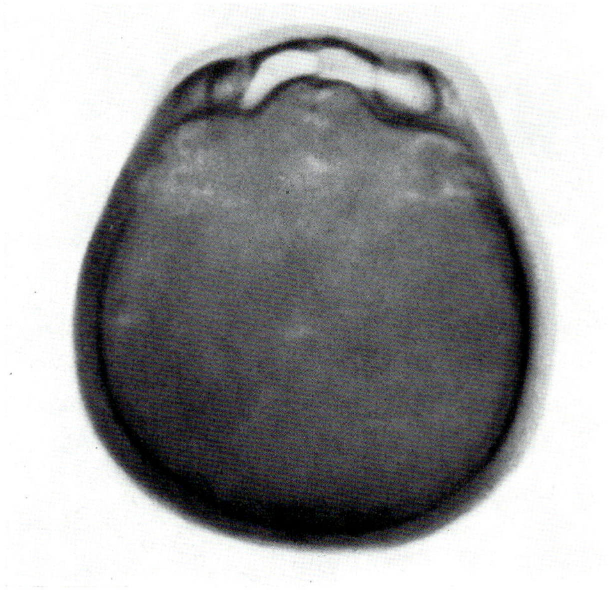

Fig. 51. Axial transverse tomogram

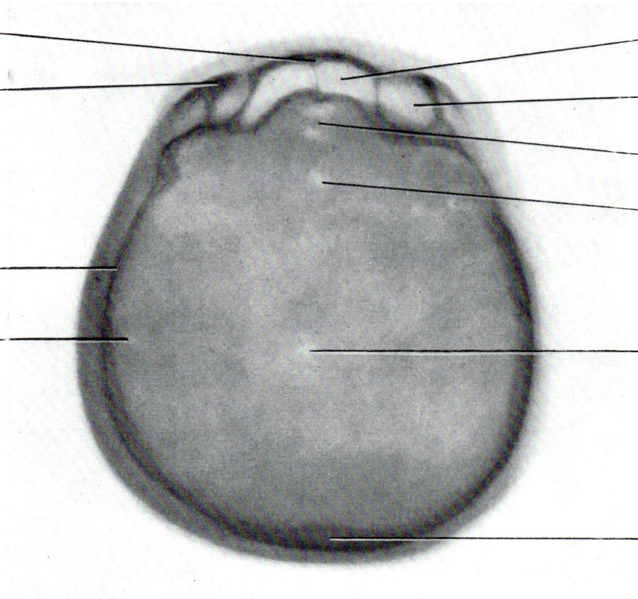

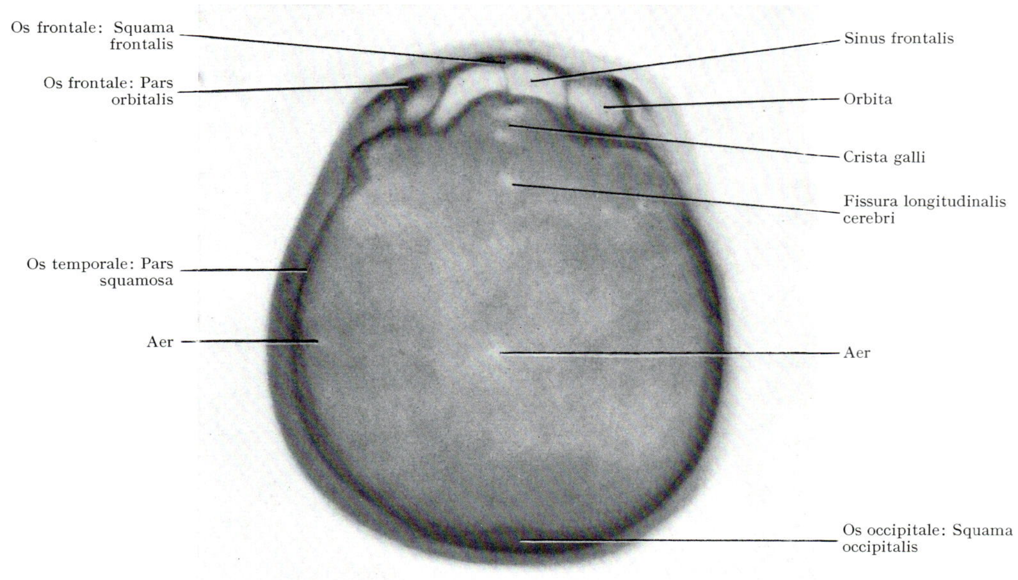

Fig. 52. Interpretation

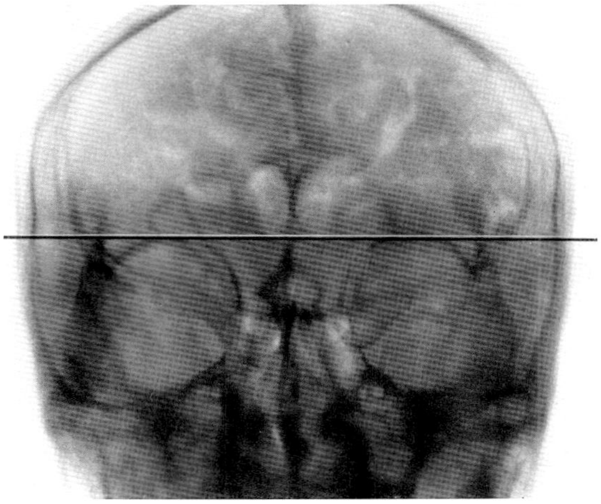

Fig. 53. Normal roentgenogram. Horizontal line showing the level tomographed

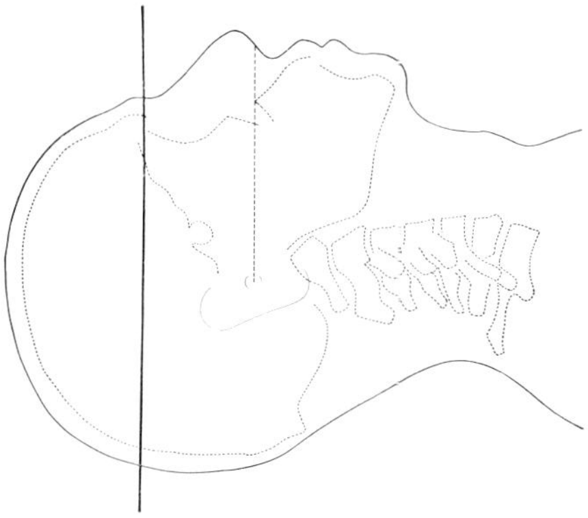

Fig. 54. Schema of tomographed level (solid line) 5 cm above the acanthiomeatal line (dashed line)

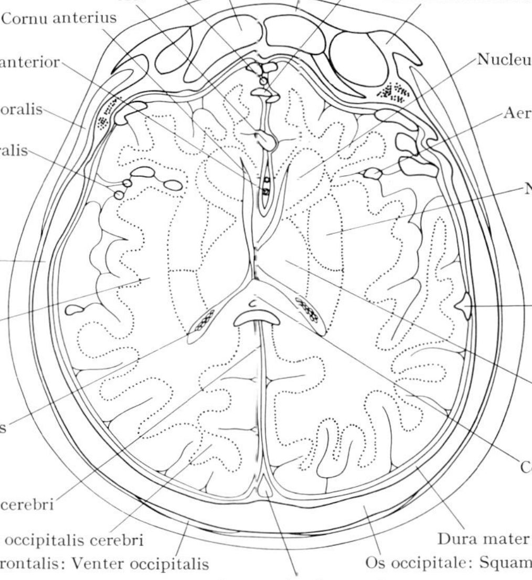

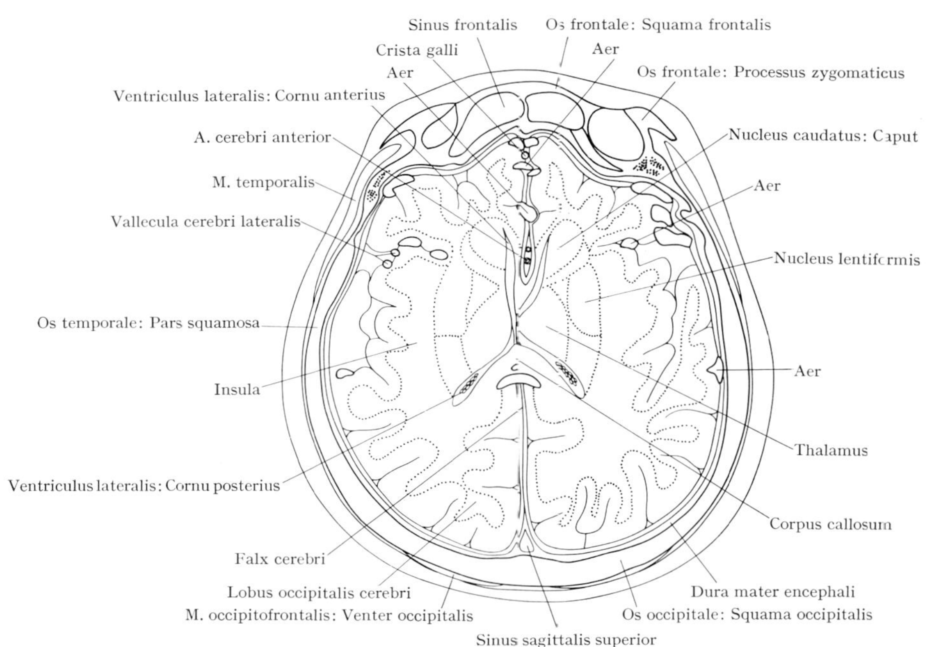

Fig. 55. Anatomical chart

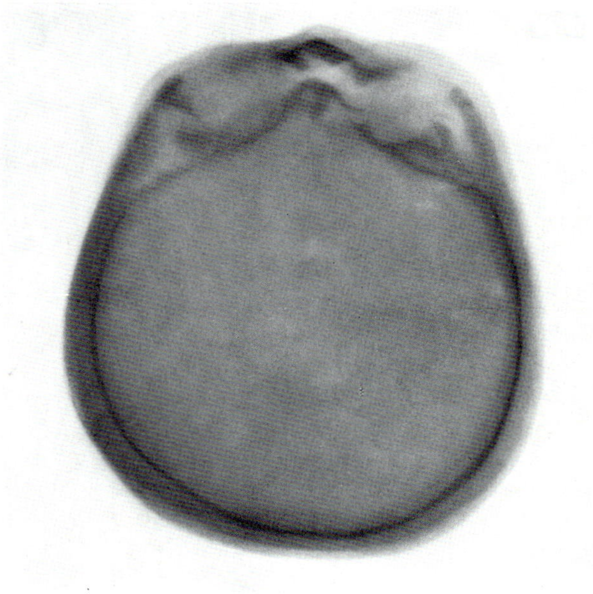

Fig. 56. Axial transverse tomogram

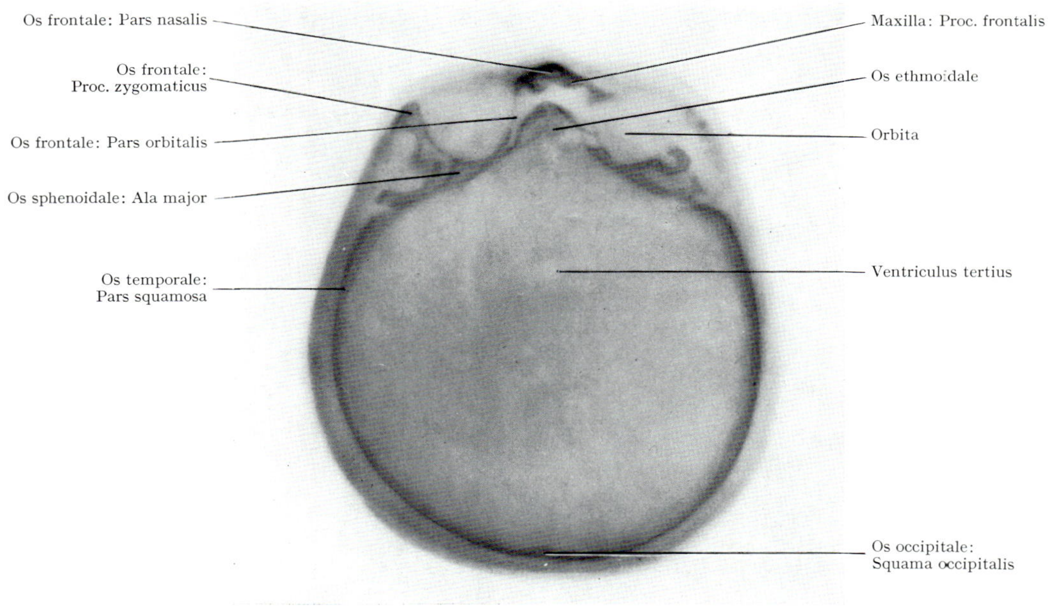

Fig. 57. Interpretation

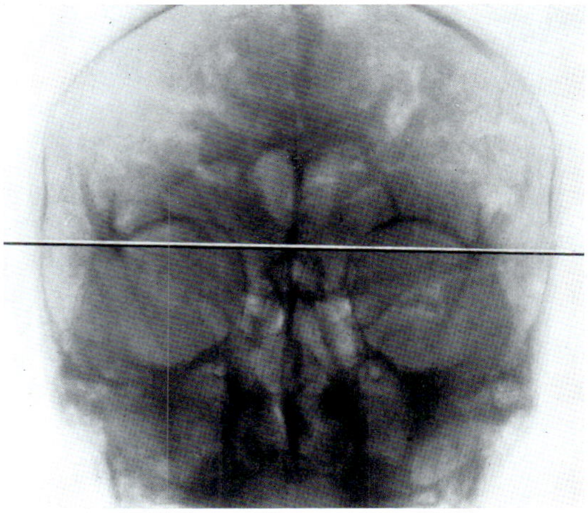

Fig. 58. Normal roentgenogram. Horizontal line showing the level tomographed

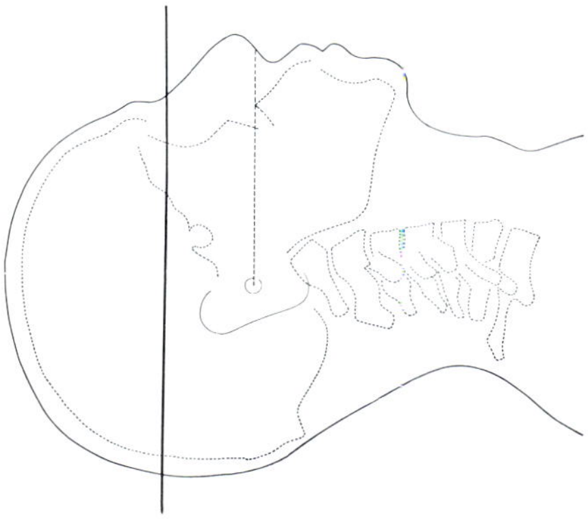

Fig. 59. Schema of tomographed level (solid line) 4 cm above the acanthiomeatal line (dashed line)

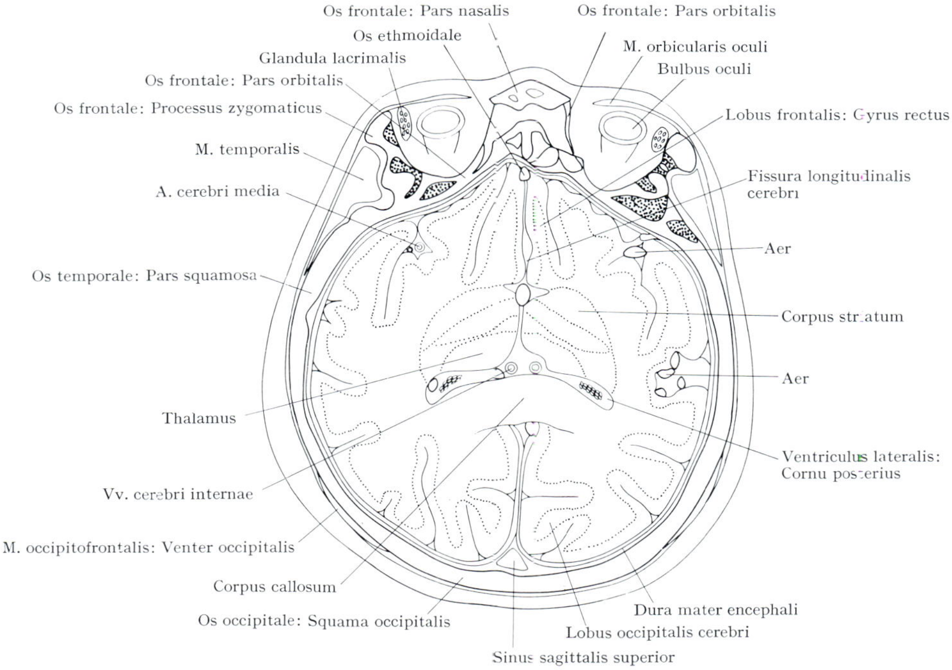

Fig. 60. Anatomical chart

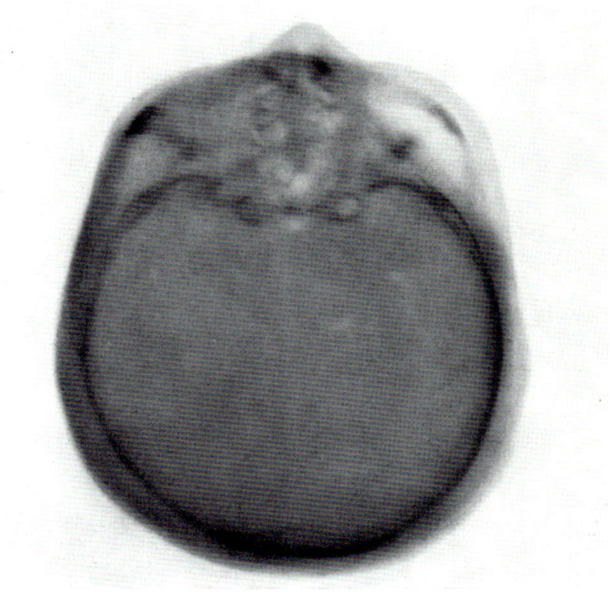

Fig. 61. Axial transverse tomogram

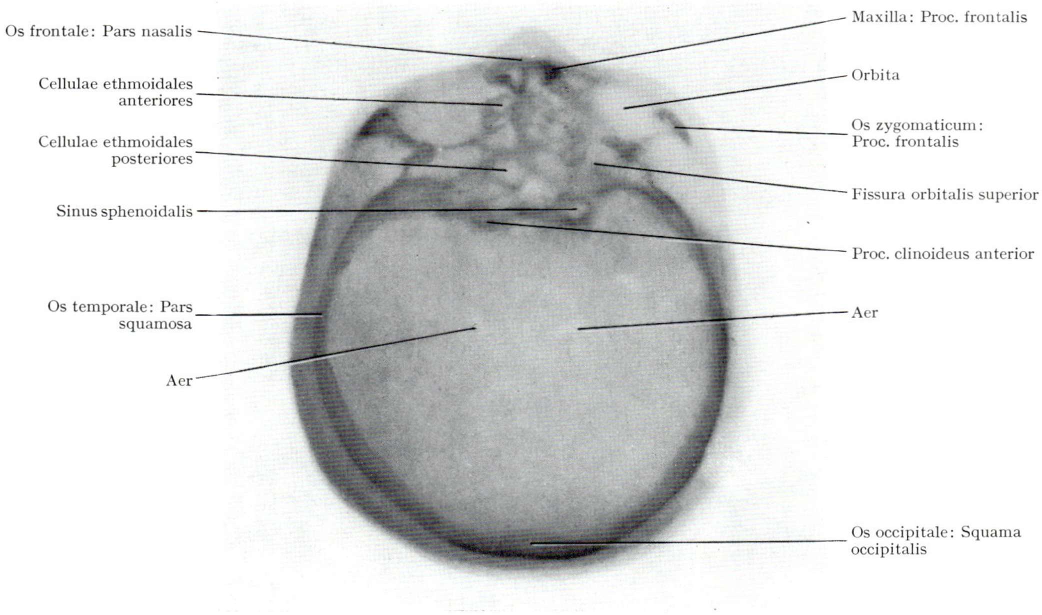

Fig. 62. Interpretation

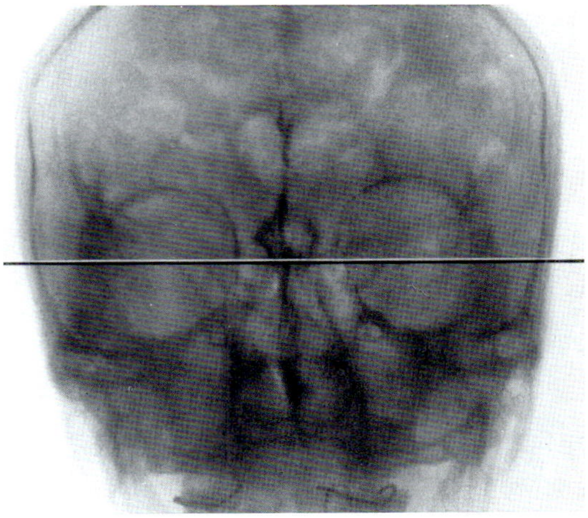

Fig. 63. Normal roentgenogram. Horizontal line showing the level tomographed

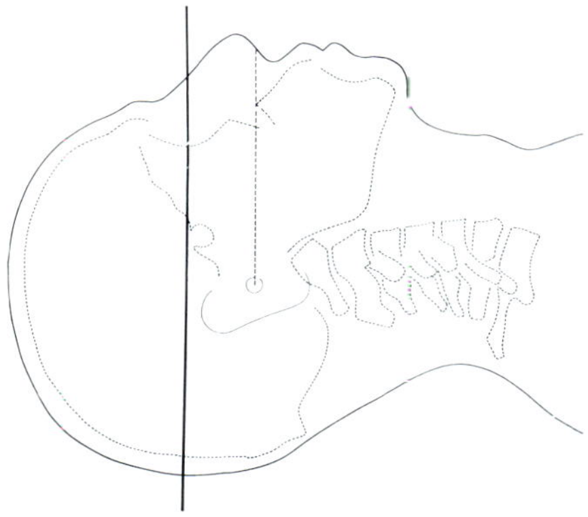

Fig. 64. Schema of tomographed level (solid line) 3 cm above the acanthiomeatal line (dashed line)

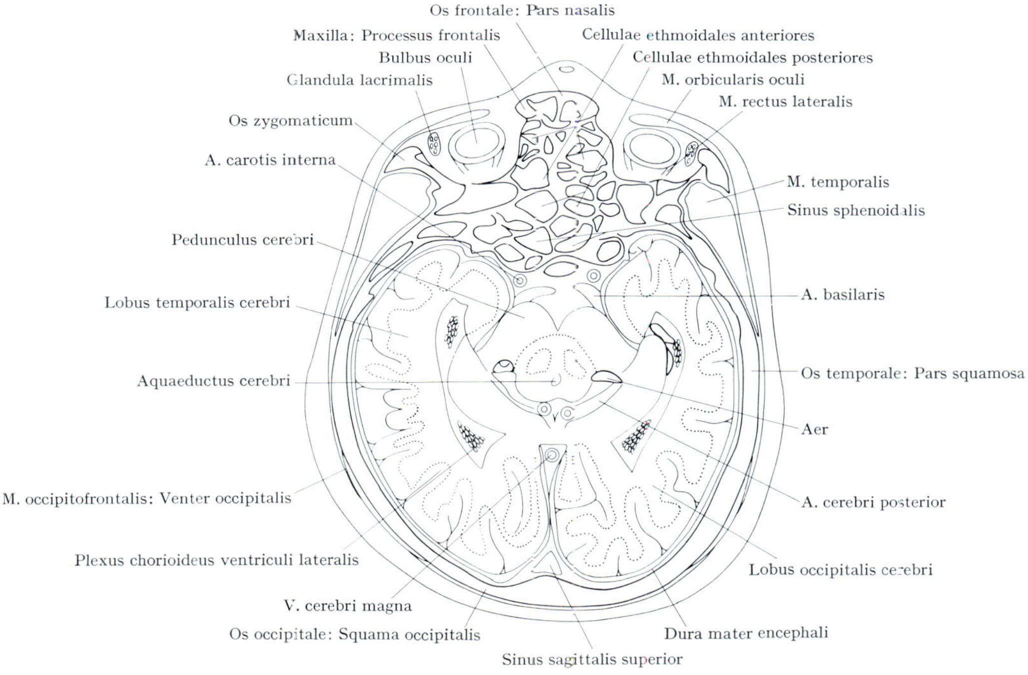

Fig. 65. Anatomical chart

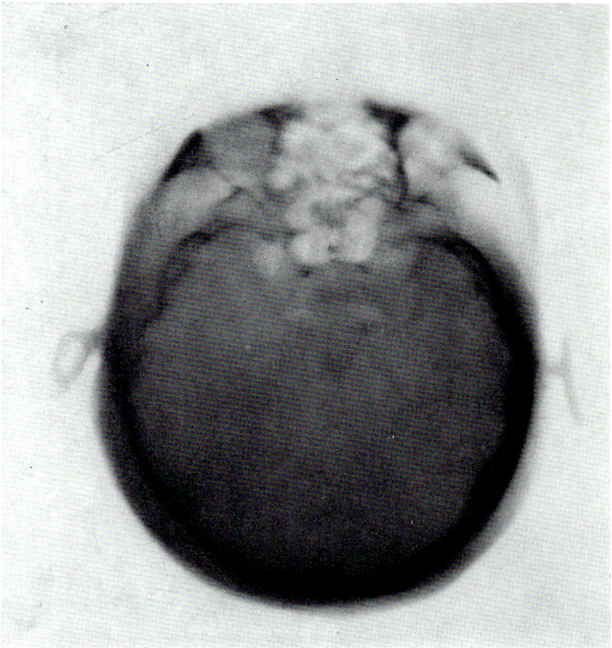

Fig. 66. Axial transverse tomogram

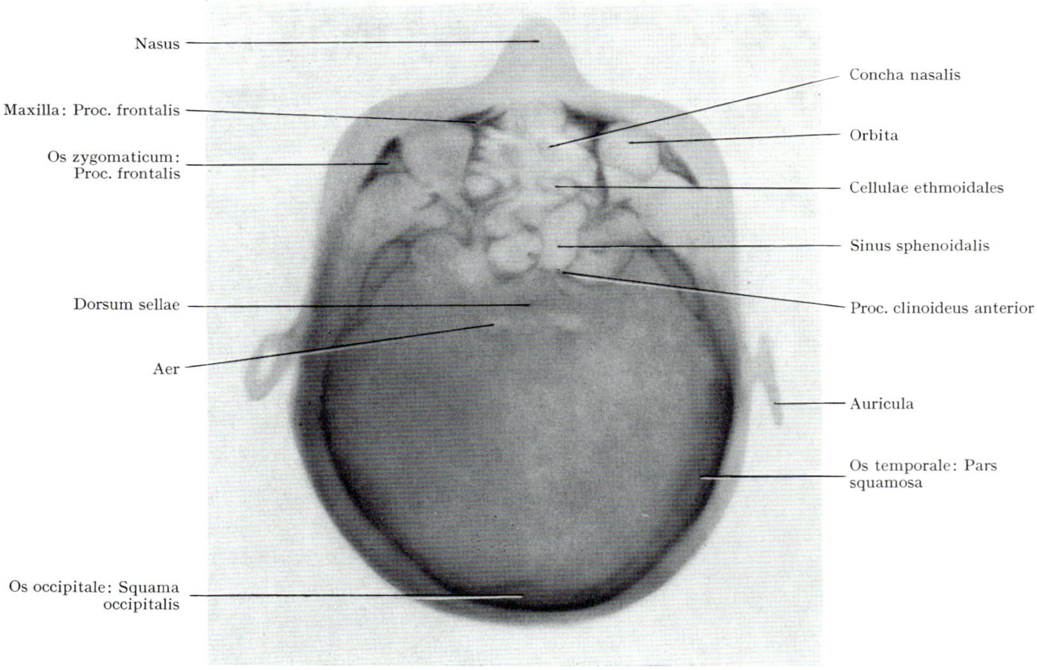

Fig. 67. Interpretation

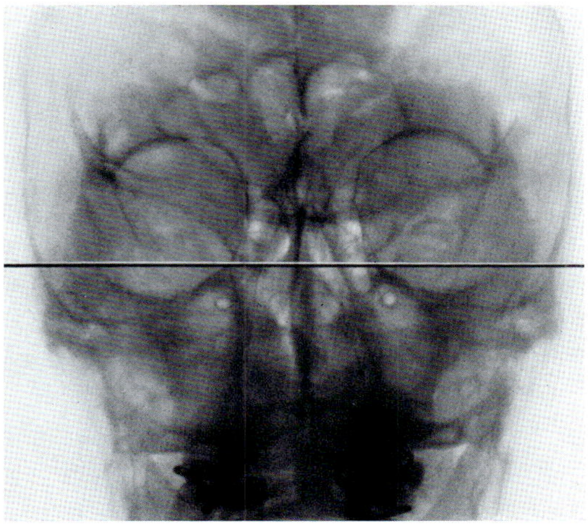

Fig. 68. Normal roentgenogram. Horizontal line showing the level tomographed

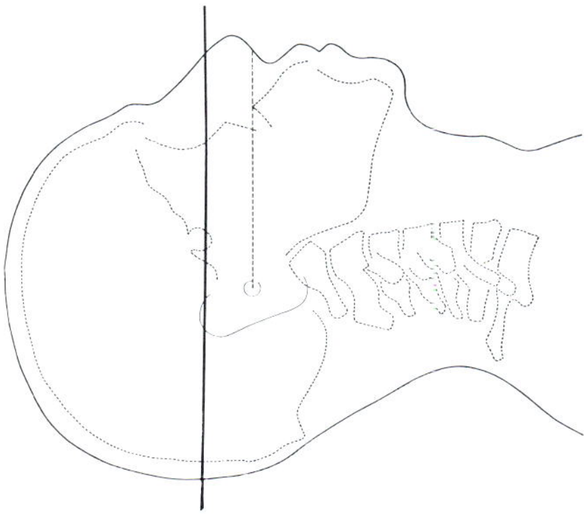

Fig. 69. Schema of tomographed level (solid line) 2 cm above the acanthiomeatal line (dashed line)

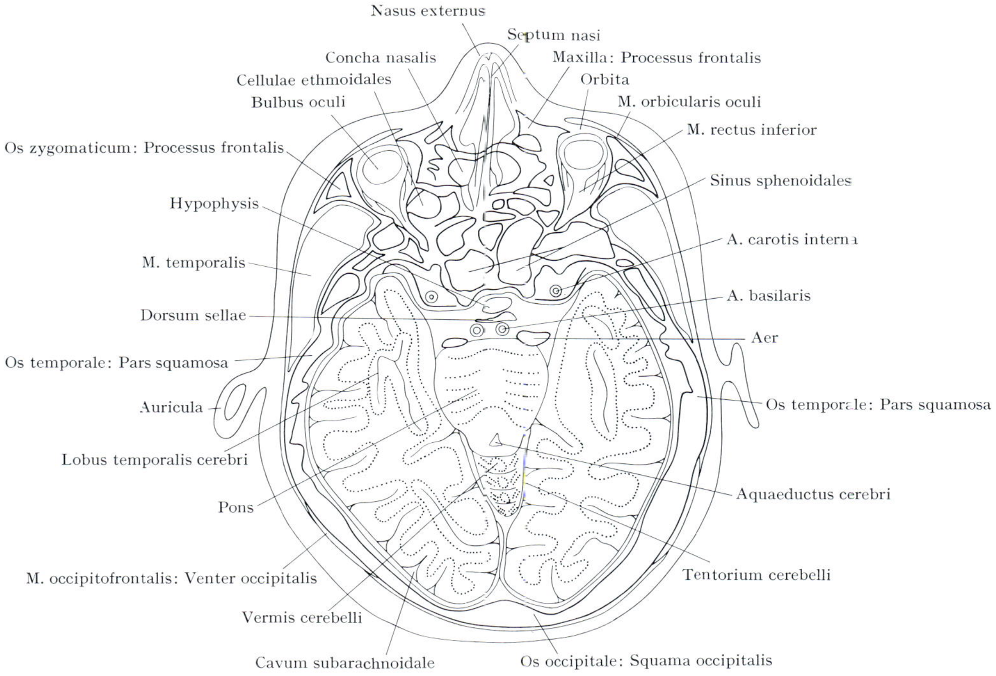

Fig. 70. Anatomical chart

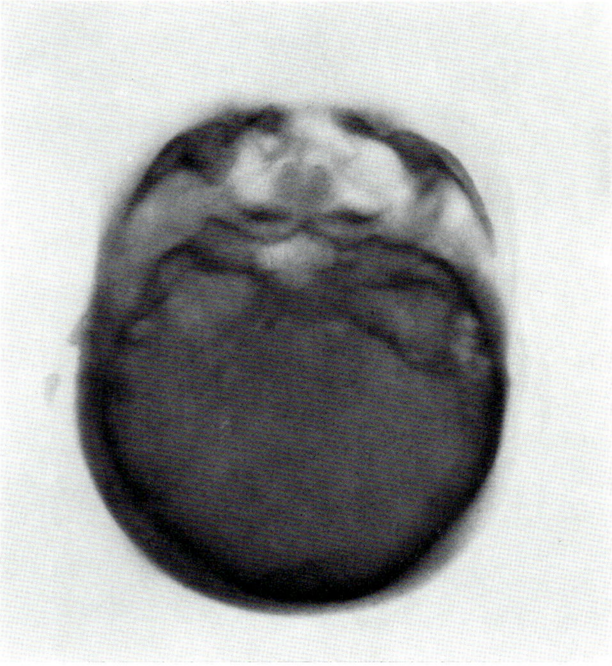

Fig. 71. Axial transverse tomogram

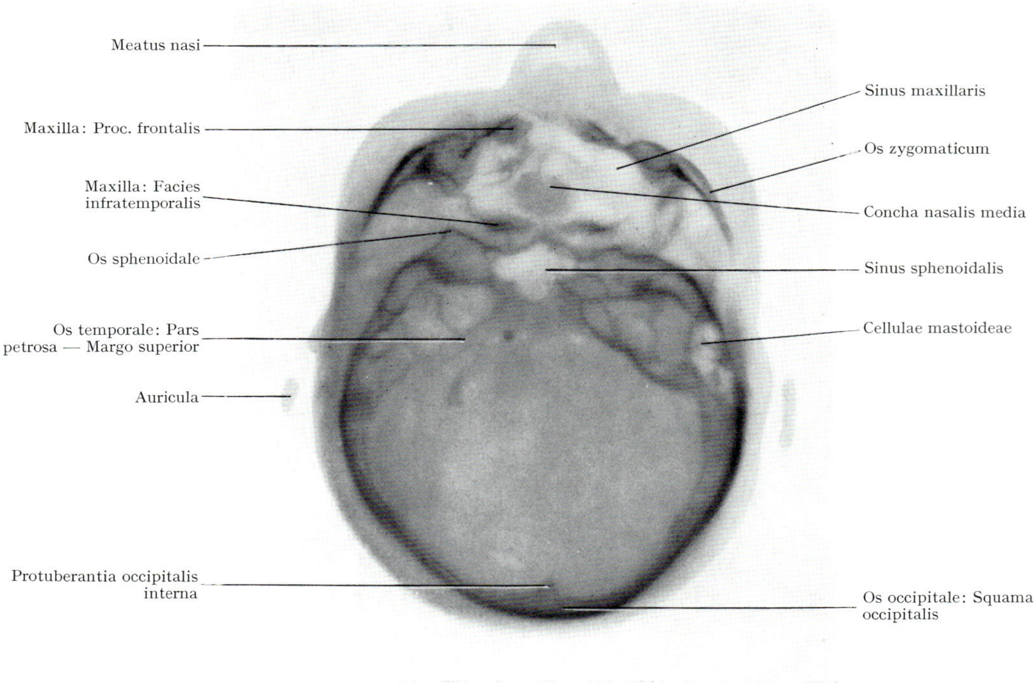

Fig. 72. Interpretation

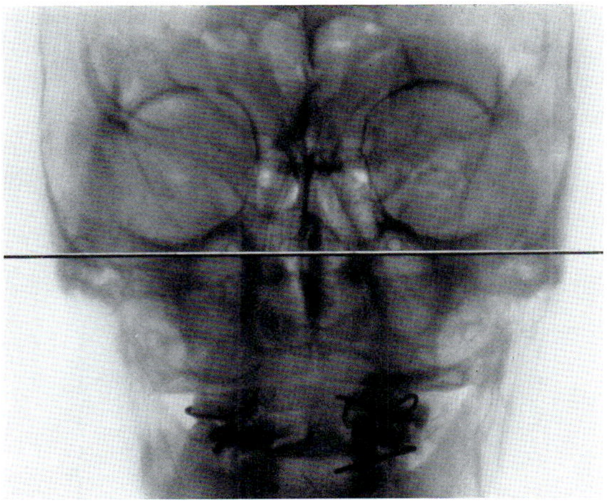

Fig. 73. Normal roentgenogram. Horizontal line showing the level tomographed

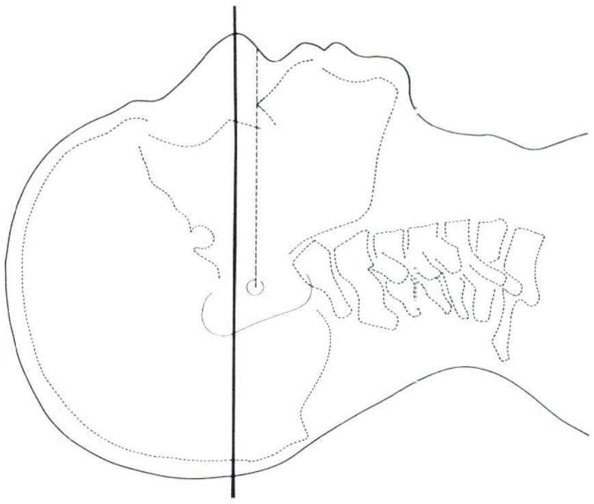

Fig. 74. Schema of tomographed level (solid line) 1 cm above the acanthiomeatal line (dashed line)

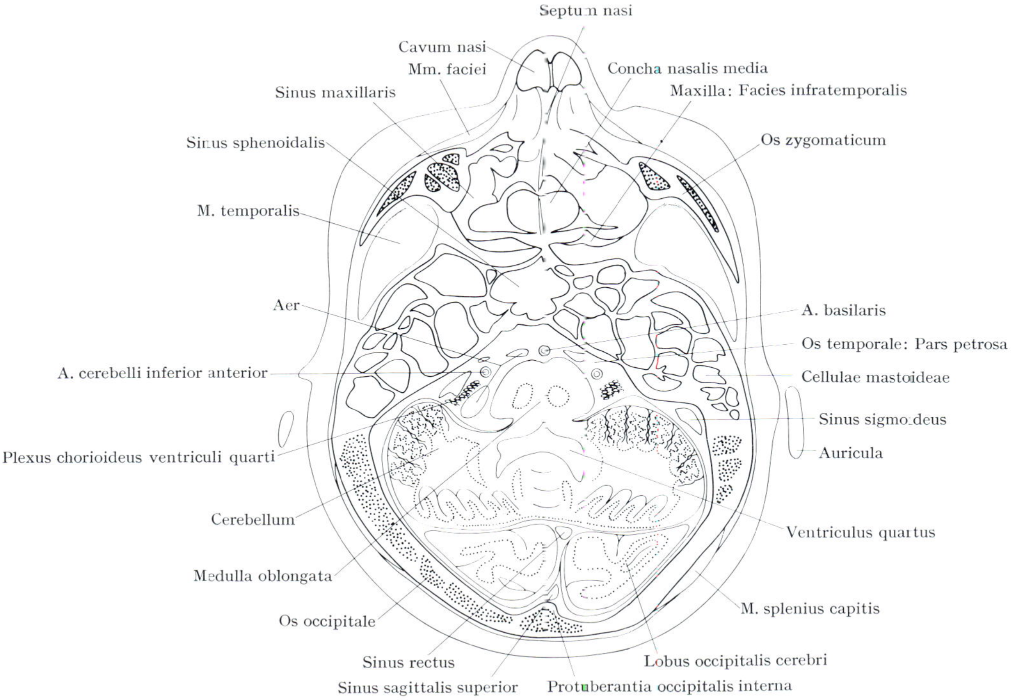

Fig. 75. Anatomical chart

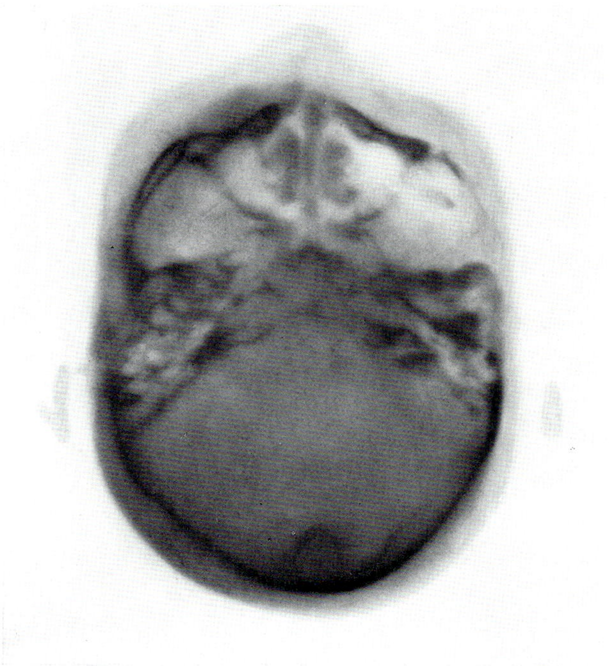

Fig. 76. Axial transverse tomogram

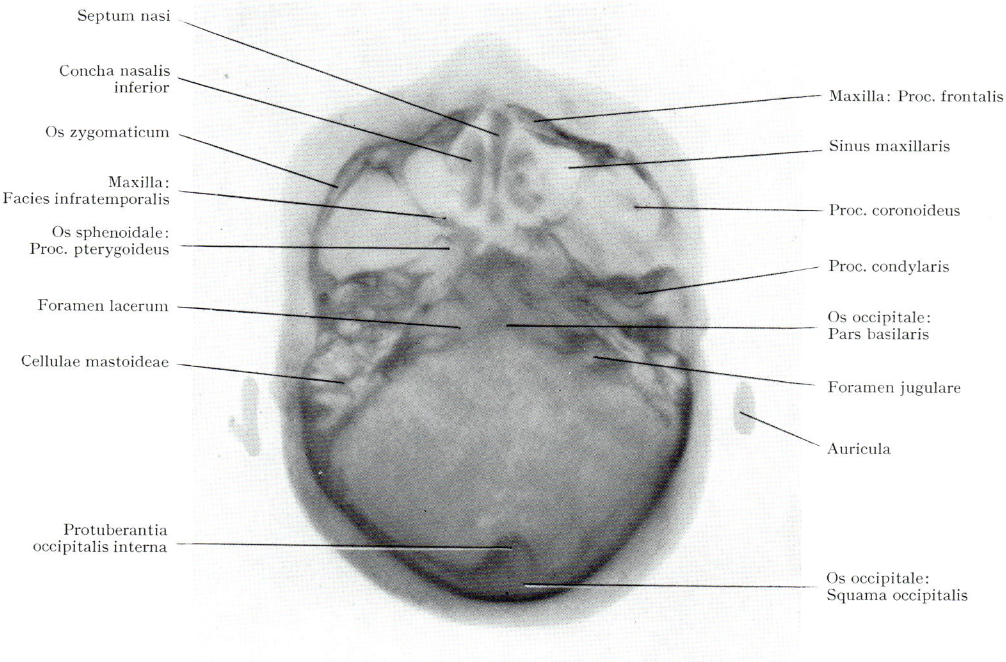

Fig. 77. Interpretation

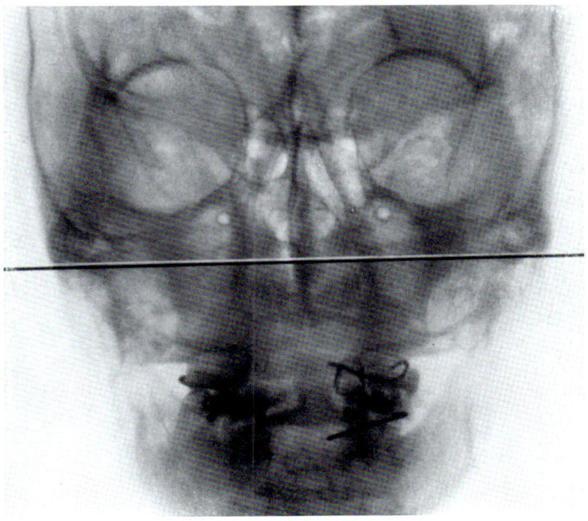

Fig. 78. Normal roentgenogram. Horizontal line showing the level tomographed

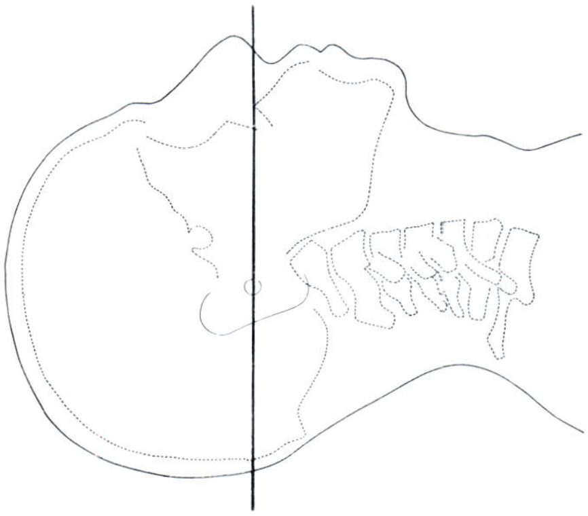

Fig. 79. Schema of tomographed level (solid line) along the acanthiomeatal line

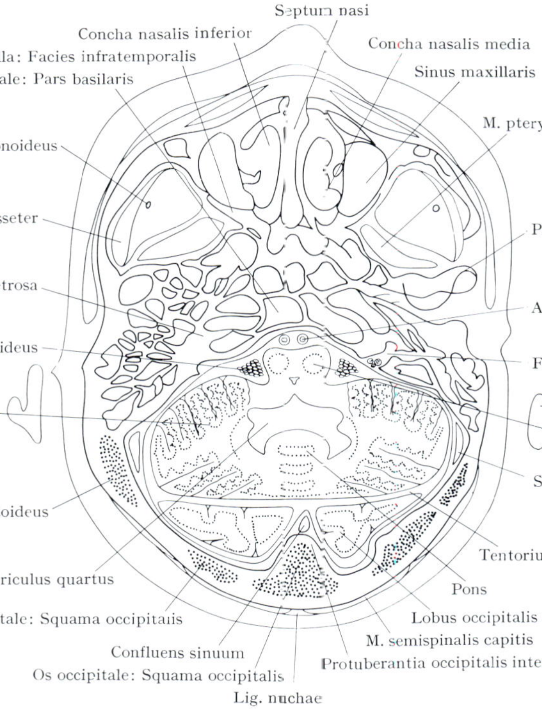

Fig. 80. Anatomical chart

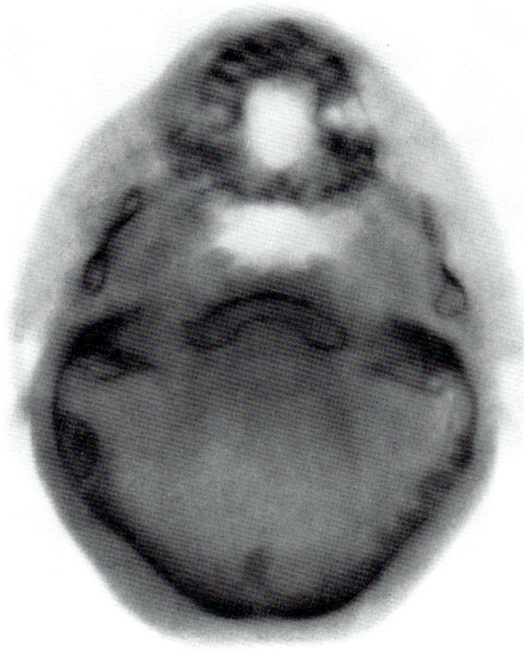

Fig. 81. Axial transverse tomogram

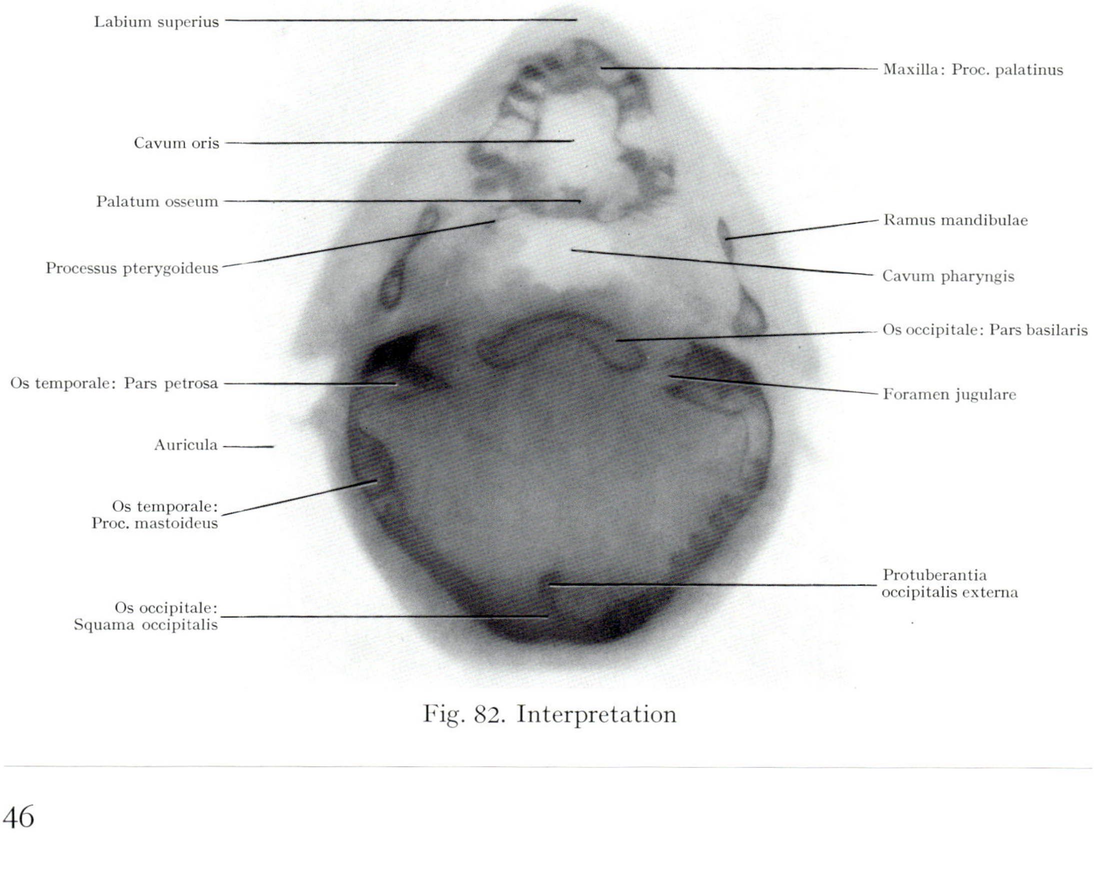

Fig. 82. Interpretation

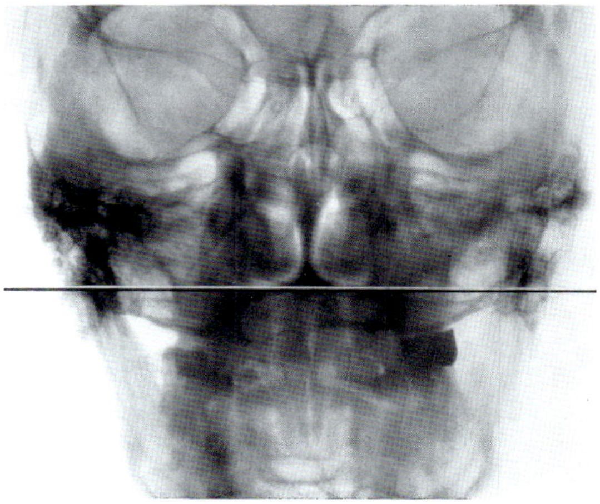

Fig. 83. Normal roentgenogram. Horizontal line showing the level tomographed

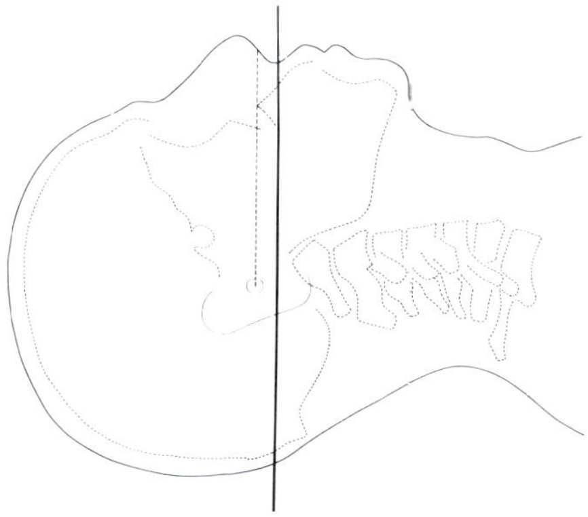

Fig. 84. Schema of tomographed level (solid line) 1 cm below the acanthiomeatal line (dashed line)

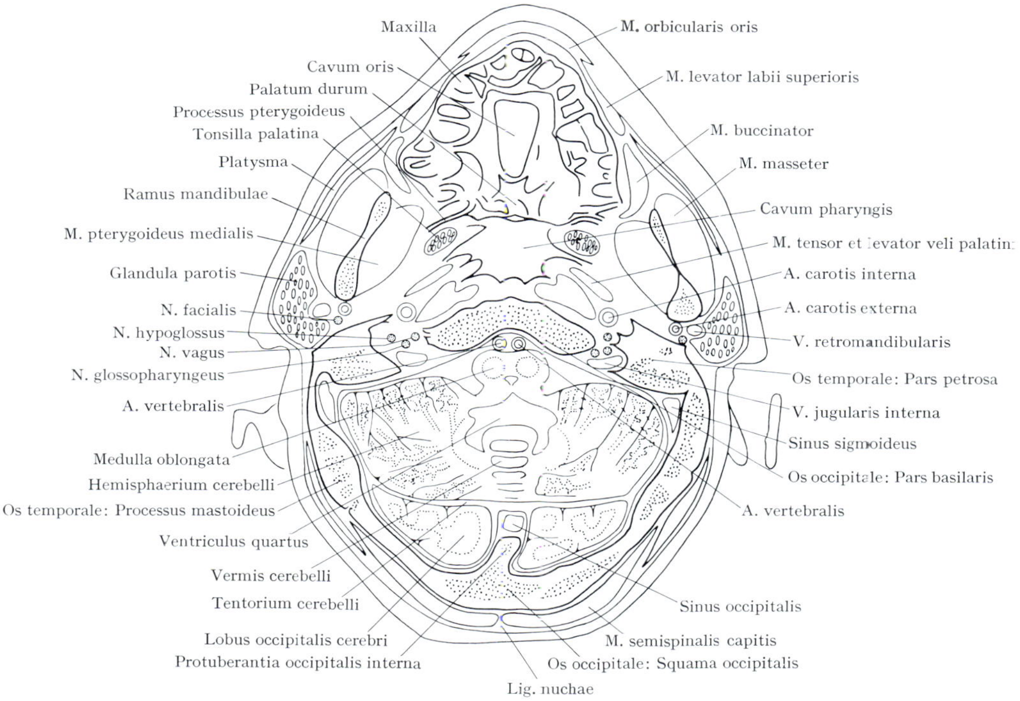

Fig. 85. Anatomical chart

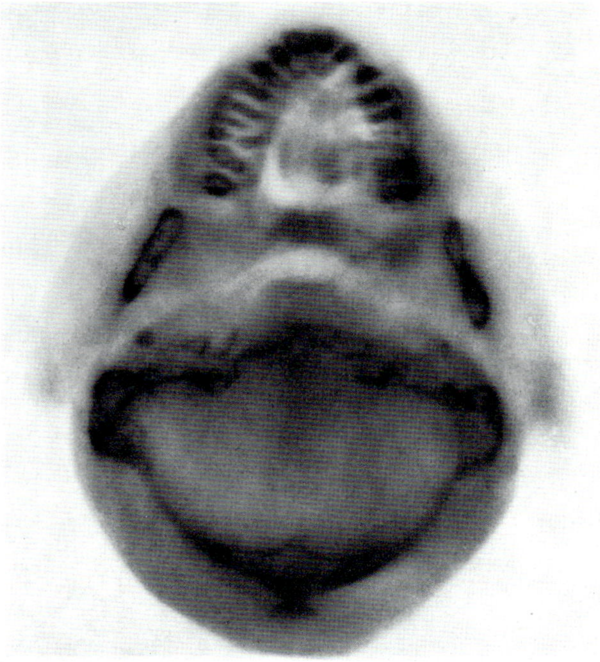

Fig. 86. Axial transverse tomogram

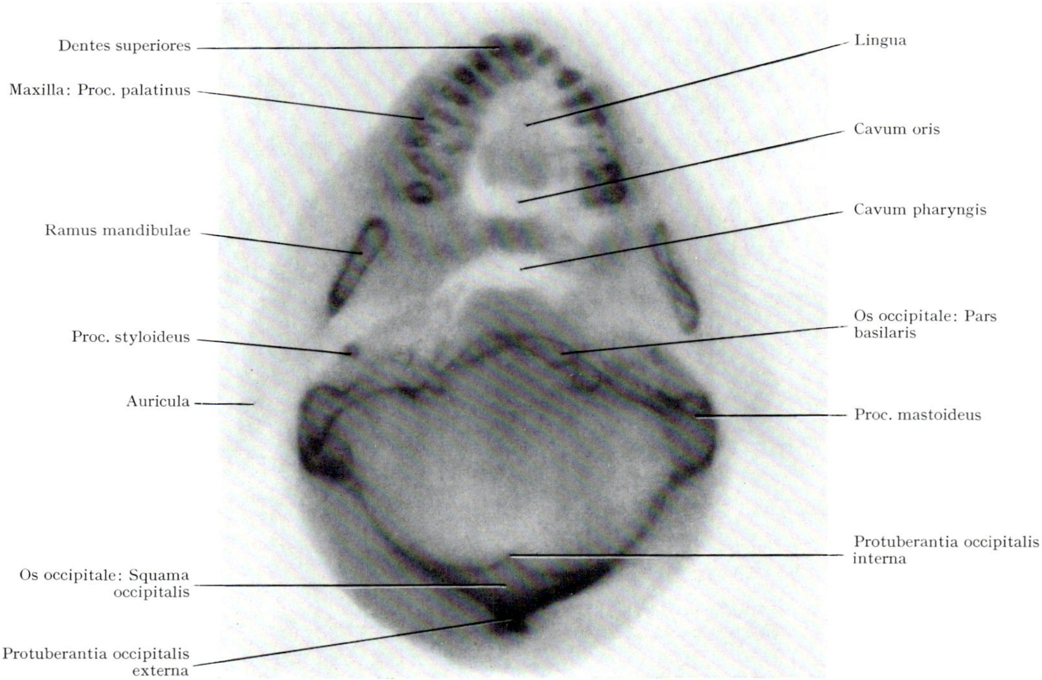

Fig. 87. Interpretation

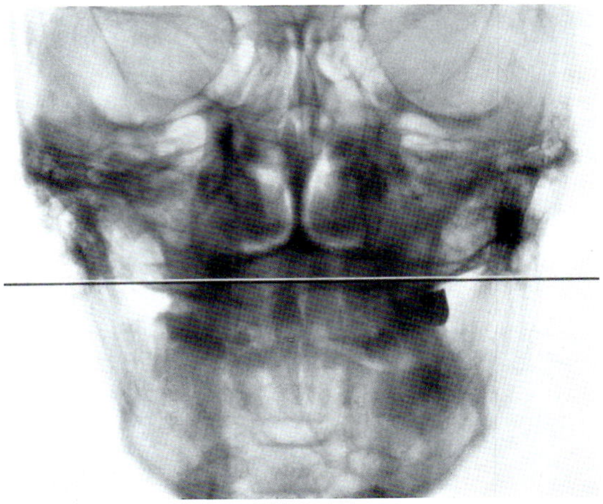

Fig. 88. Normal roentgenogram. Horizontal line showing the level tomographed

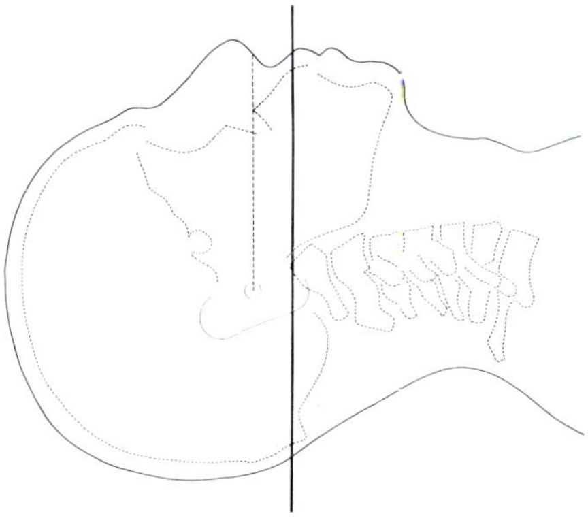

Fig. 89. Schema of tomographed level (solid line) 2 cm below the acanthiomeatal line (dashed line)

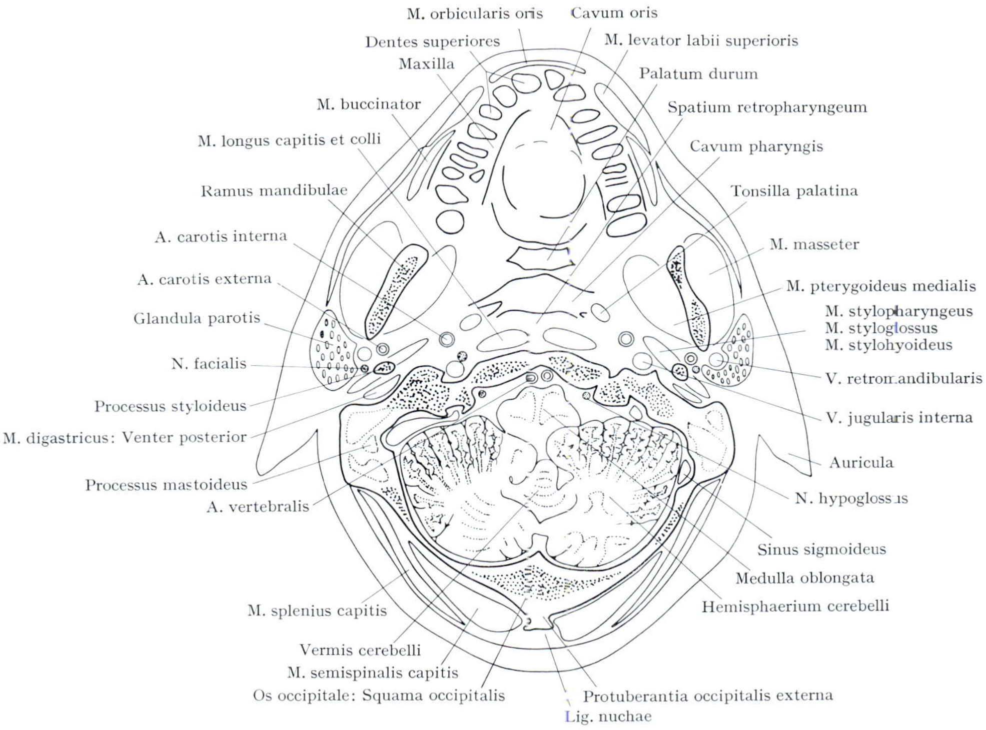

Fig. 90. Anatomical chart

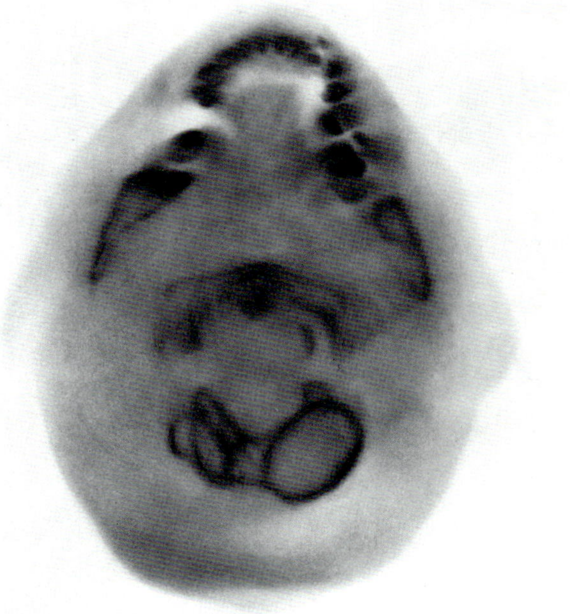

Fig. 91. Axial transverse tomogram

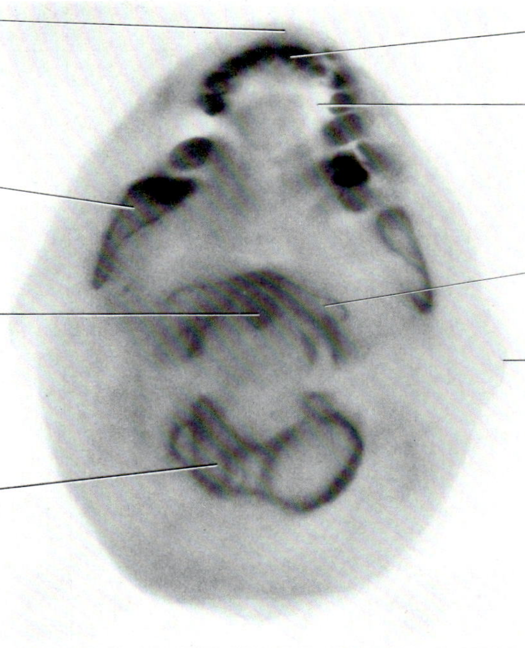

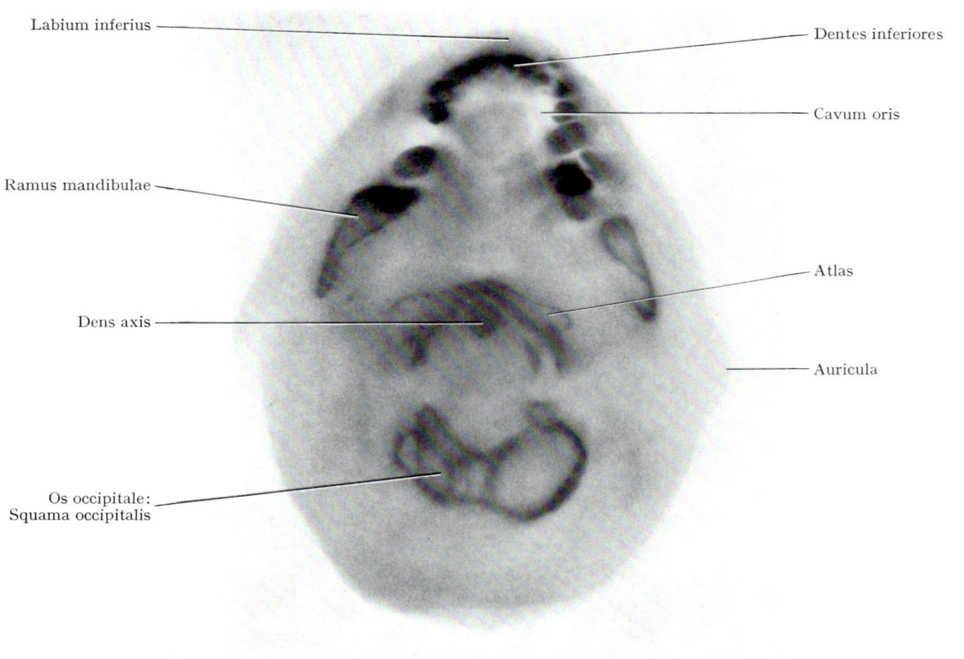

Fig. 92. Interpretation

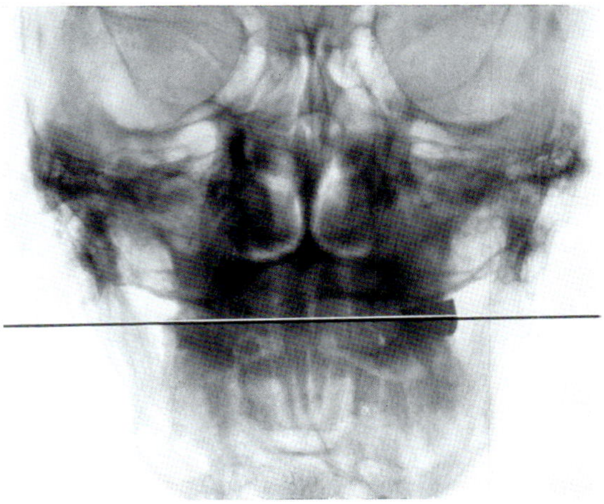

Fig. 93. Normal roentgenogram. Horizontal line showing the level tomographed

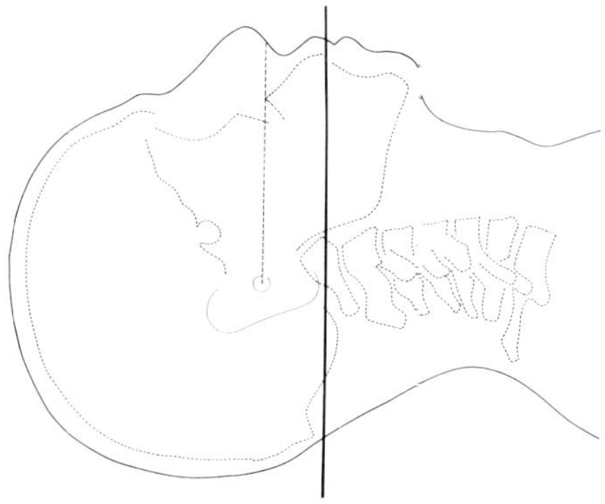

Fig. 94. Schema of tomographed level (solid line) 3 cm below the acanthiomeatal line (dashed line)

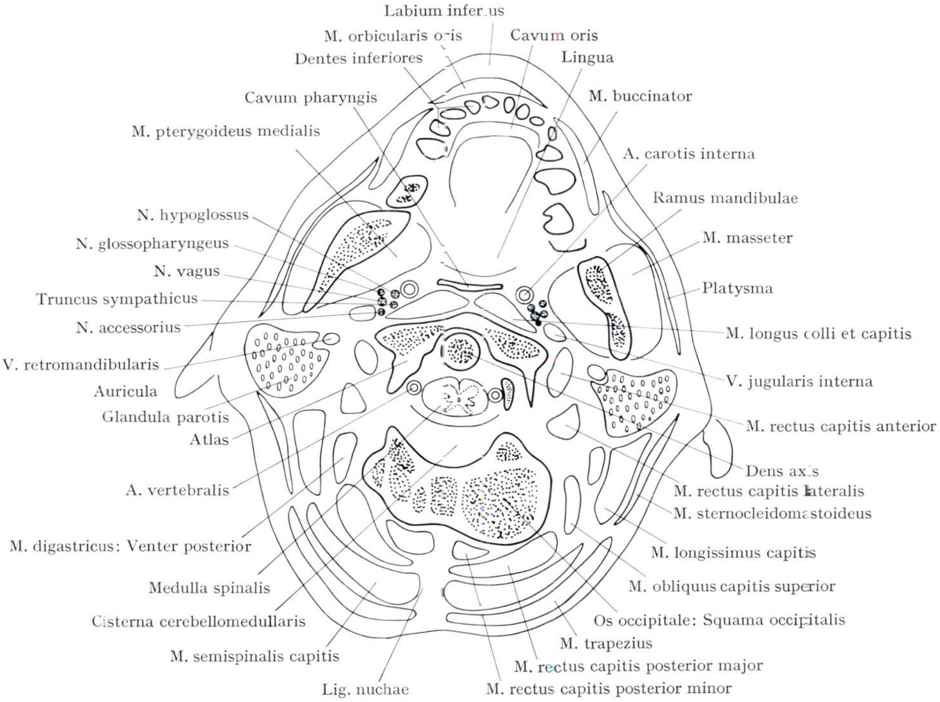

Fig. 95. Anatomical chart

Neck

Eleven axial transverse tomograms of the subject with air insufflated into the subdermal space.

Appendices:
1. Axial transverse tomograms of the parotis.
2. Axial transverse tomograms of the neck without contrast medium.

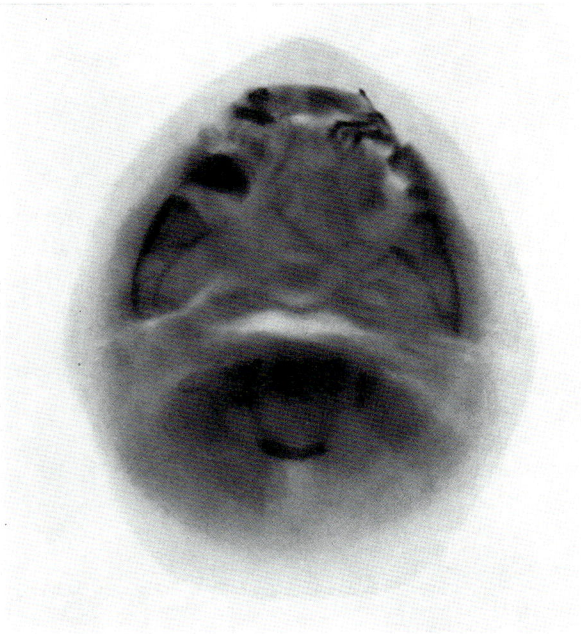

Fig. 96. Axial transverse tomogram

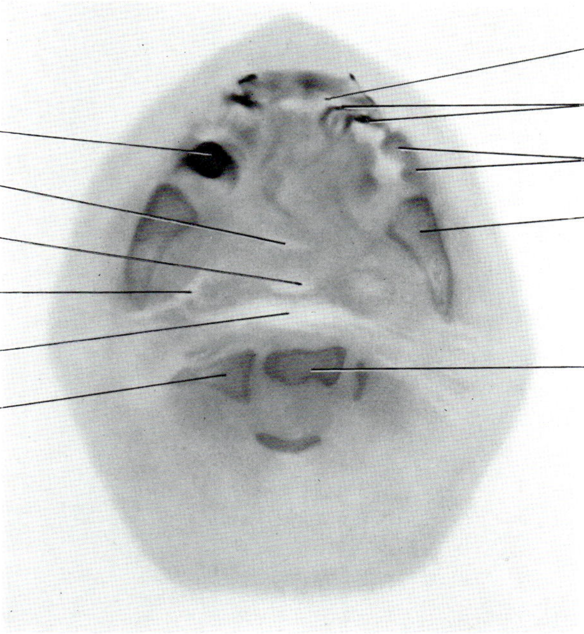

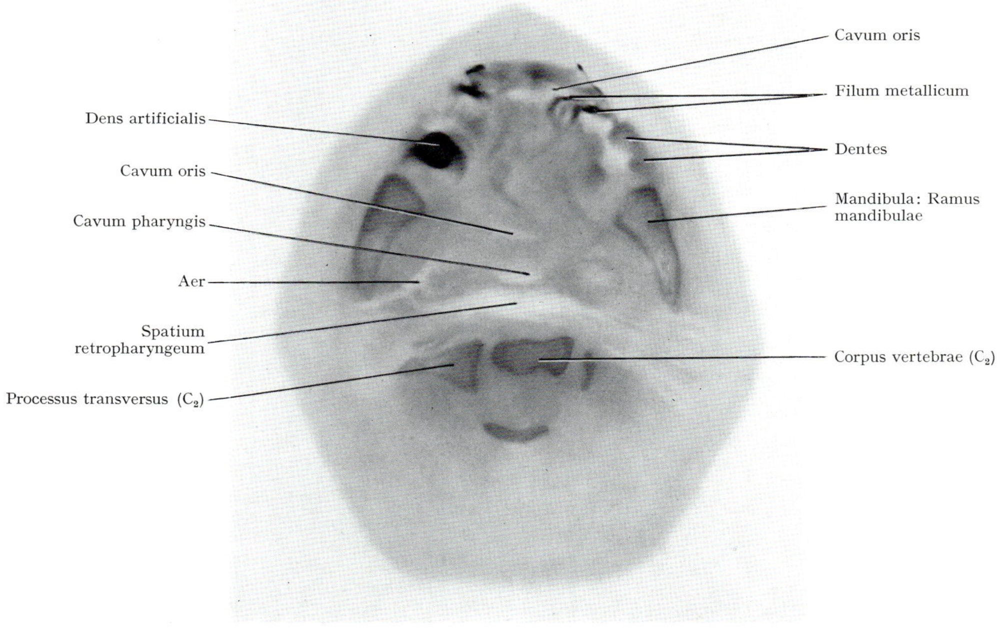

Fig. 97. Interpretation

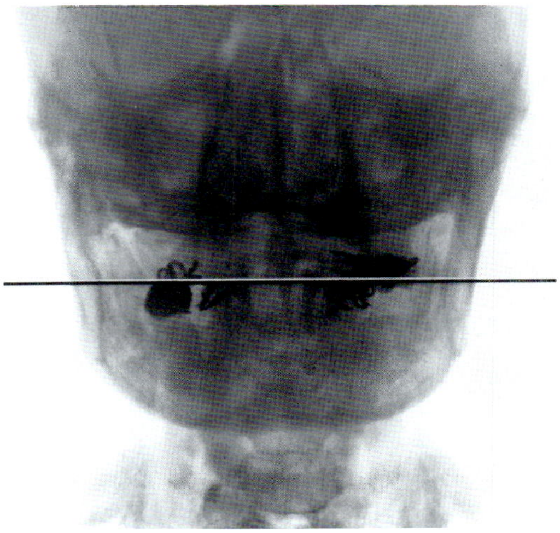

Fig. 98. Normal roentgenogram. Horizontal line showing the level tomographed

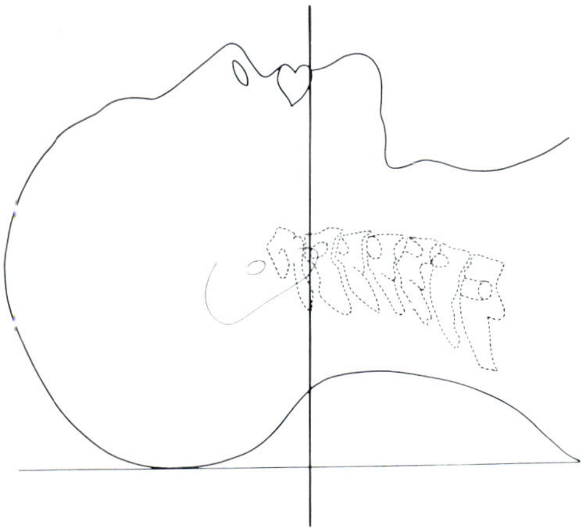

Fig 99. Schematic drawing of the level tomographed

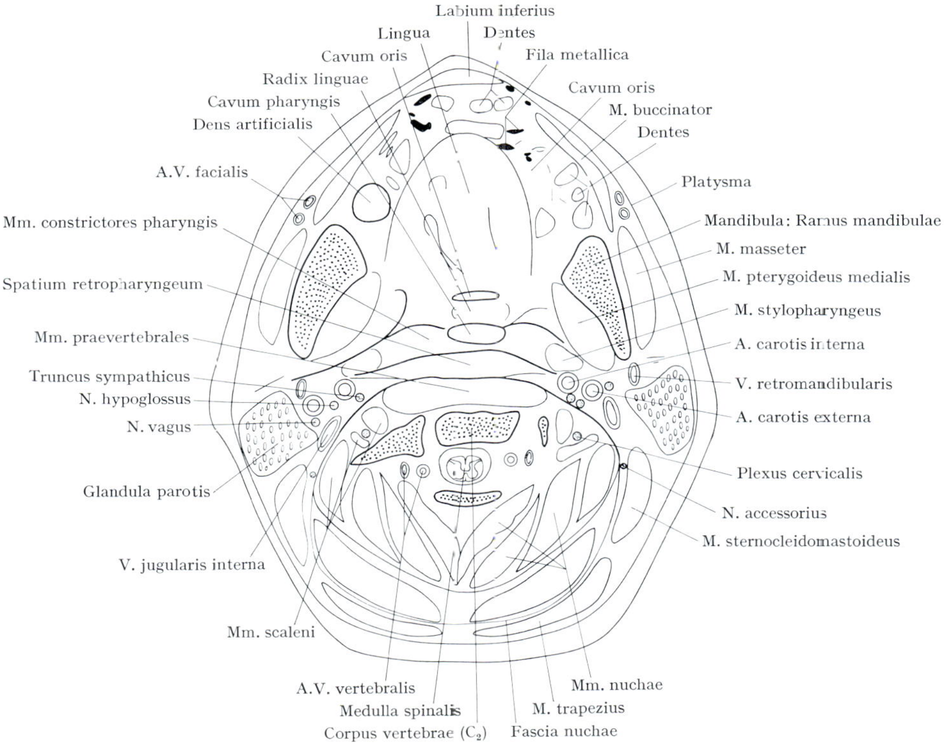

Fig. 100. Anatomical chart

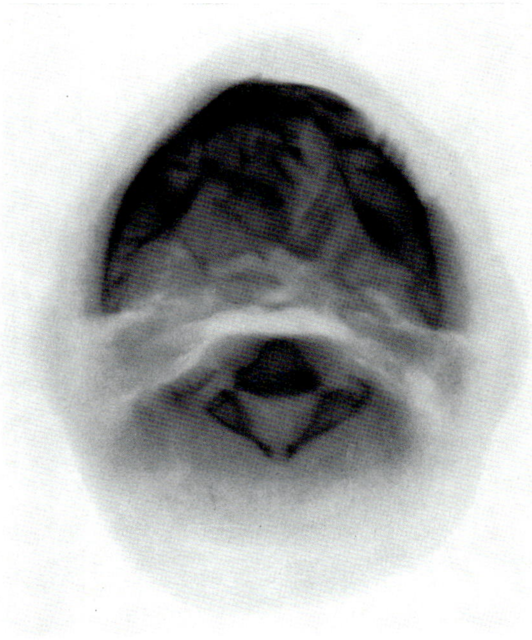

Fig. 101. Axial transverse tomogram

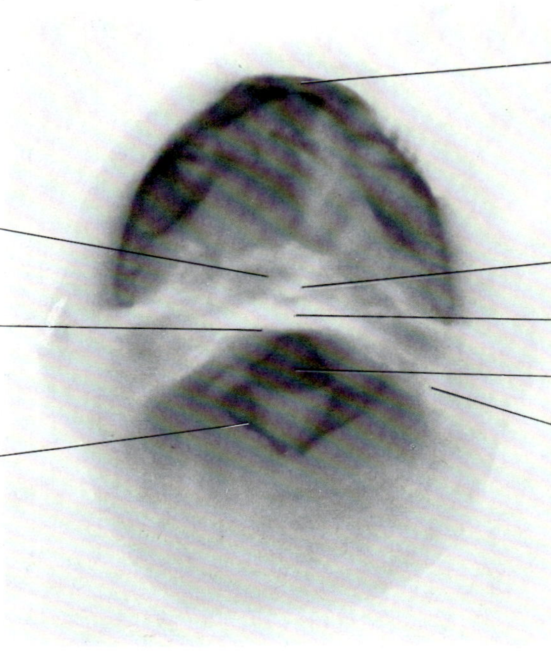

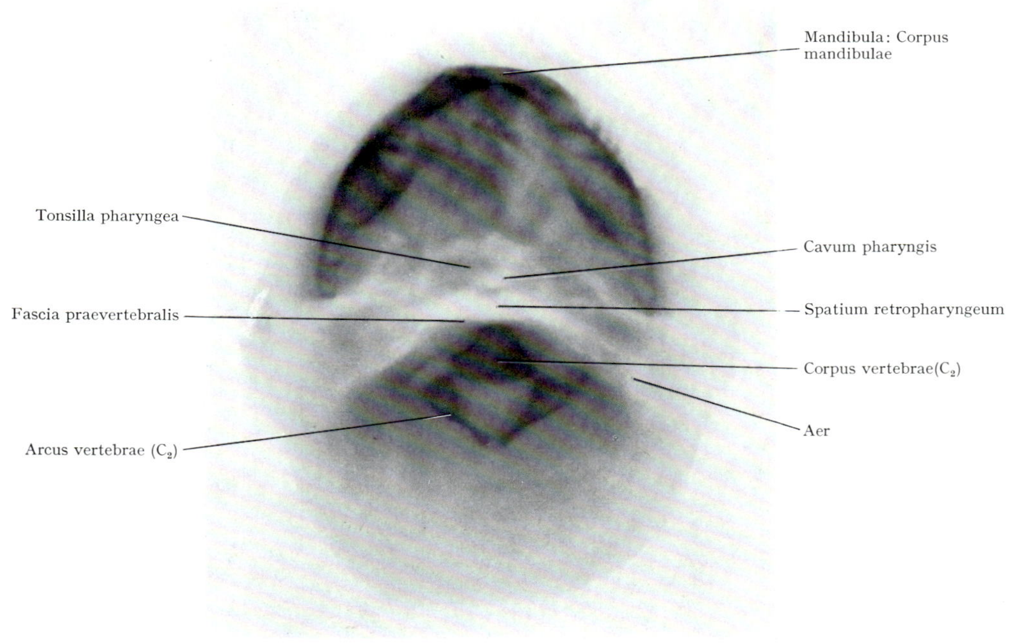

Fig. 102. Interpretation

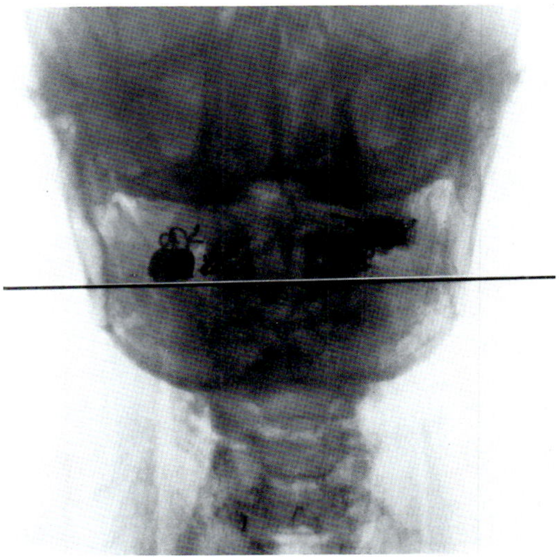

Fig. 103. Normal roentgenogram. Horizontal line showing the level tomographed

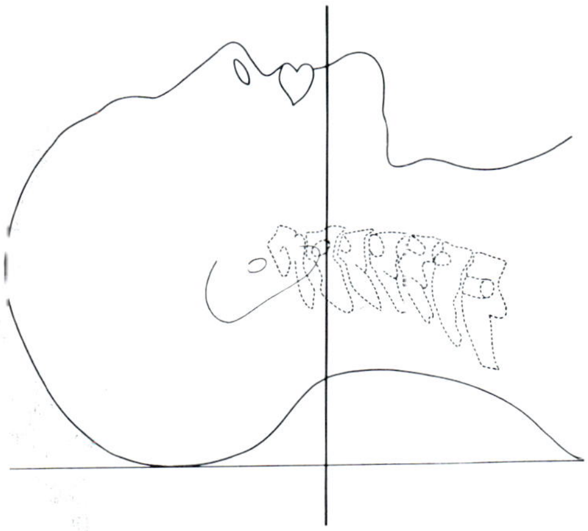

Fig. 104. Schematic drawing of the level tomographed

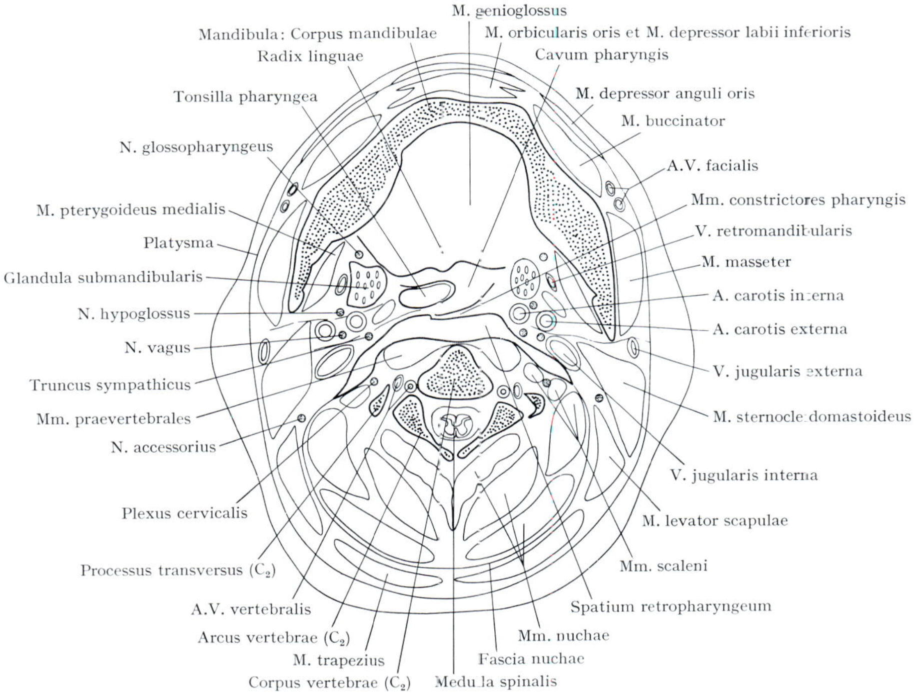

Fig. 105. Anatomical chart

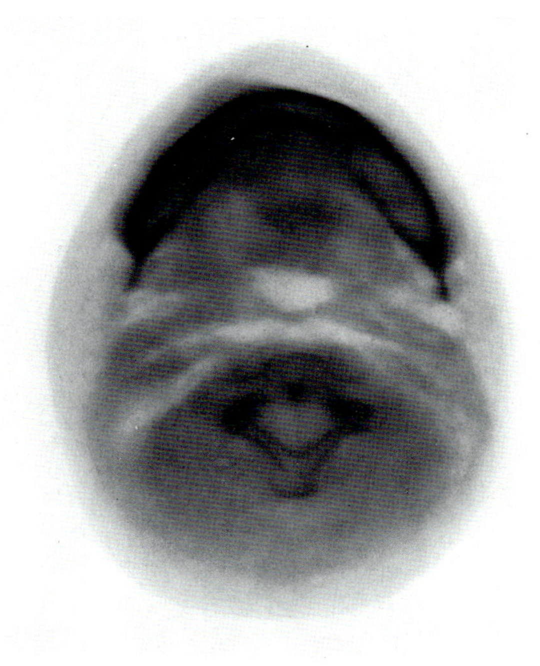

Fig. 106. Axial transverse tomogram

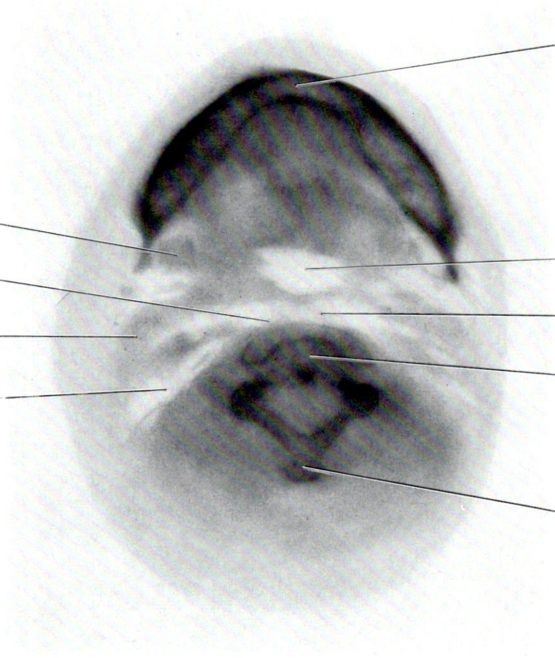

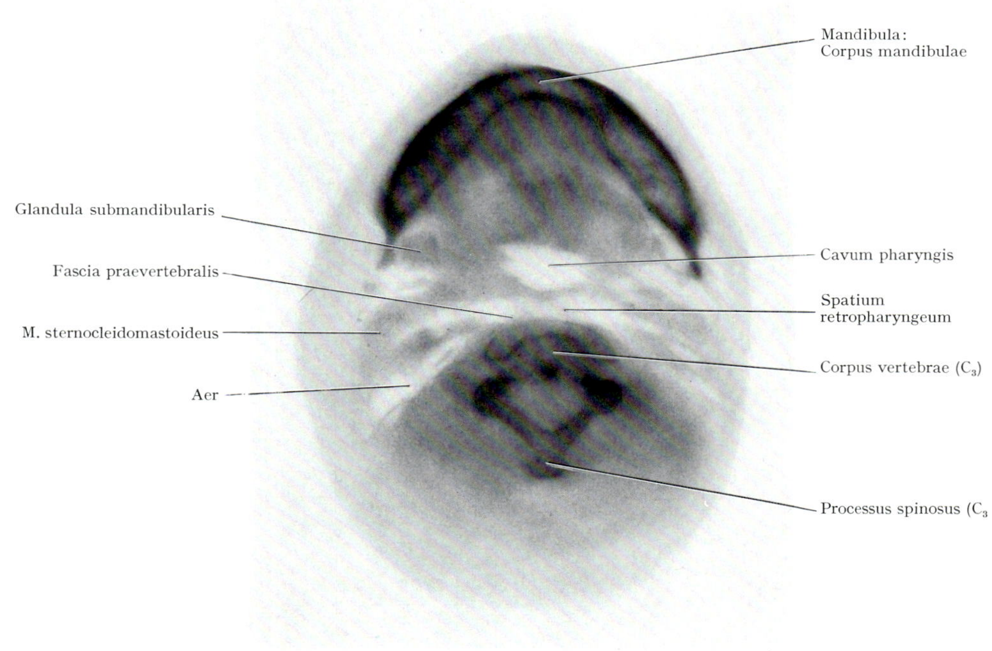

Fig. 107. Interpretation

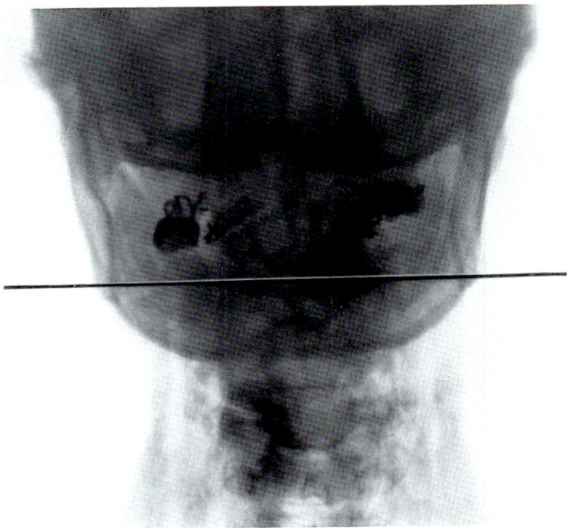

Fig. 108. Normal roentgenogram. Horizontal line showing the level tomographed

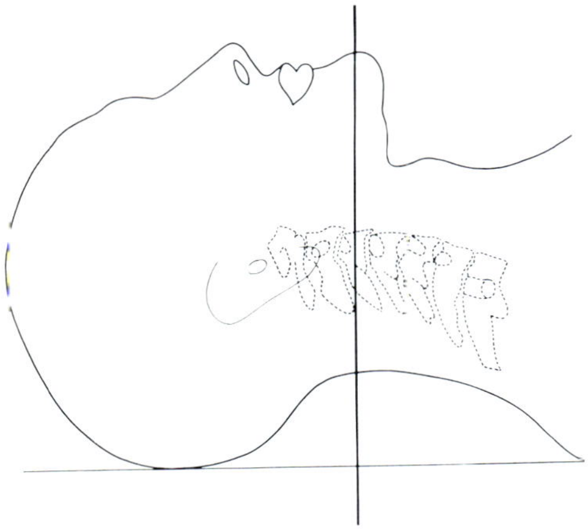

Fig. 109. Schematic drawing of the level tomographed

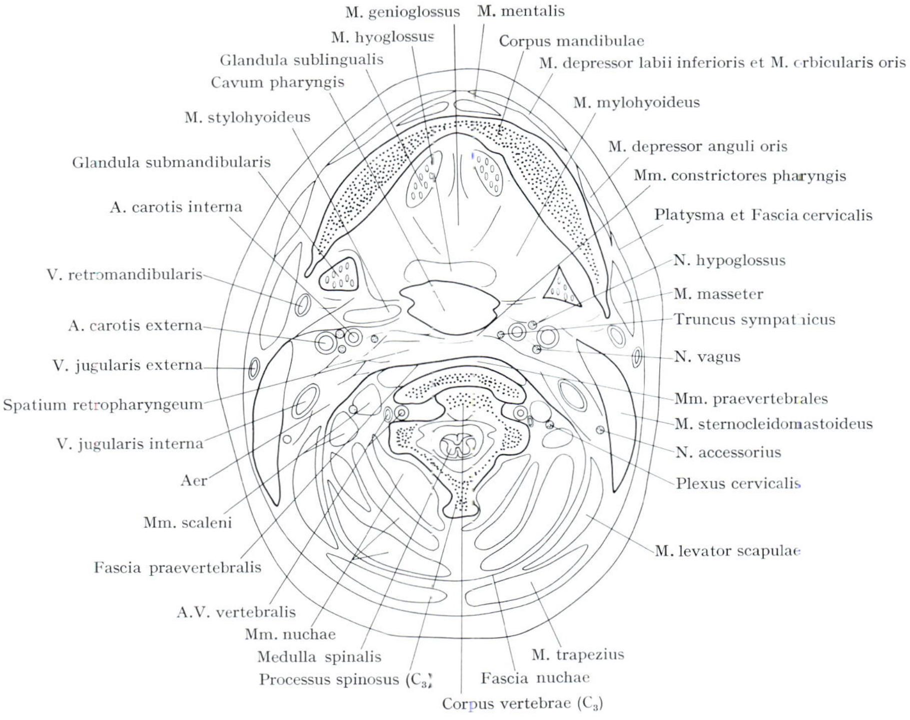

Fig. 110. Anatomical chart

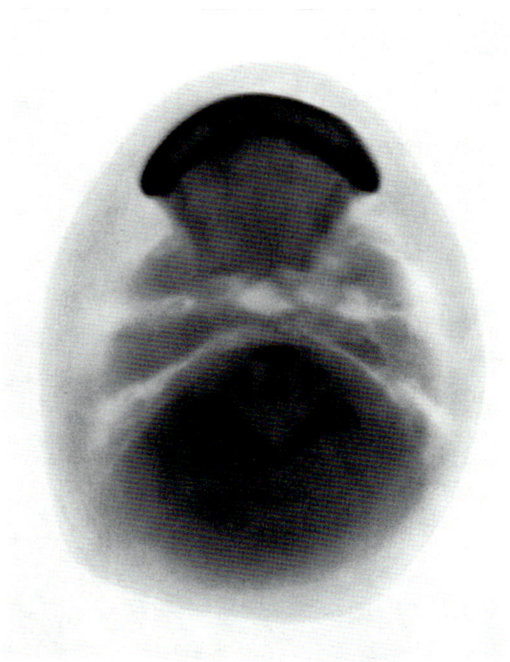

Fig. 111. Axial transverse tomogram

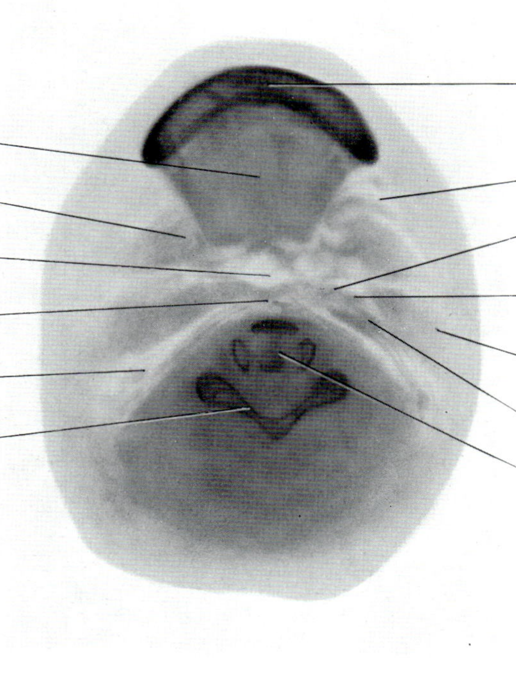

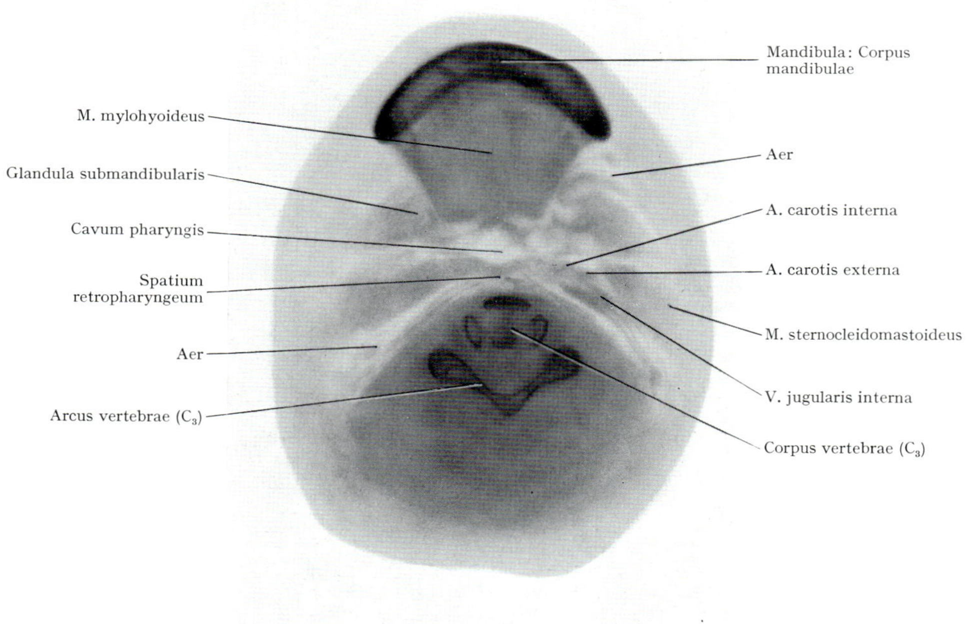

Fig. 112. Interpretation

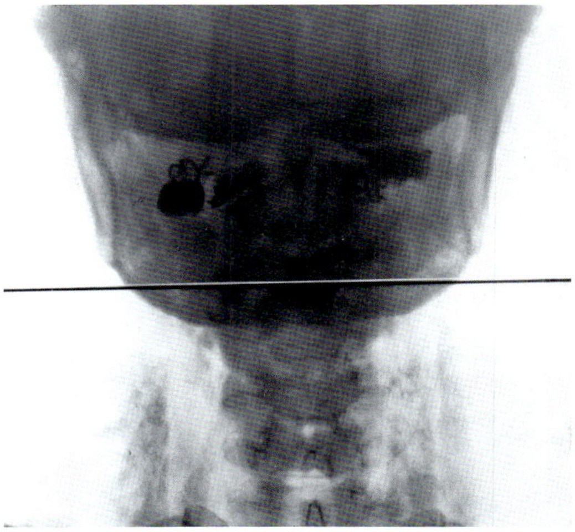

Fig. 113. Normal roentgenogram. Horizontal line showing the level tomographed

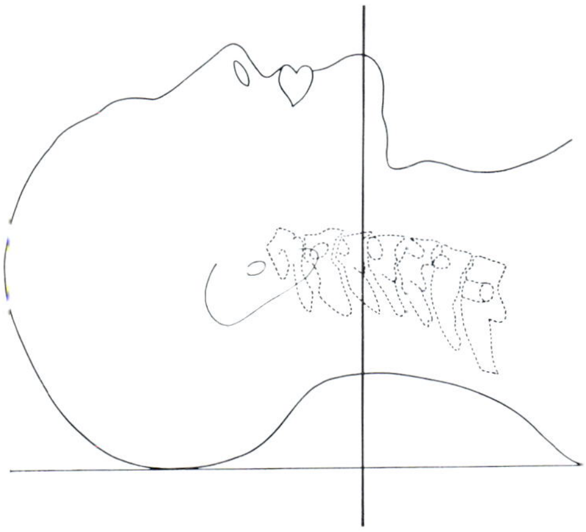

Fig. 114. Schematic drawing of the level tomographed

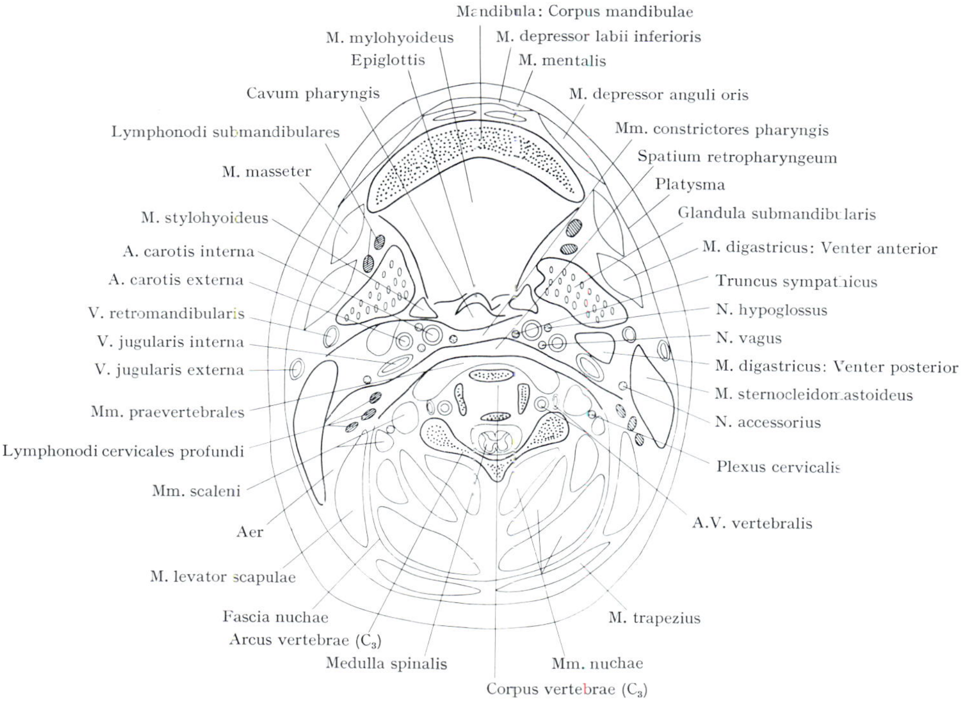

Fig. 115. Anatomical chart

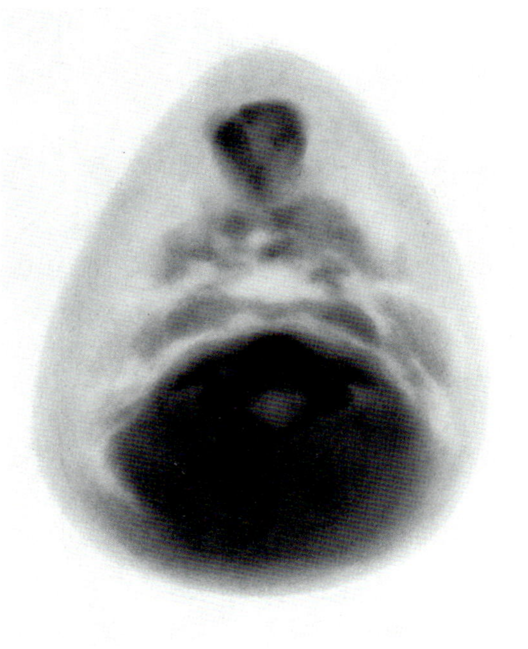

Fig. 116. Axial transverse tomogram

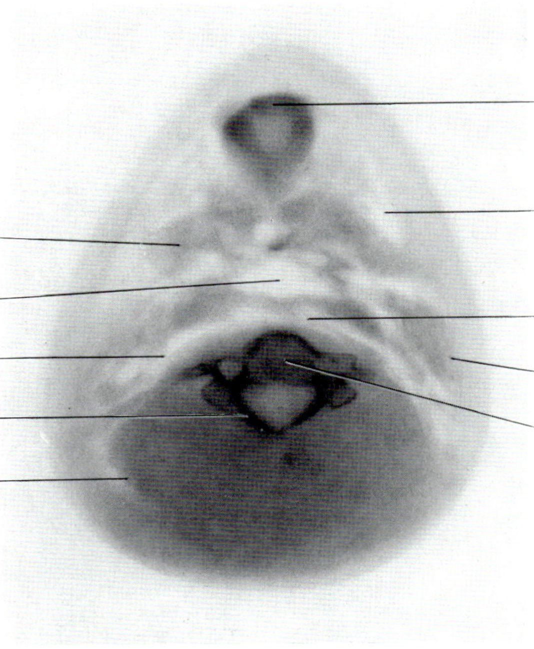

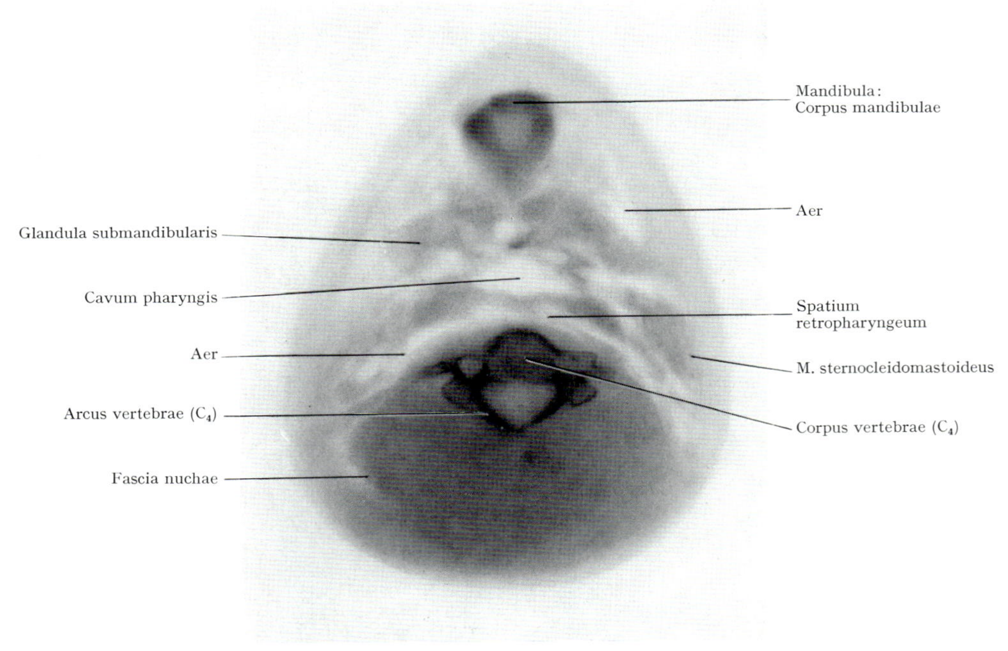

Fig. 117. Interpretation

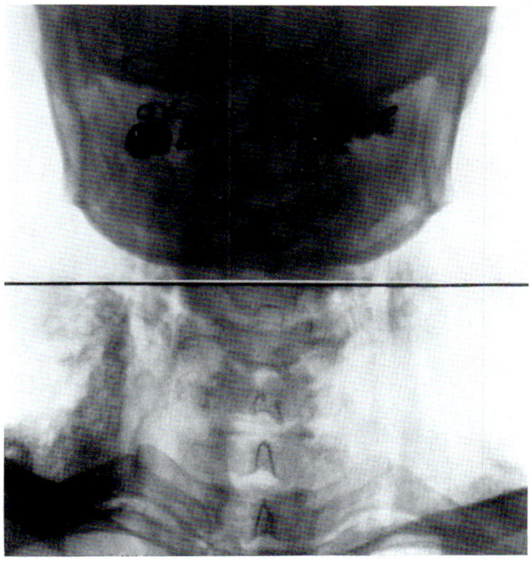

Fig. 118. Normal roentgenogram. Horizontal line showing the level tomographed

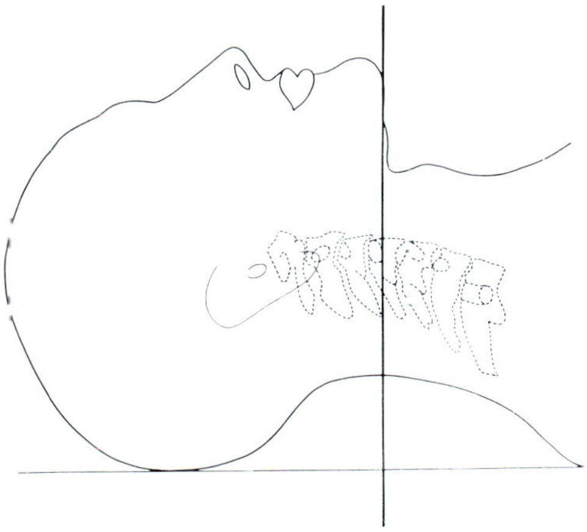

Fig. 119. Schematic drawing of the level tomographed

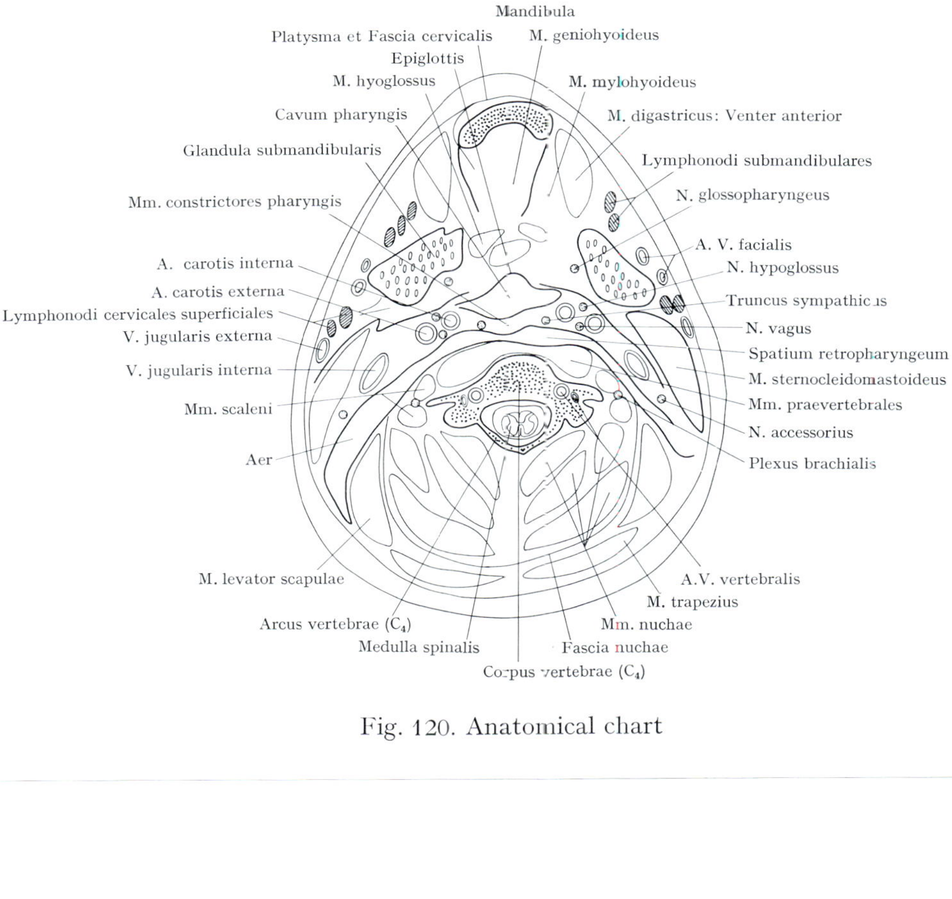

Fig. 120. Anatomical chart

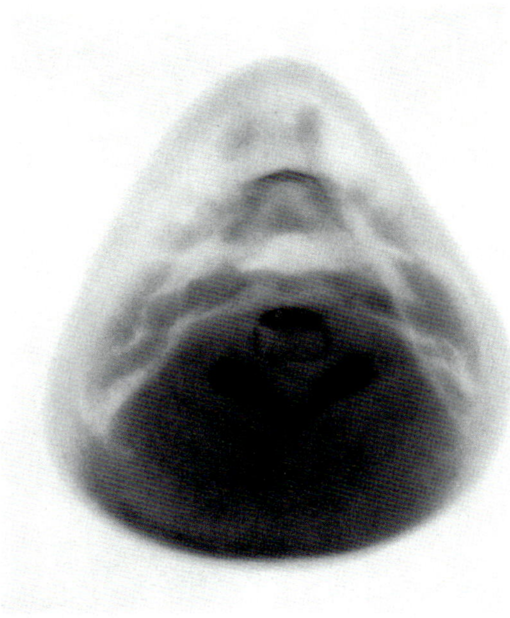

Fig. 121. Axial transverse tomogram

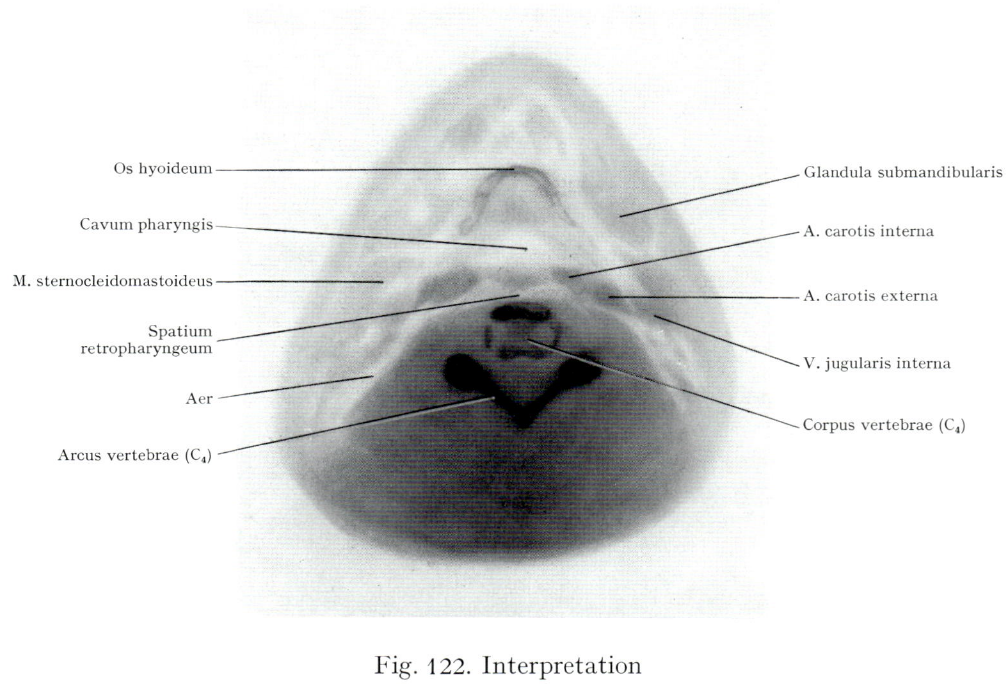

Fig. 122. Interpretation

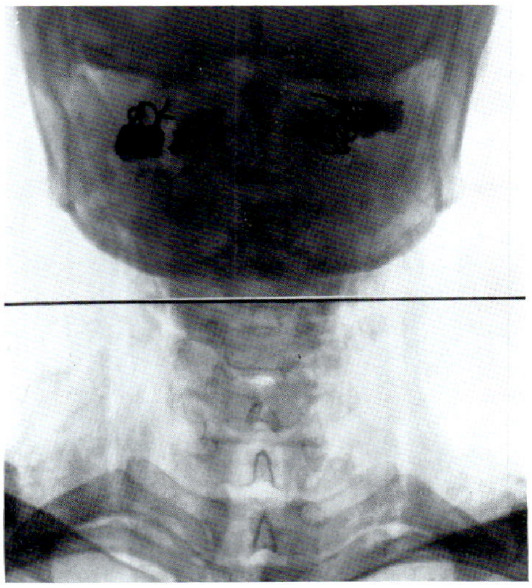

Fig. 123. Normal roentgenogram. Horizontal line showing the level tomographed

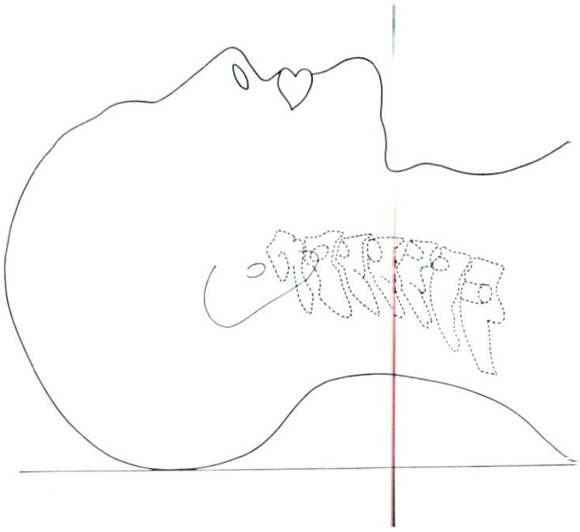

Fig. 124. Schematic drawing of the level tomographed

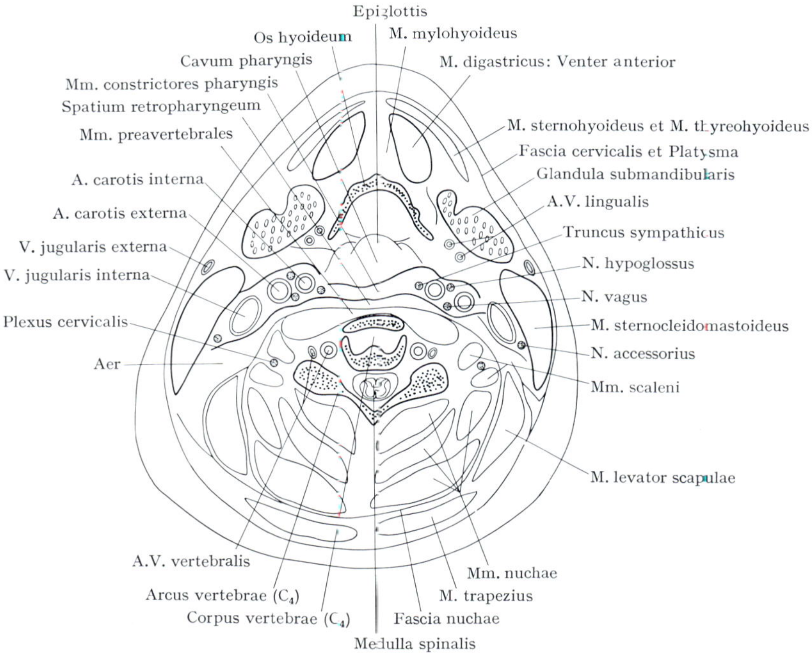

Fig. 125. Anatomical chart

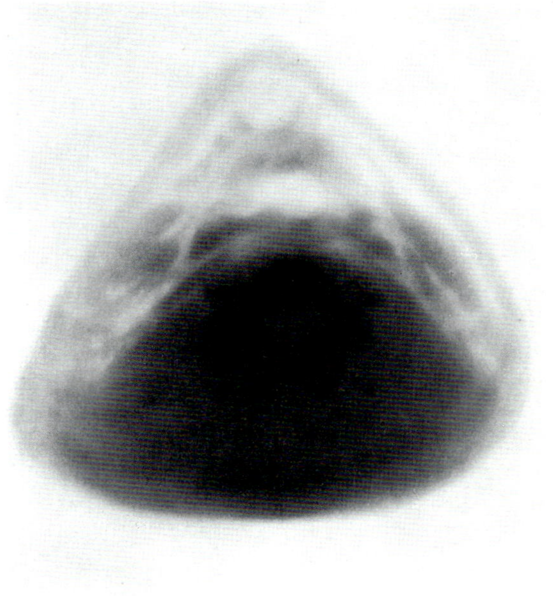

Fig. 126. Axial transverse tomogram

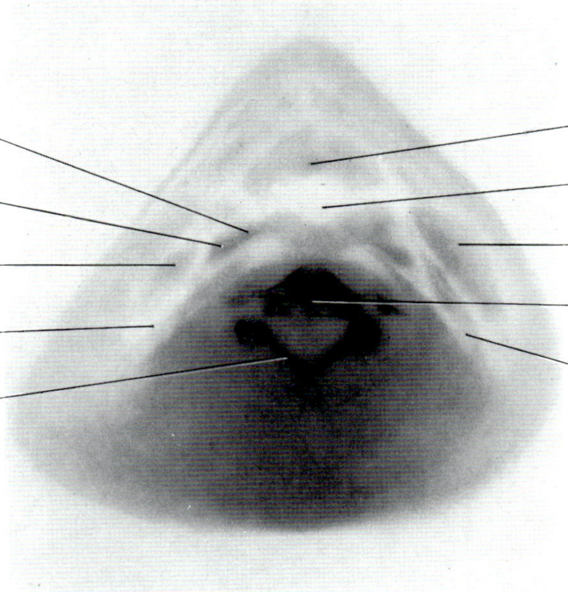

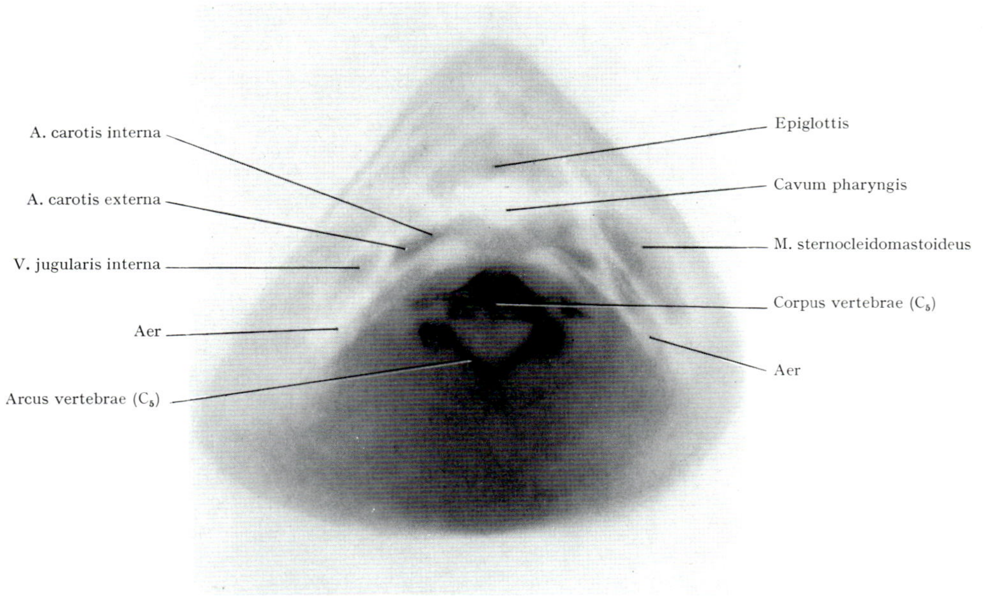

Fig. 127. Interpretation

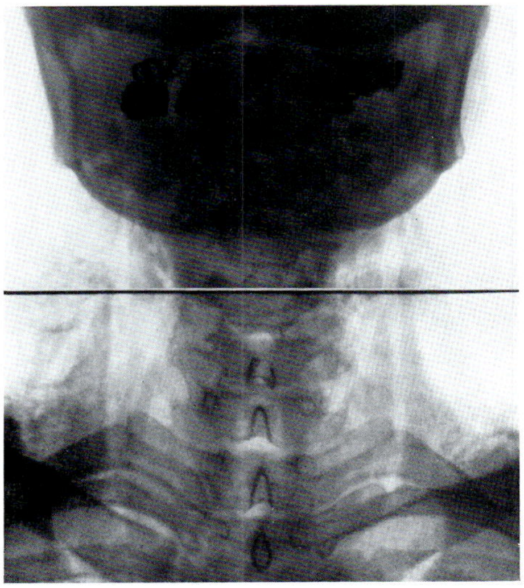

Fig. 128. Normal roentgenogram. Horizontal line showing the level tomographed

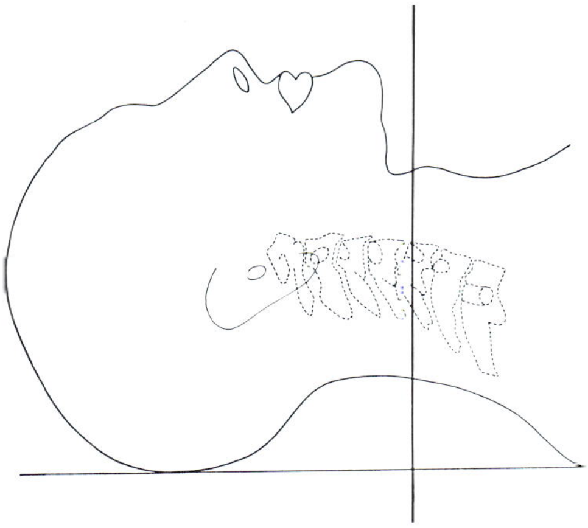

Fig. 129. Schematic drawing of the level tomographed

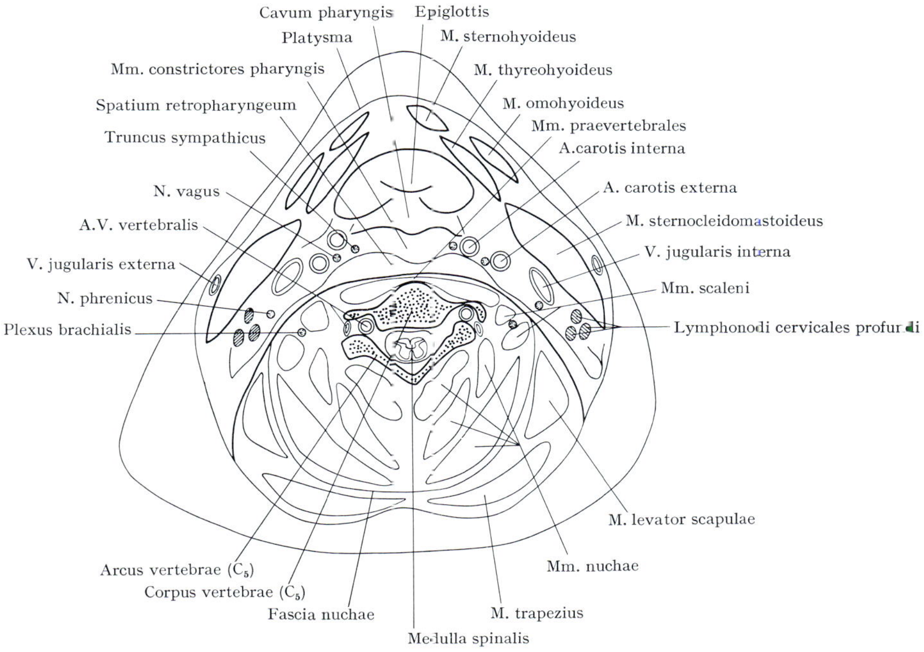

Fig. 130. Anatomical chart

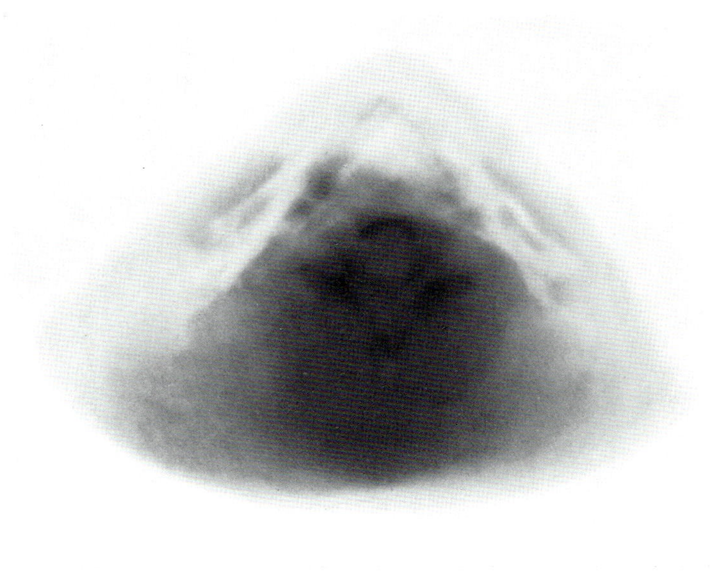

Fig. 131. Axial transverse tomogram

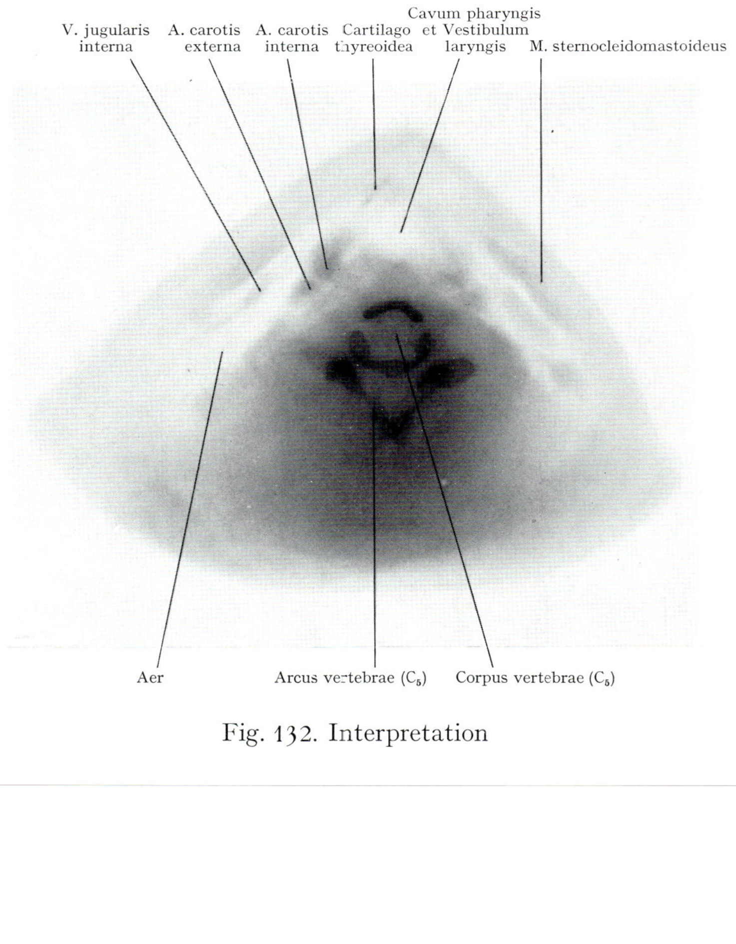

Fig. 132. Interpretation

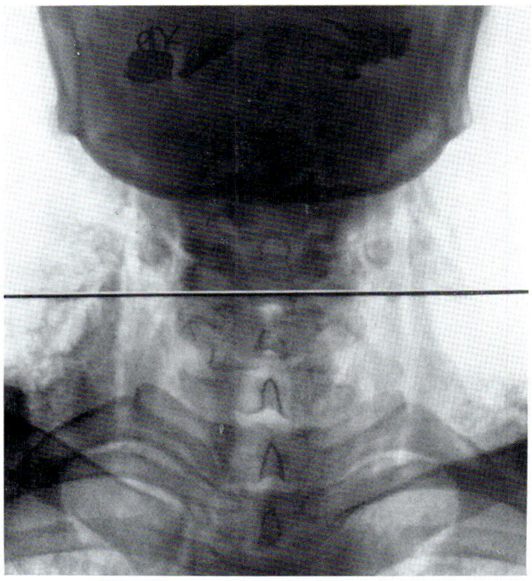

Fig. 133. Normal roentgenogram. Horizontal line showing the level tomographed

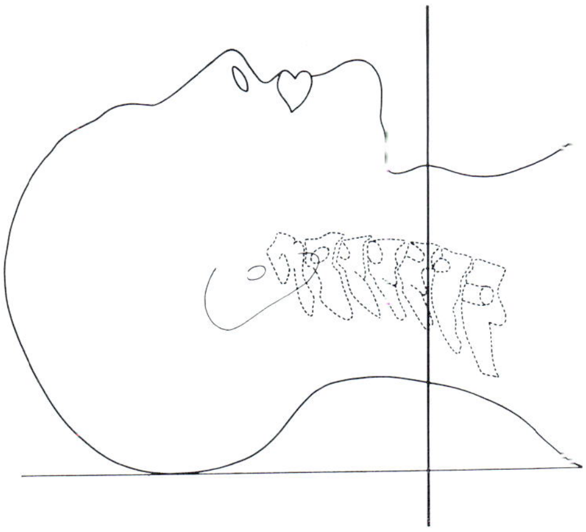

Fig. 134. Schematic drawing of the level tomographed

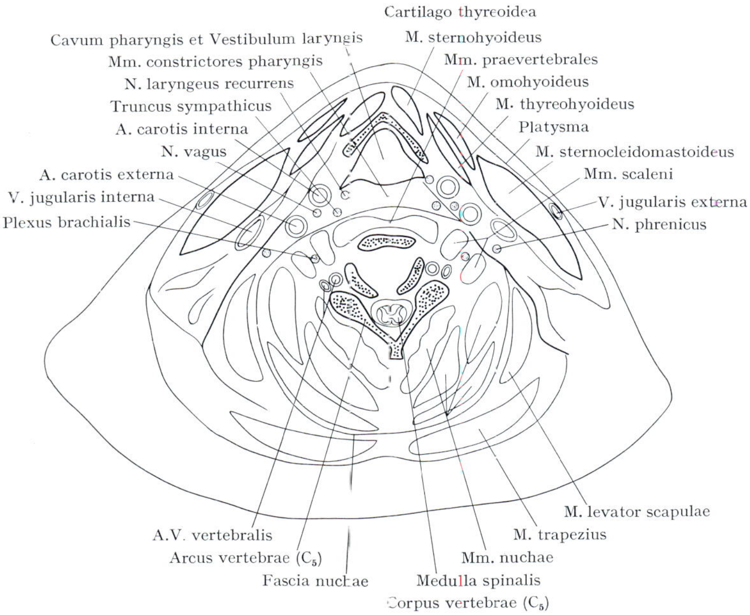

Fig. 135. Anatomical chart

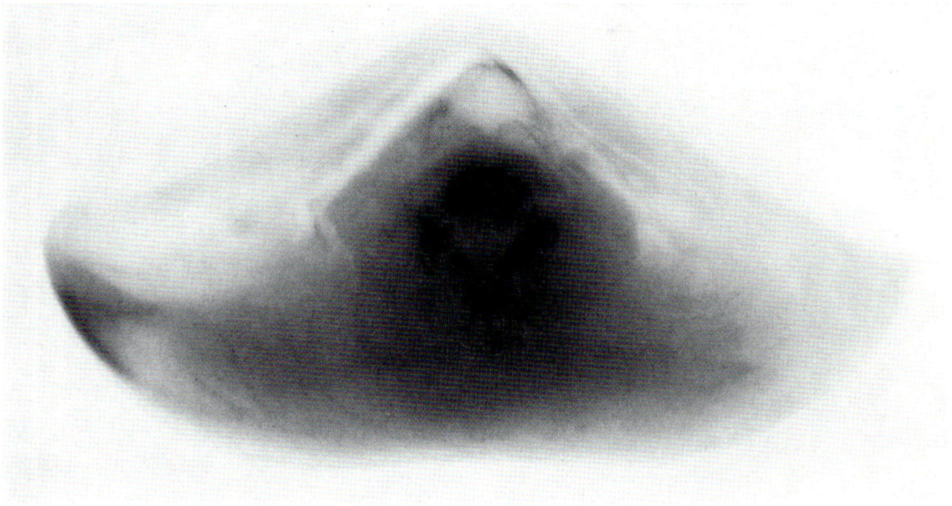

Fig. 136. Axial transverse tomogram

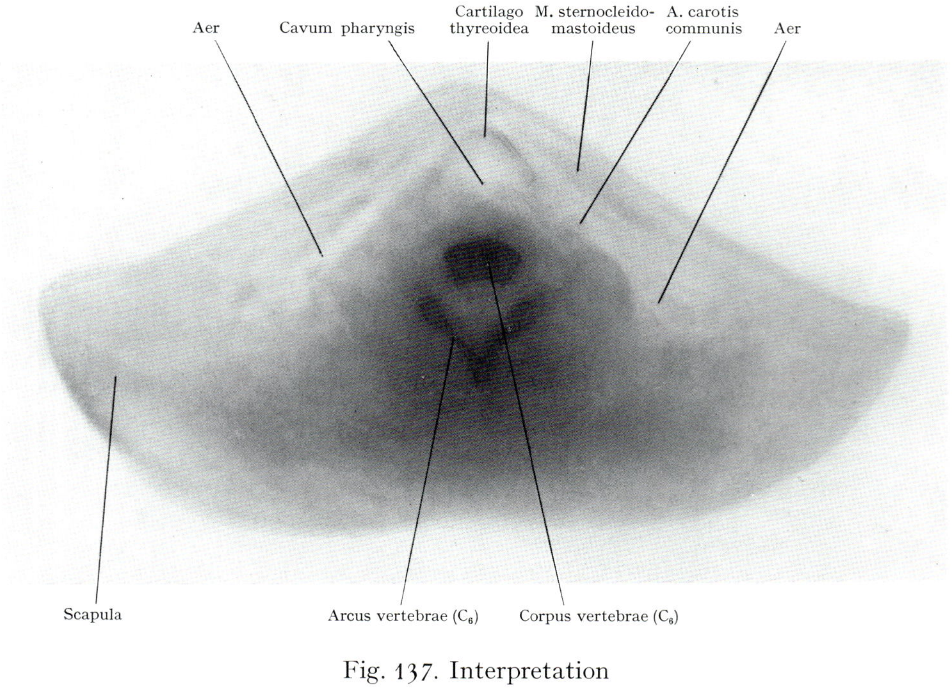

Fig. 137. Interpretation

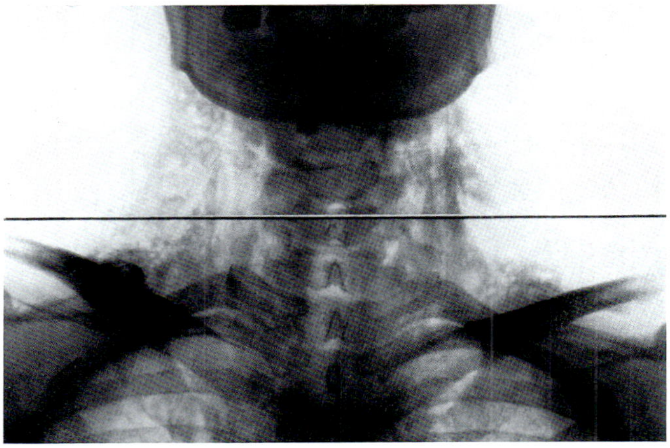

Fig. 138. Normal roentgenogram. Horizontal line showing the level tomographed

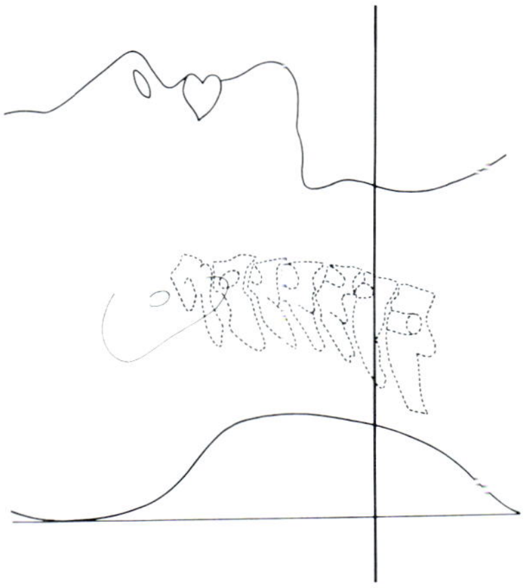

Fig. 139. Schematic drawing of the level tomographed

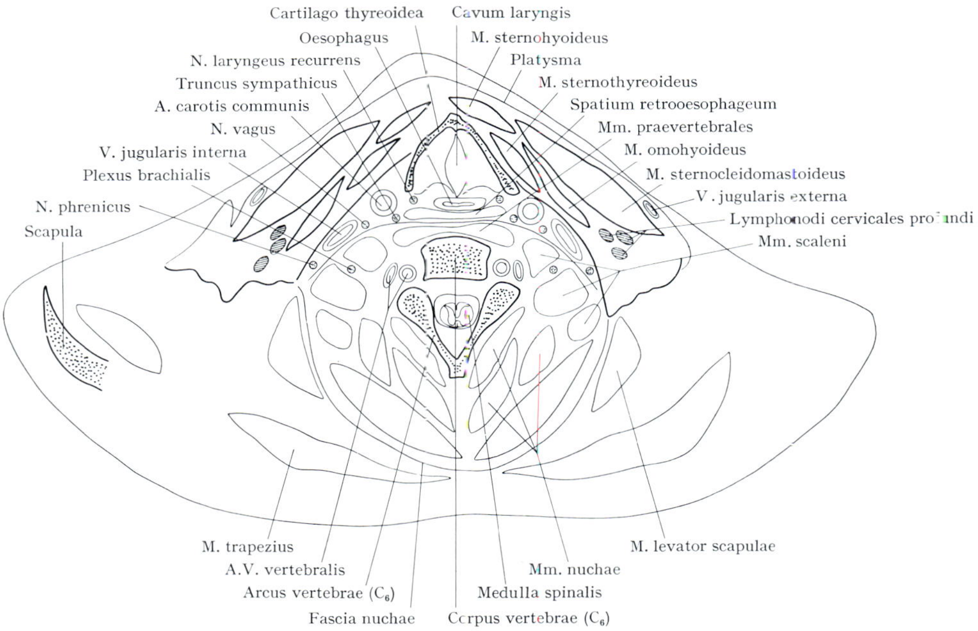

Fig. 140. Anatomical chart

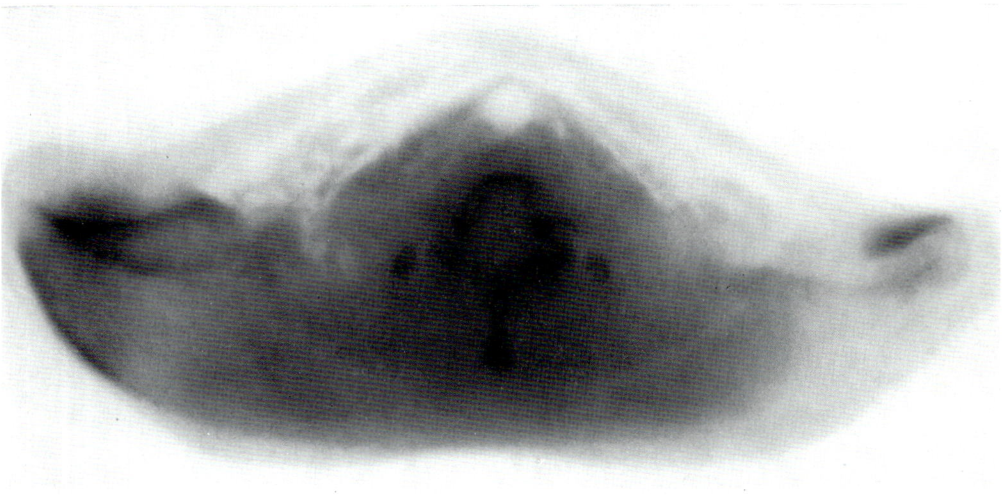

Fig. 141. Axial transverse tomogram

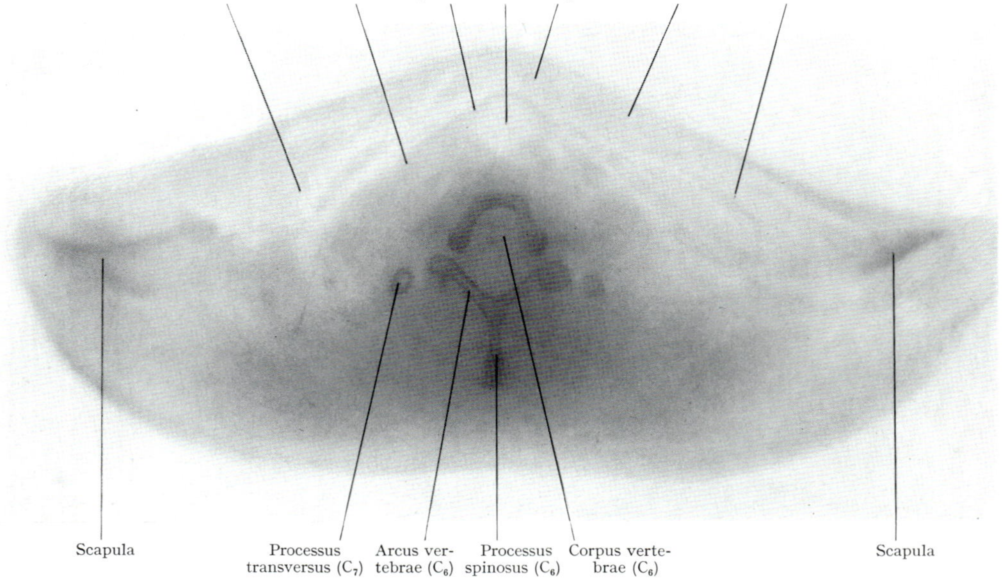

Fig. 142. Interpretation

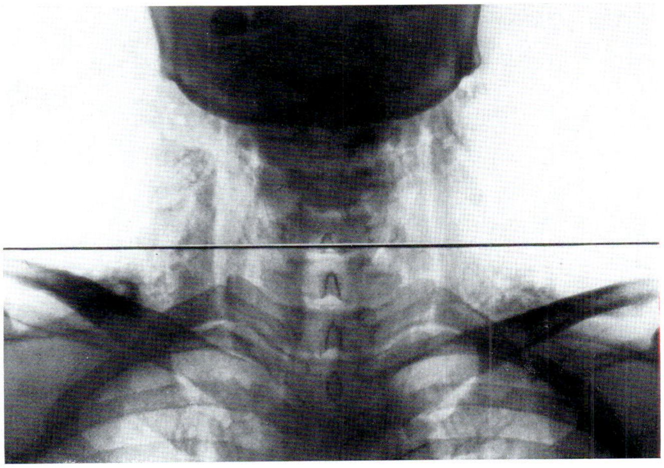

Fig. 143. Normal roentgenogram. Horizontal line showing the level tomographed

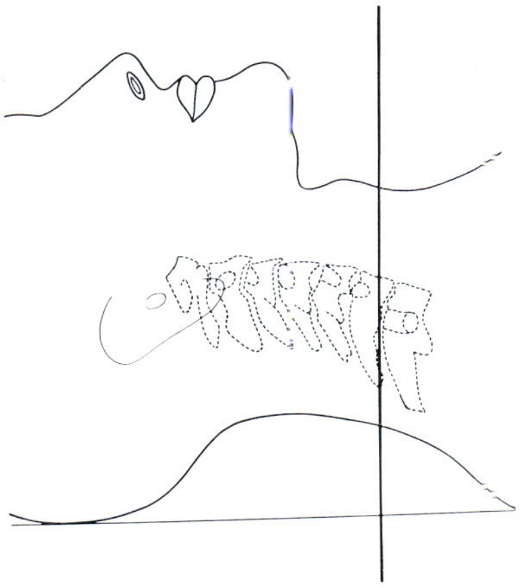

Fig. 144. Schematic drawing of the level tomographed

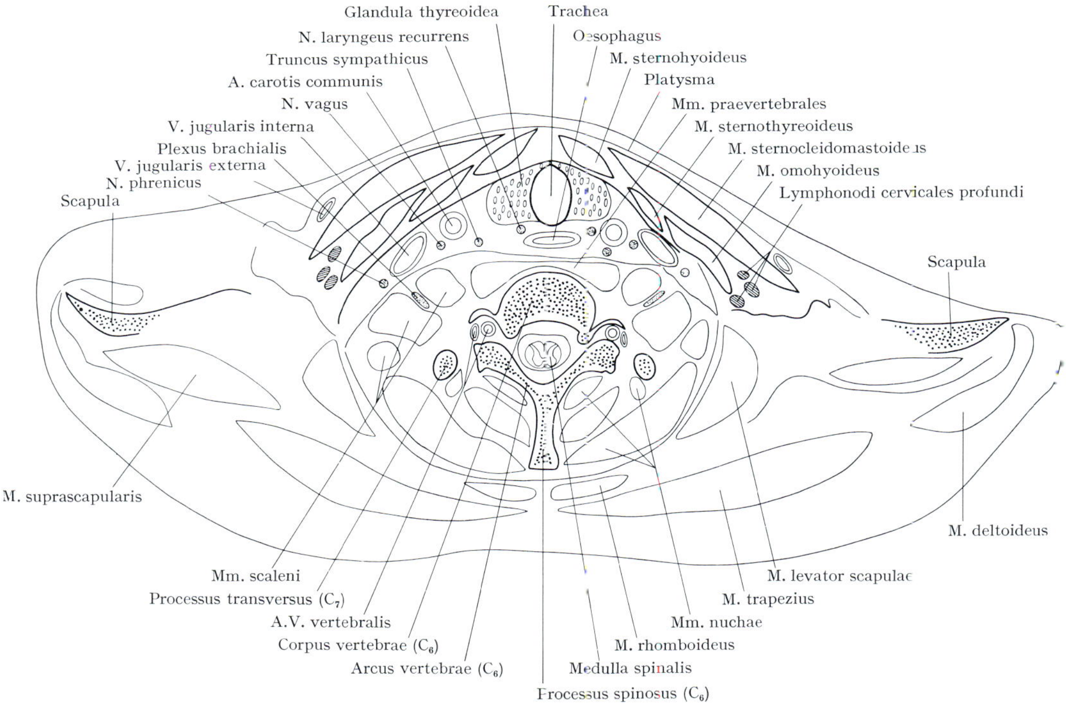

Fig. 145. Anatomical chart

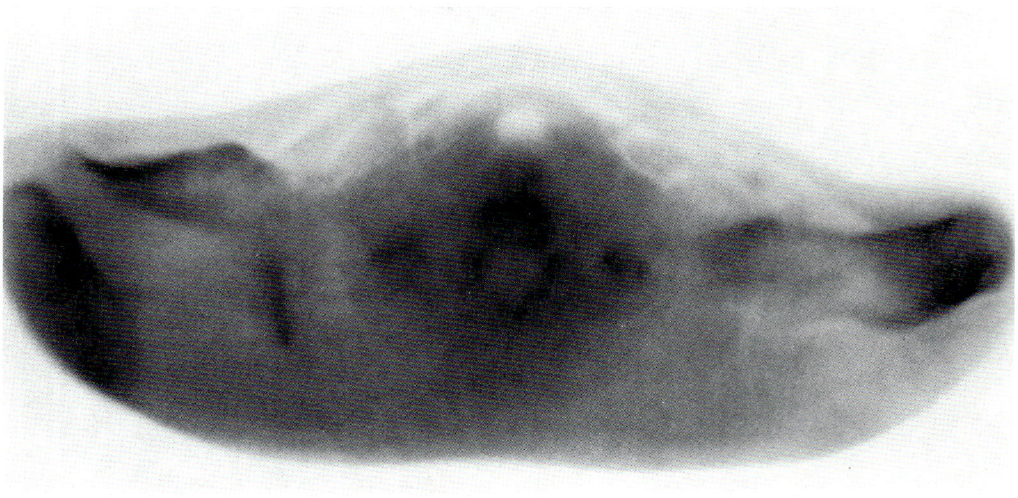

Fig. 146. Axial transverse tomogram

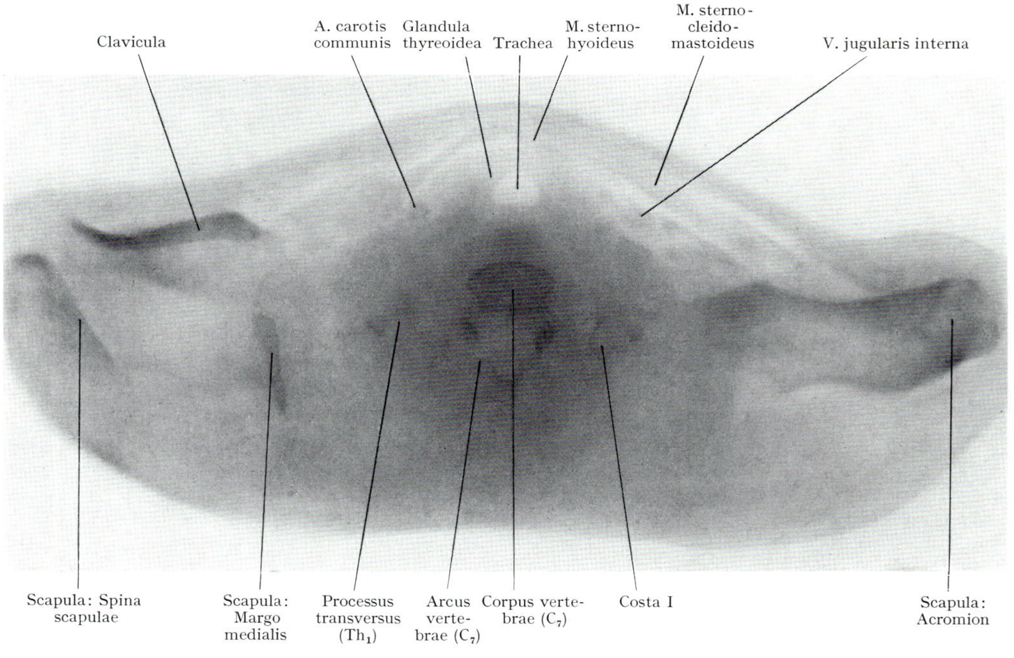

Fig. 147. Interpretation

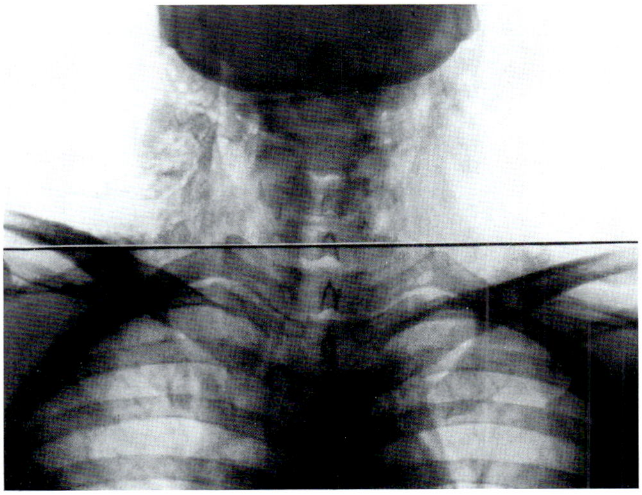

Fig. 148. Normal roentgenogram. Horizontal line showing the level tomographed

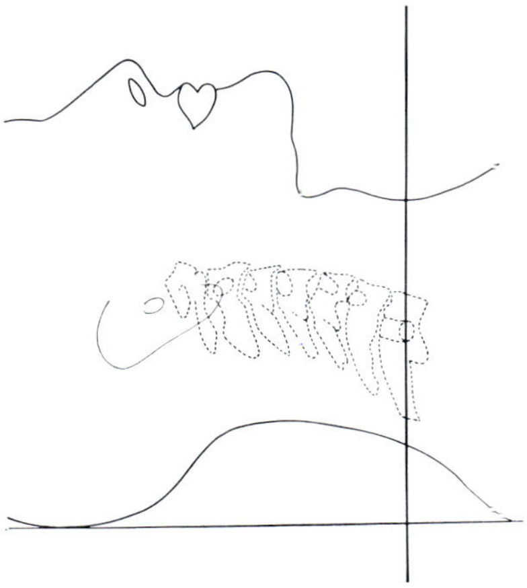

Fig. 149. Schematic drawing of the level tomographed

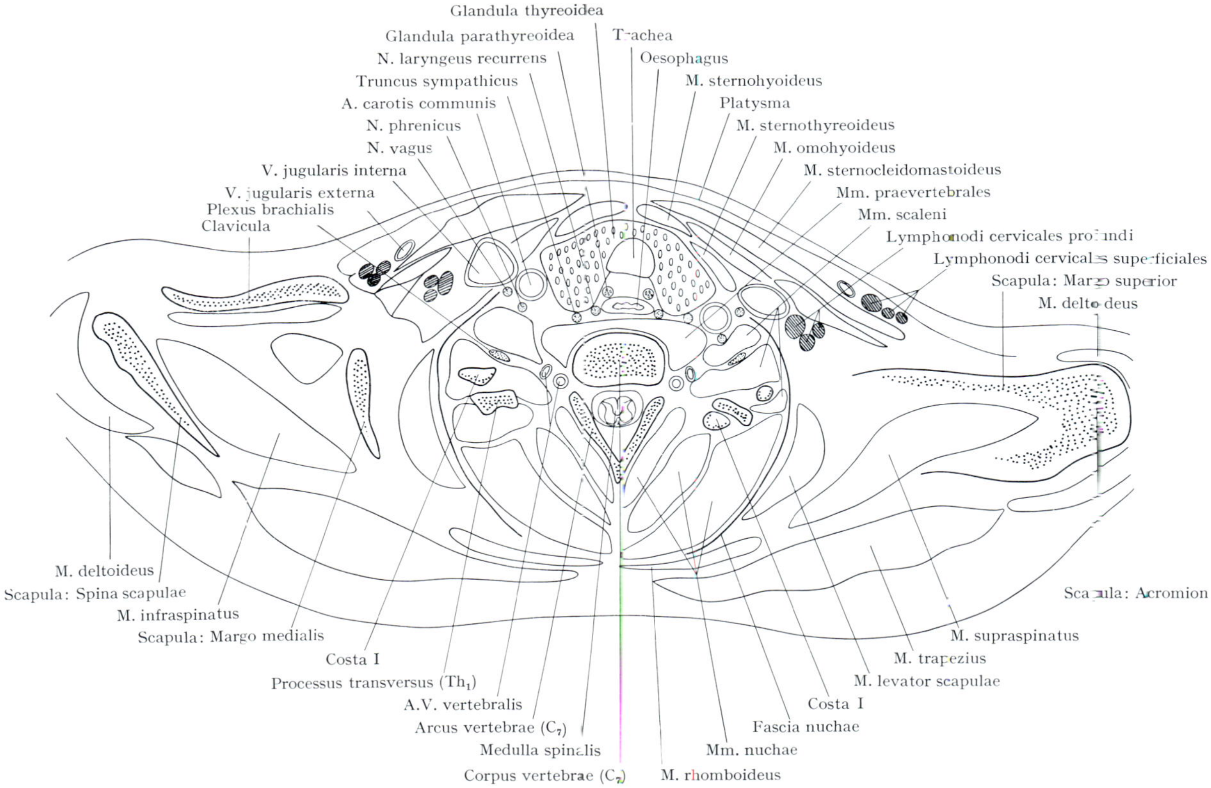

Fig. 150. Anatomical chart

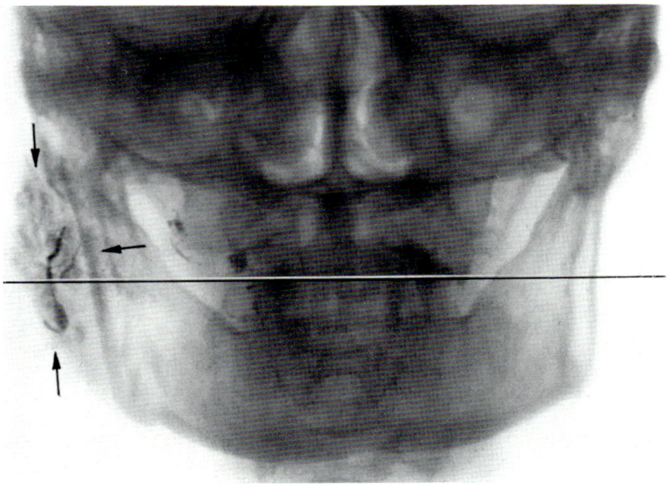

Fig. 151. Normal roentgenogram of the parotis (↗). Horizontal line showing the level tomographed

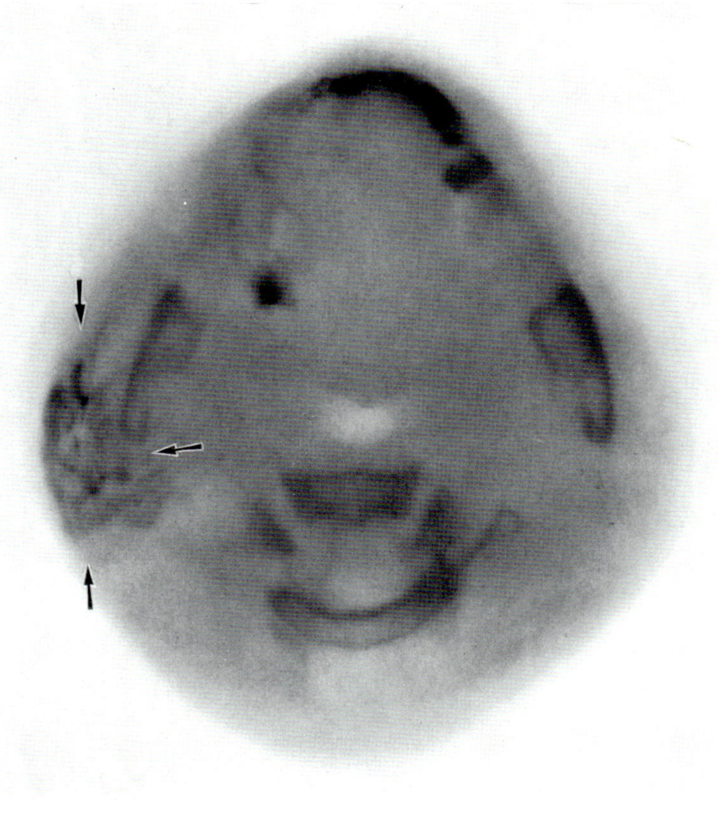

Fig. 152. Axial transverse tomogram of the parotis (↗) (see Figs. 96 and 97)

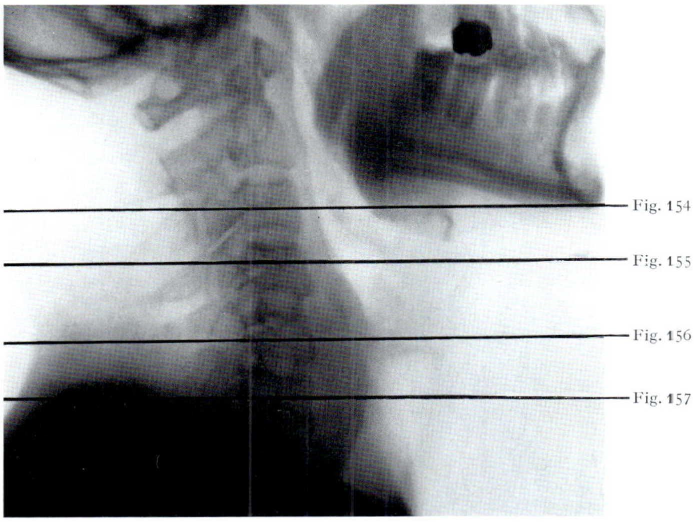

Fig. 153. Normal roentgenogram of the neck without contrast medium. Horizontal lines showing the level tomographed

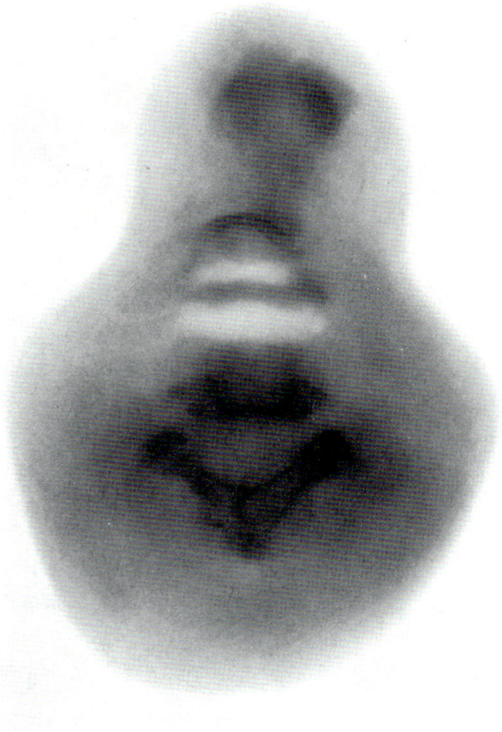

Fig. 154. Axial transverse tomogram of the neck (see Figs. 121 and 122)

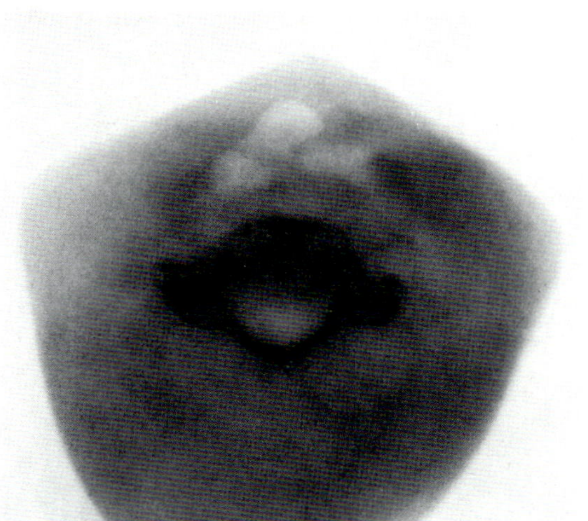

Fig. 155. Axial transverse tomogram of the neck (see Figs. 126 and 127)

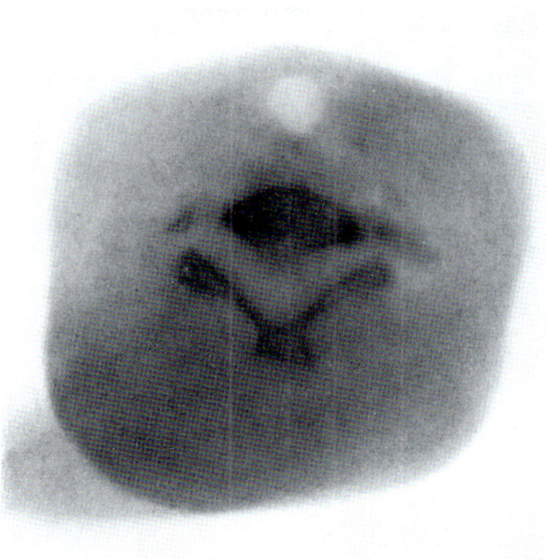

Fig. 156. Axial transverse tomogram of the neck (see Figs. 141 and 142)

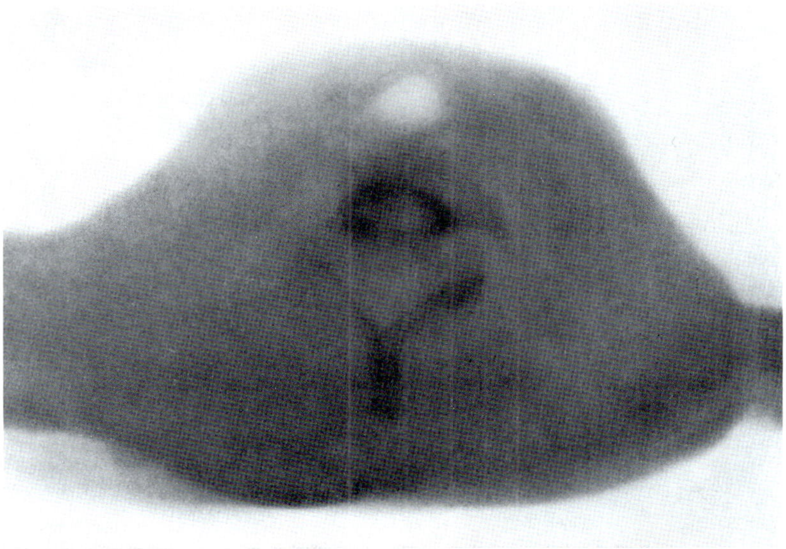

Fig. 157. Axial transverse tomogram of the neck (see Figs. 142 and 147)

Chest

Twenty three axial transverse tomograms.

Appendices:

1. Axial transverse tomograms of the esophagus.
2. Axial transverse tomograms of the thoracic duct and lymph nodes.

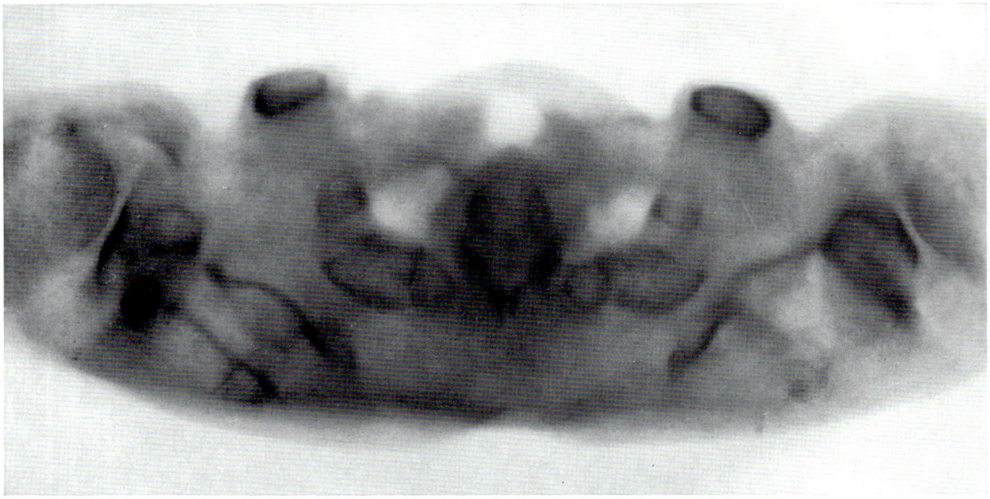

Fig. 158. Axial transverse tomogram

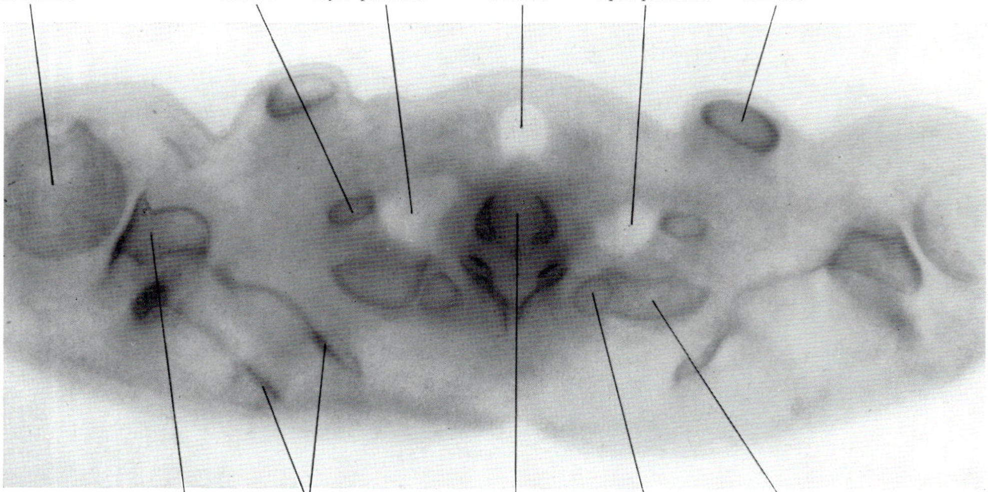

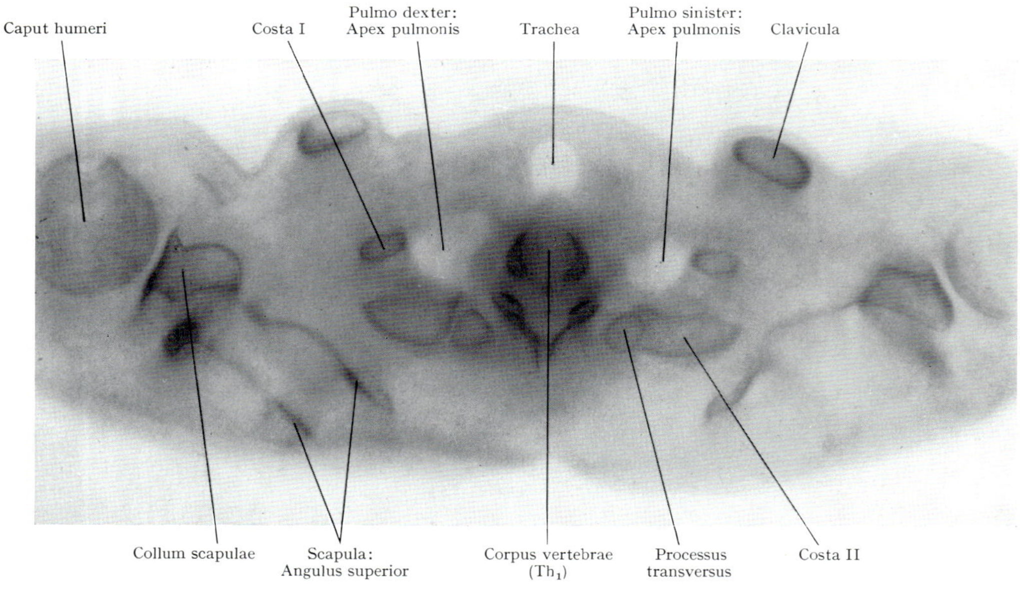

Fig. 159. Interpretation

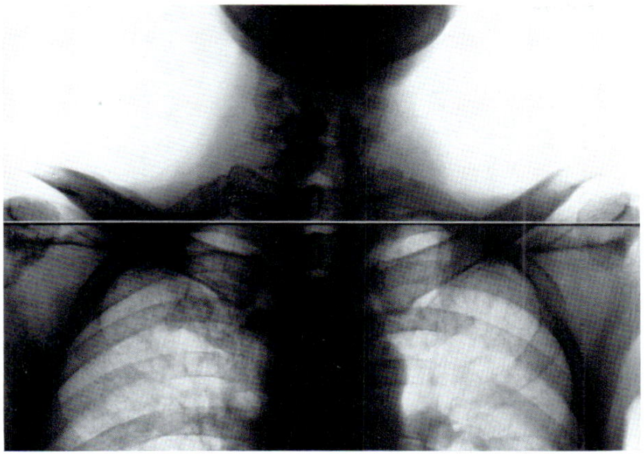

Fig. 160. Normal roentgenogram. Horizontal line showing the level tomographed

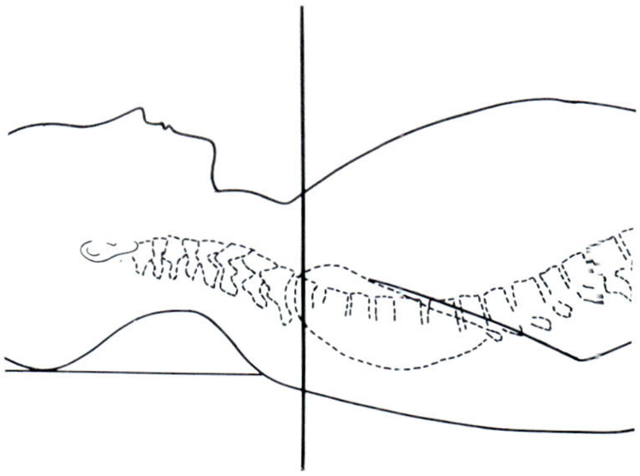

Fig. 161. Schematic drawing of the level tomographed. Subject supine with arms parallel to body axis

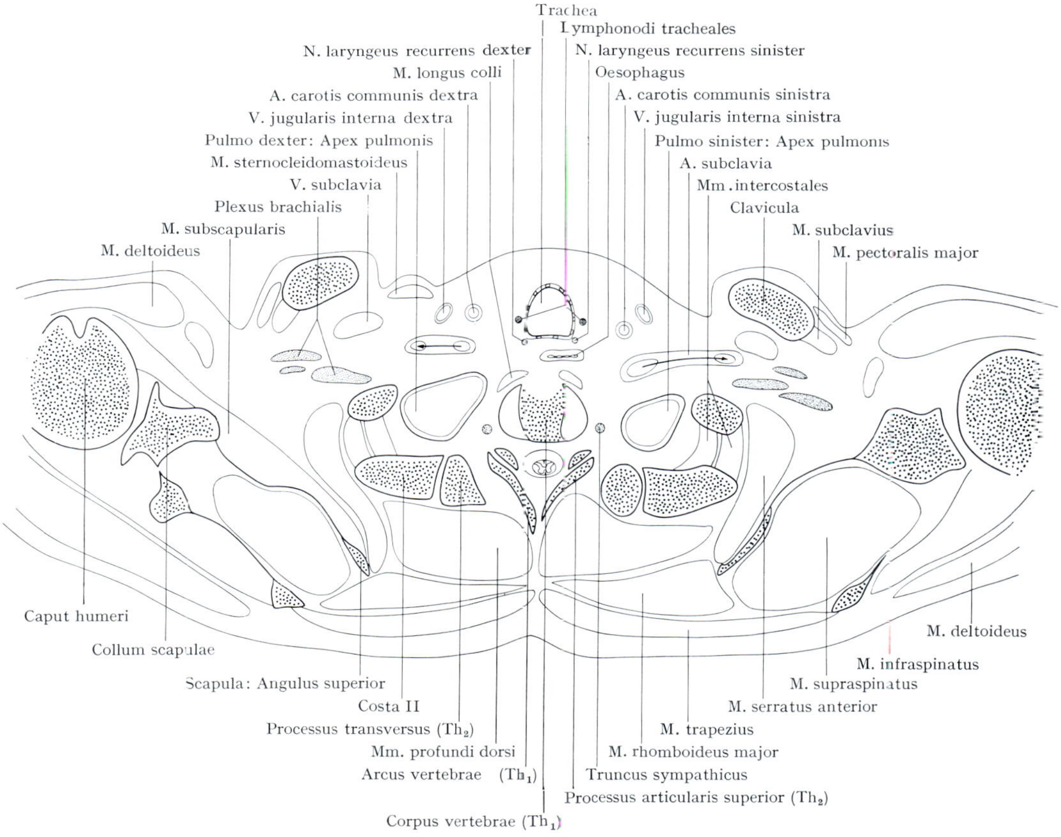

Fig. 162. Anatomical chart

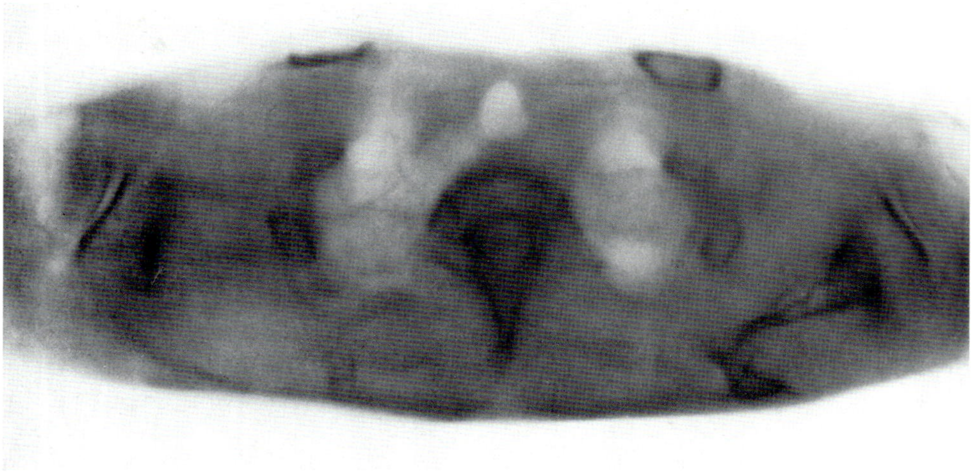

Fig. 163. Axial transverse tomogram

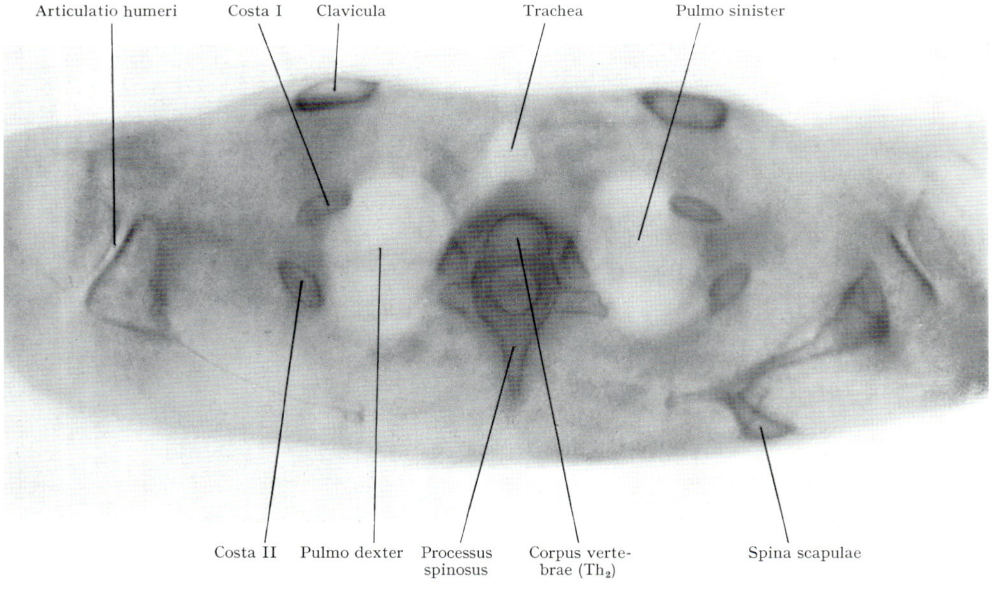

Fig. 164. Interpretation

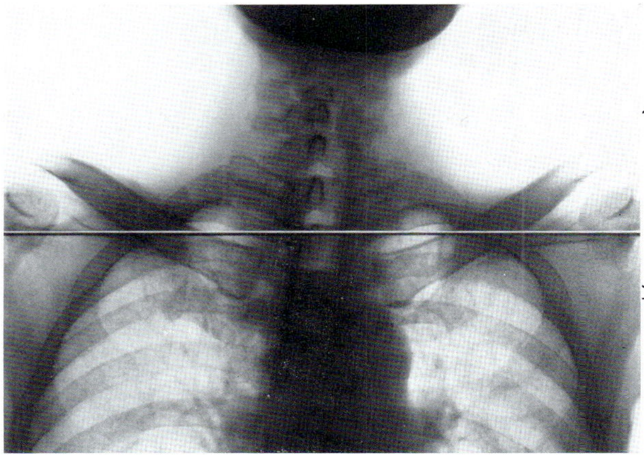

Fig. 165. Normal roentgenogram. Horizontal line showing the level tomographed

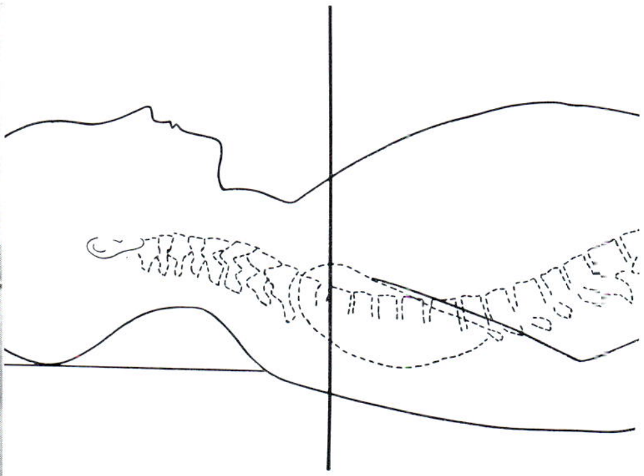

Fig. 166. Schematic drawing of the level tomographed. Subject supine with arms parallel to body axis

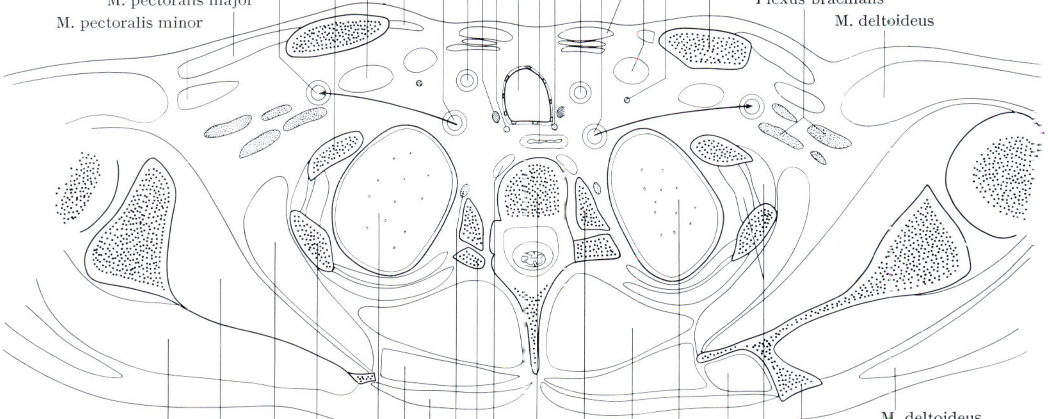

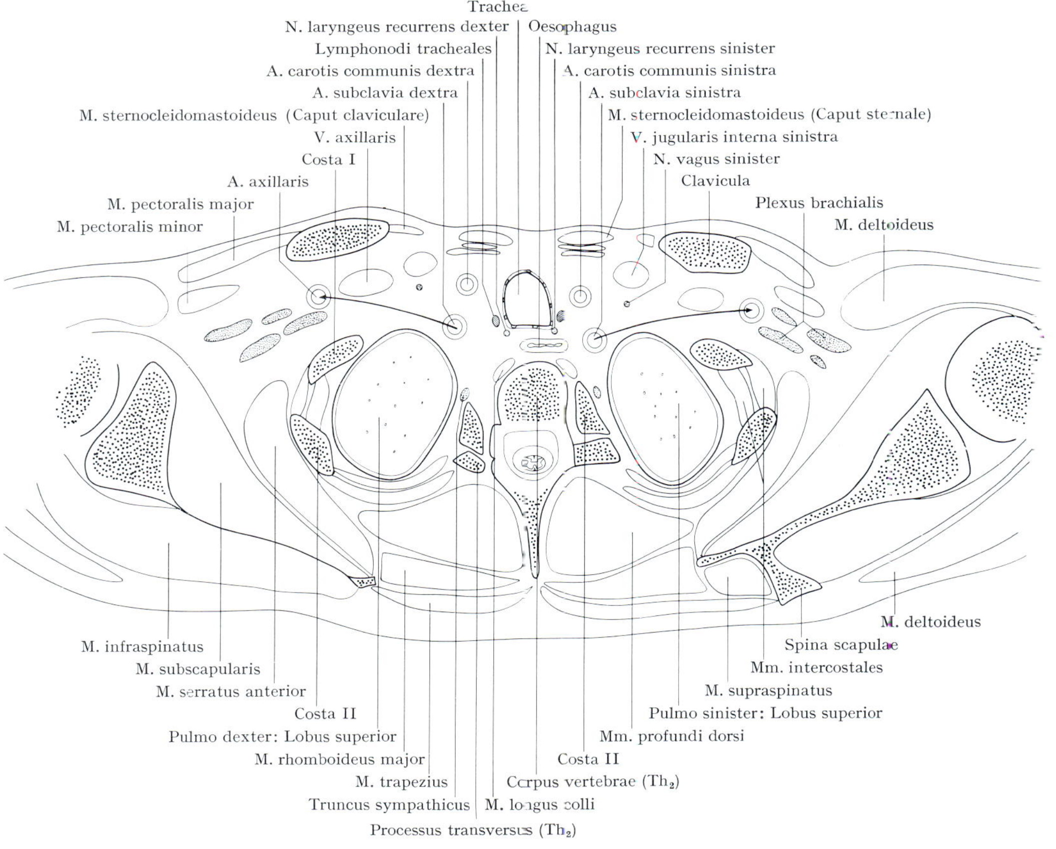

Fig. 167. Anatomical chart

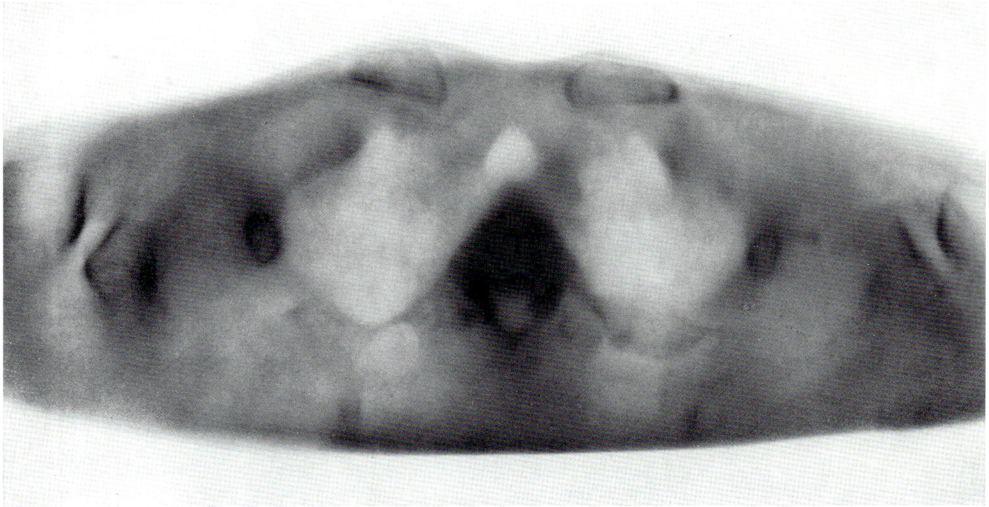

Fig. 168. Axial transverse tomogram

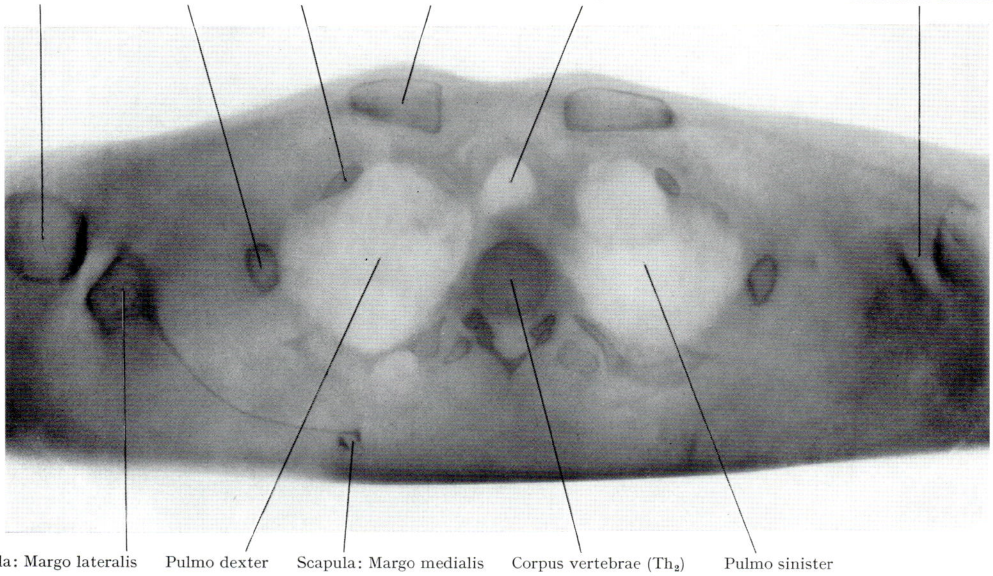

Fig. 169. Interpretation

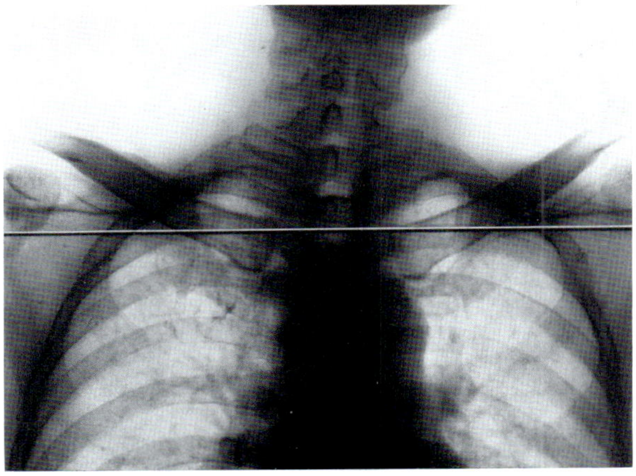

Fig. 170. Normal roentgenogram. Horizontal line showing the level tomographed

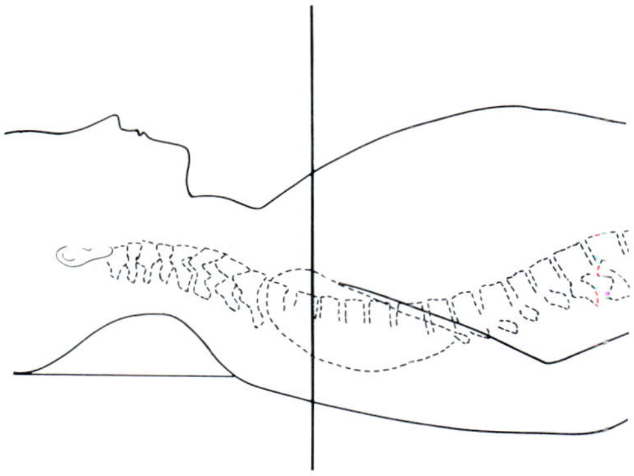

Fig. 171. Schematic drawing of the level tomographed. Subject supine with arms parallel to body axis

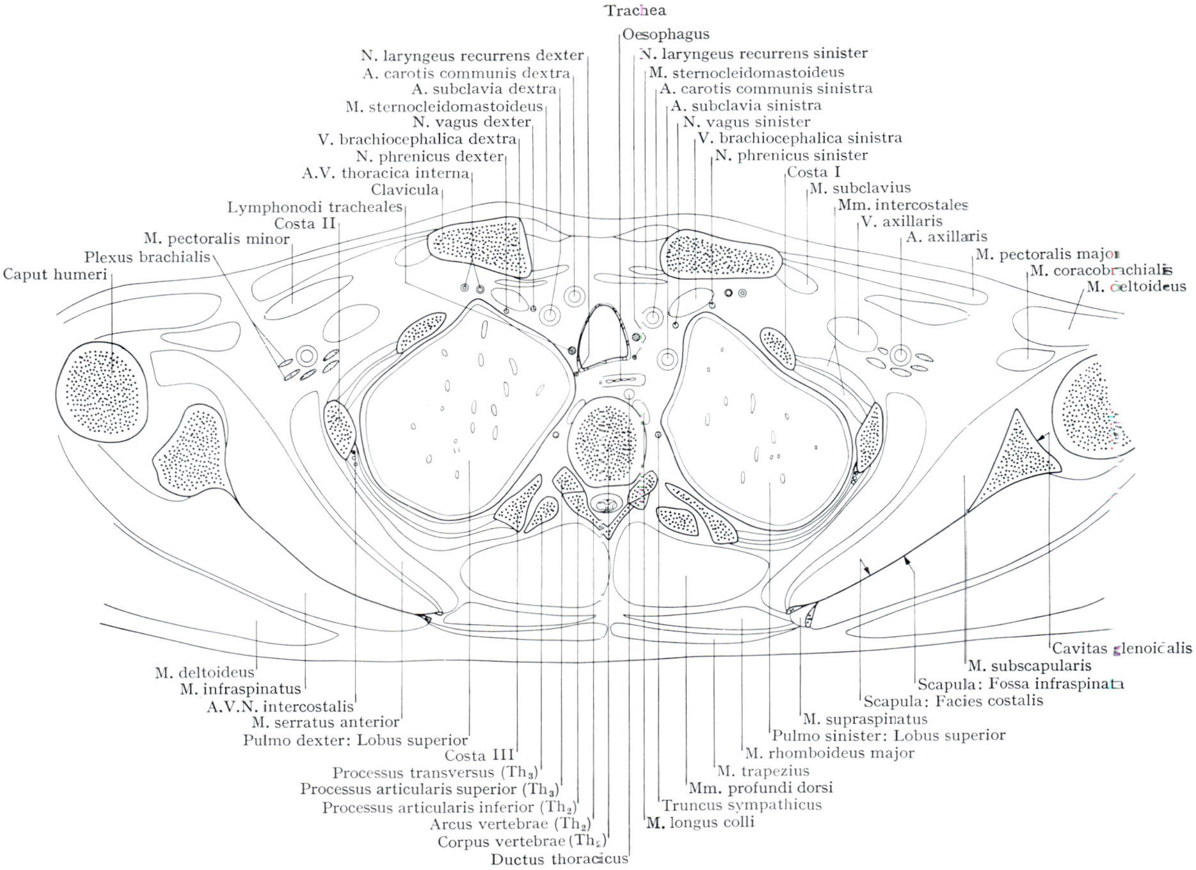

Fig. 172. Anatomical chart

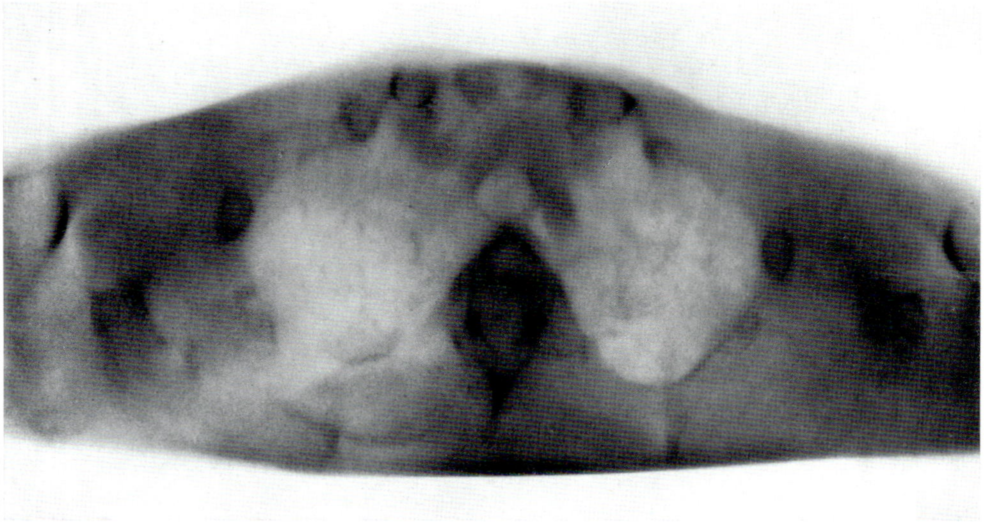

Fig. 173. Axial transverse tomogram

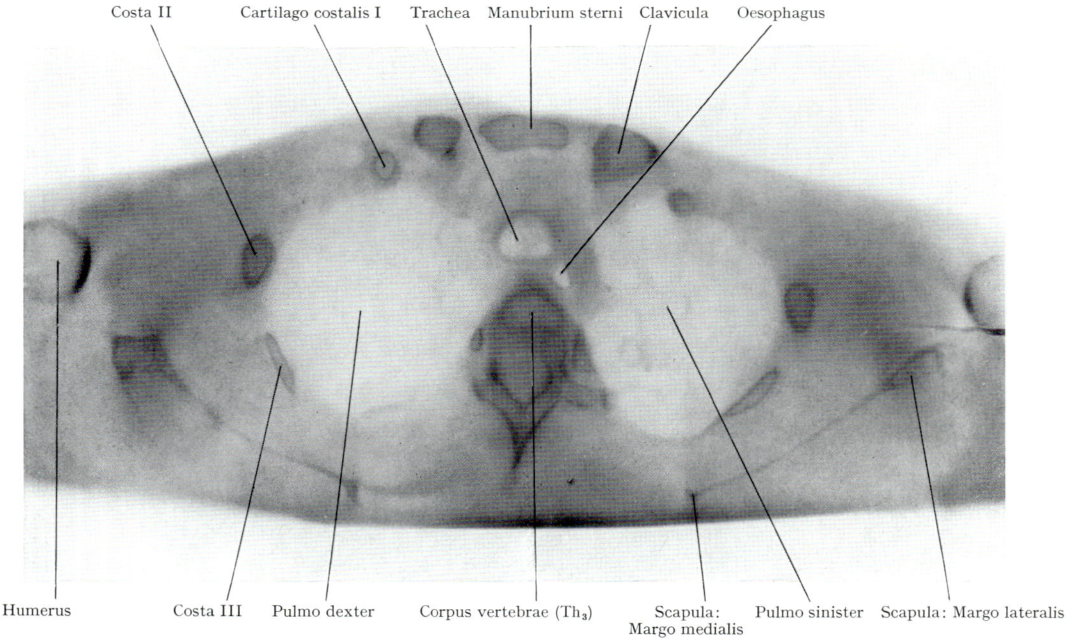

Fig. 174. Interpretation

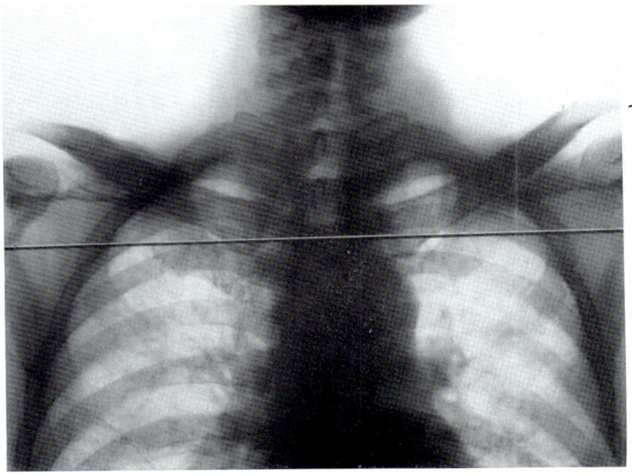

Fig. 175. Normal roentgenogram. Horizontal line showing the level tomographed

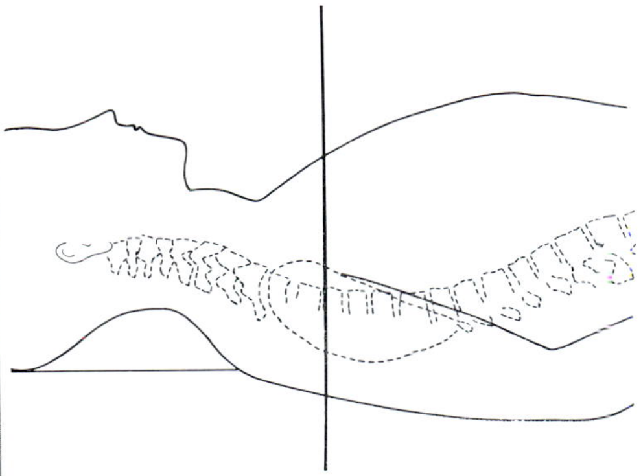

Fig. 176. Schematic drawing of the level tomographed. Subject supine with arms parallel to body axis

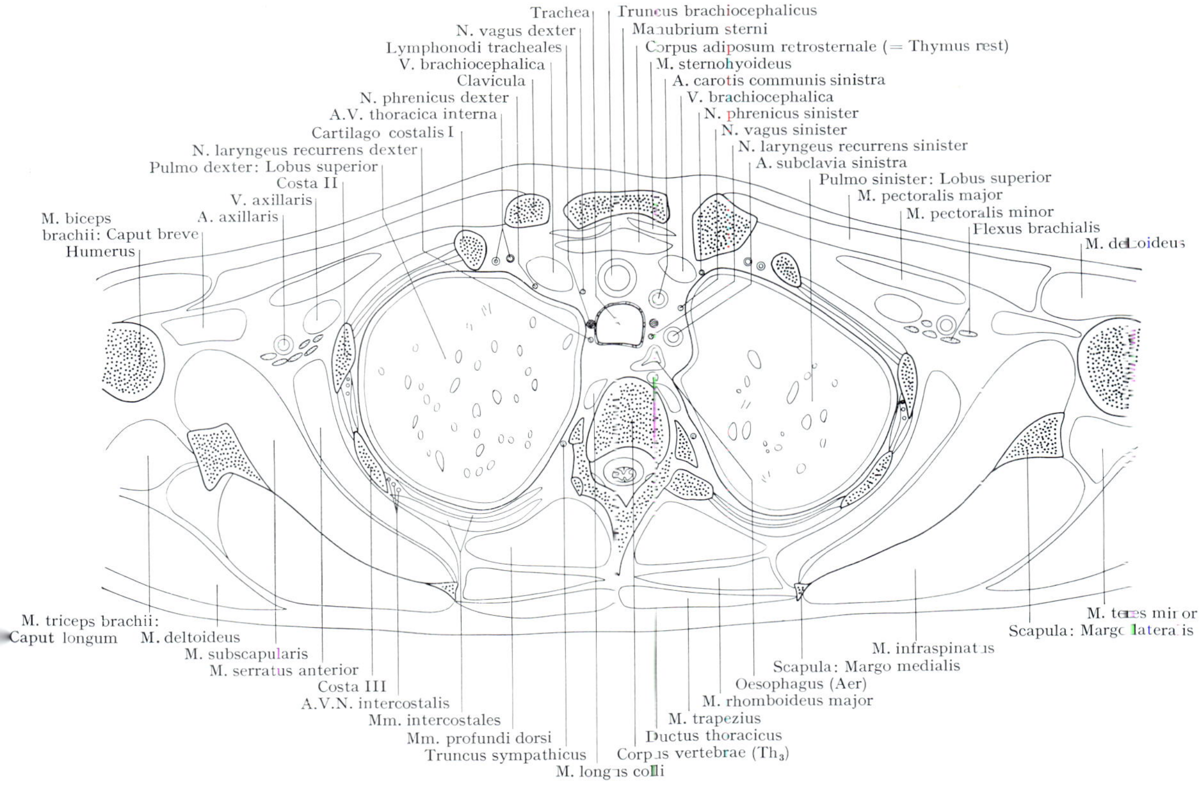

Fig. 177. Anatomical chart

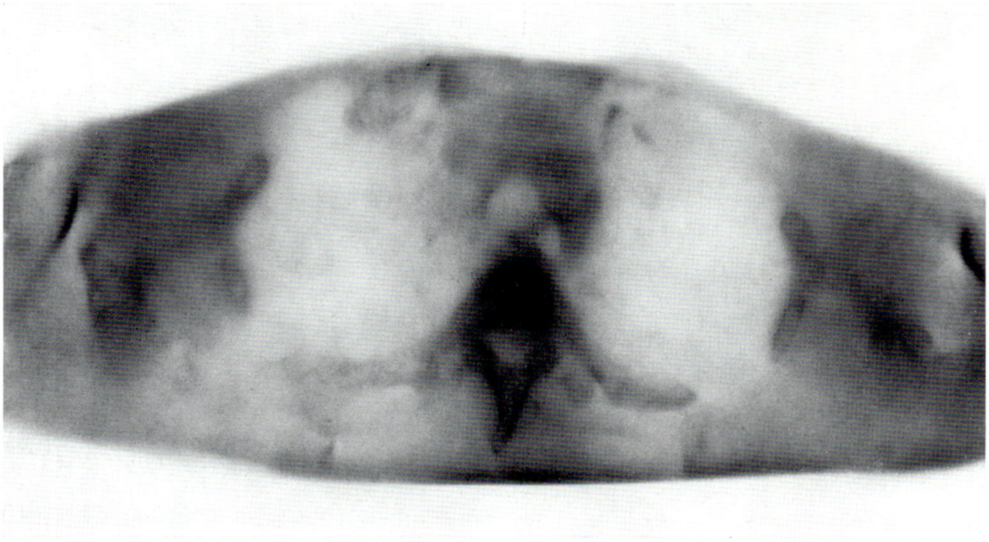

Fig. 178. Axial transverse tomogram

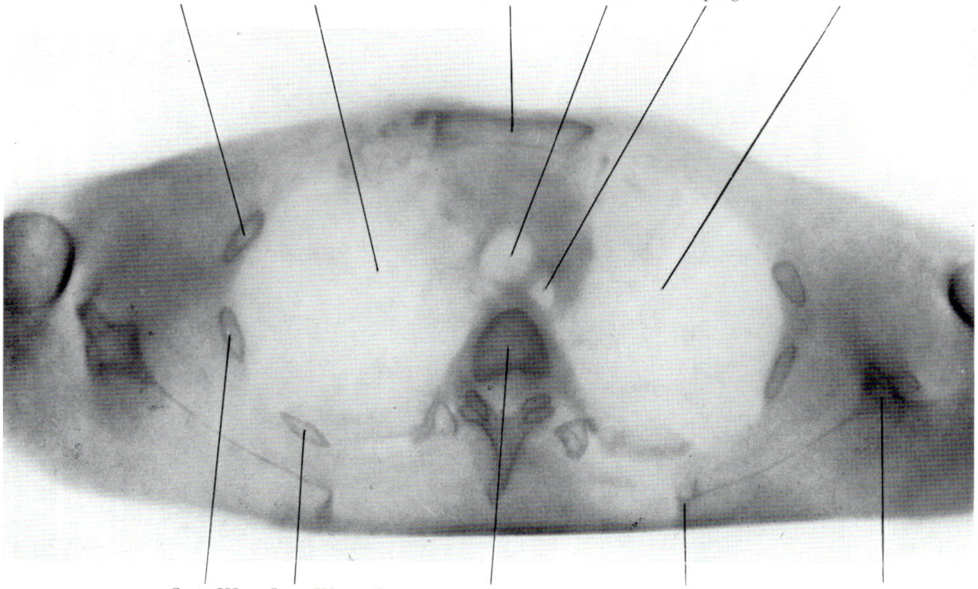

Fig. 179. Interpretation

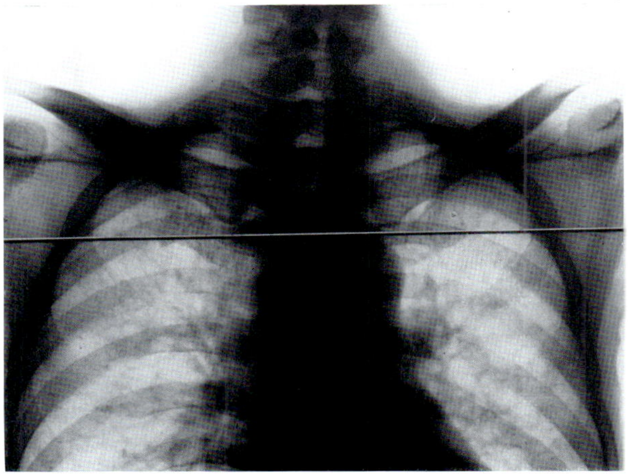

Fig. 180. Normal roentgenogram. Horizontal line showing the level tomographed

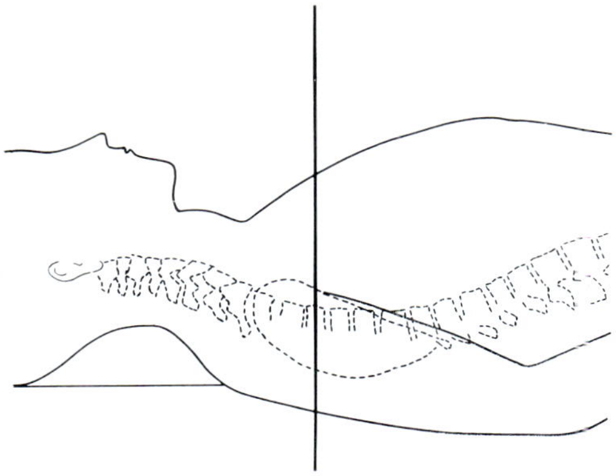

Fig. 181. Schematic drawing of the level tomographed. Subject supine with arms parallel to body axis

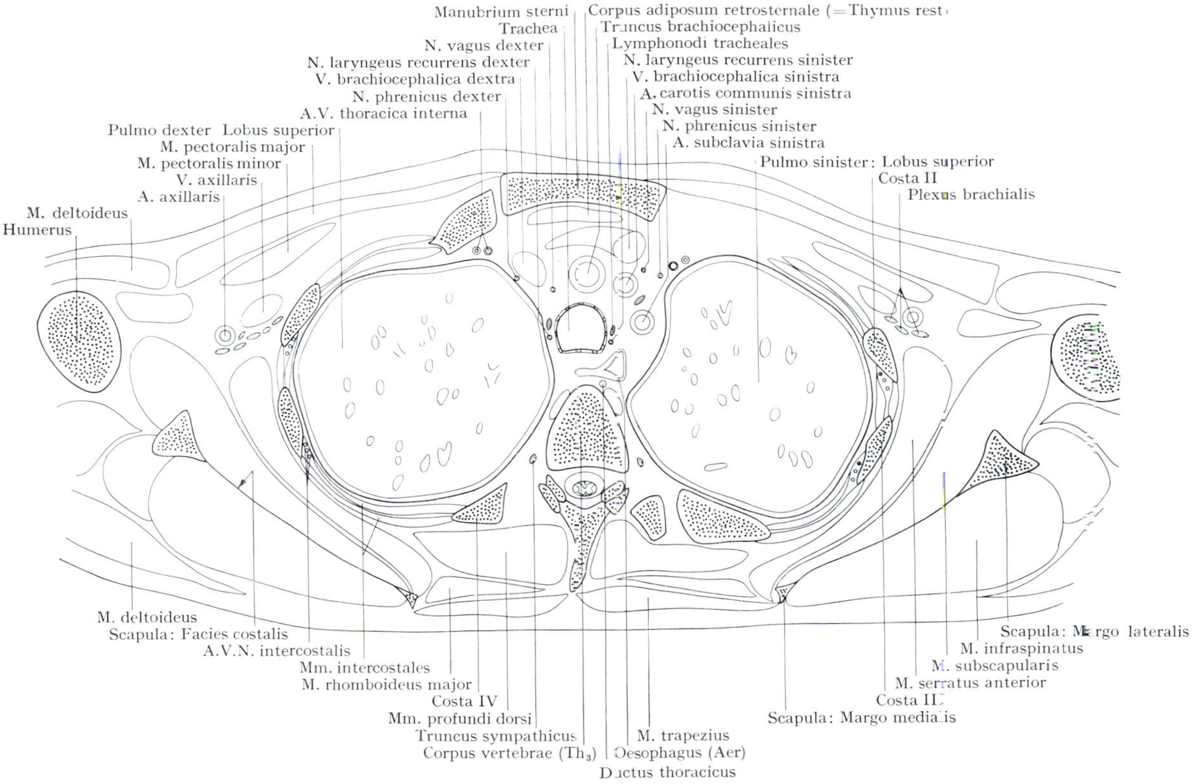

Fig. 182. Anatomical chart

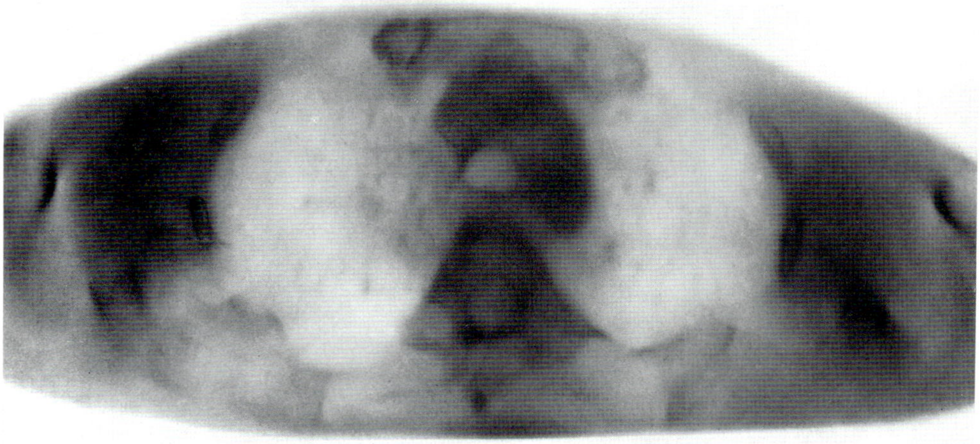

Fig. 183. Axial transverse tomogram

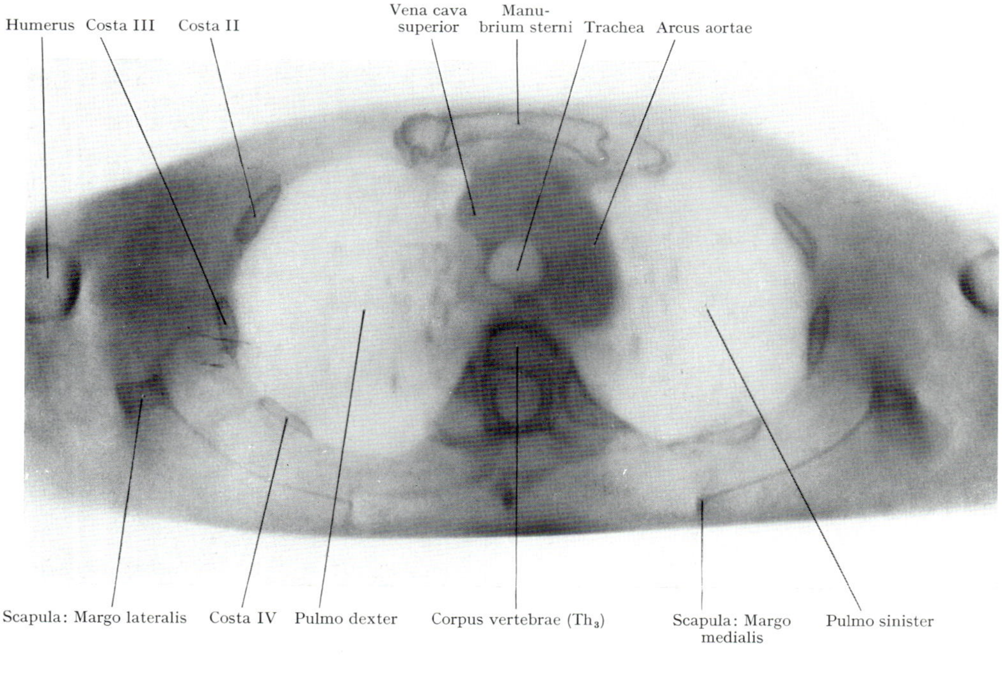

Fig. 184. Interpretation

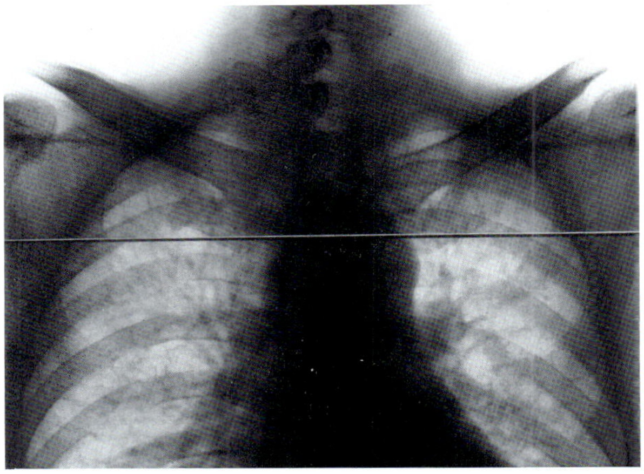

Fig. 185. Normal roentgenogram. Horizontal line showing the level tomographed

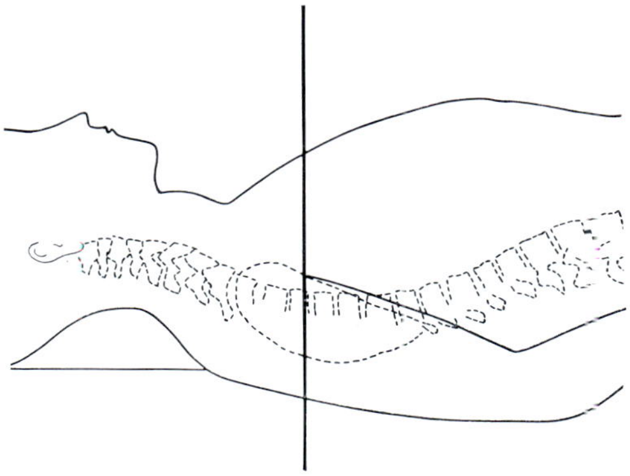

Fig. 186. Schematic drawing of the level tomographed. Subject supine with arms parallel to body axis

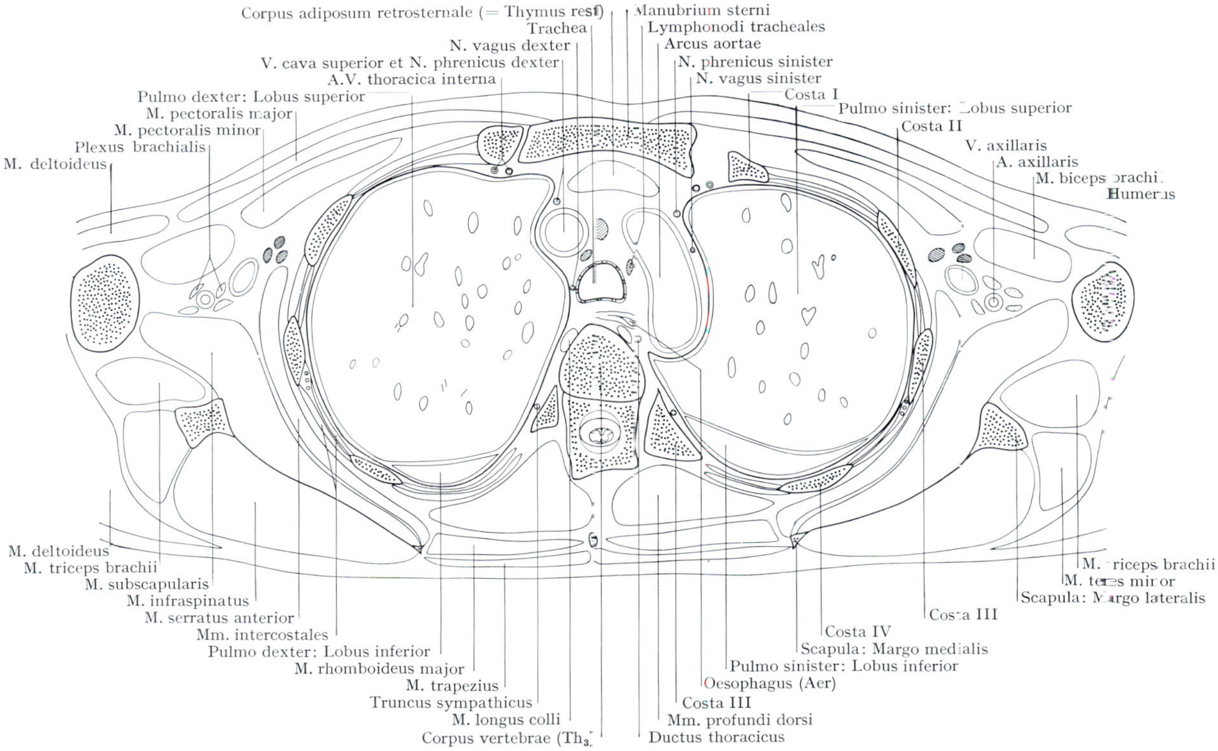

Fig. 187. Anatomical chart

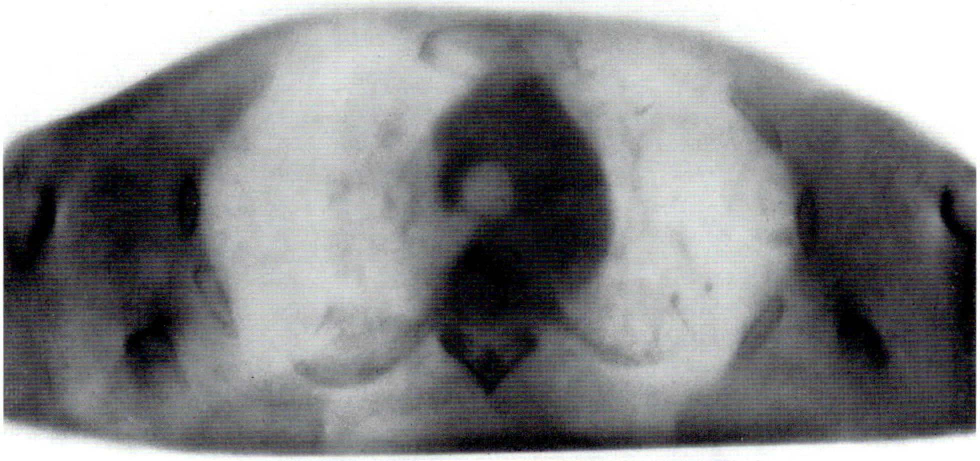

Fig. 188. Axial transverse tomogram

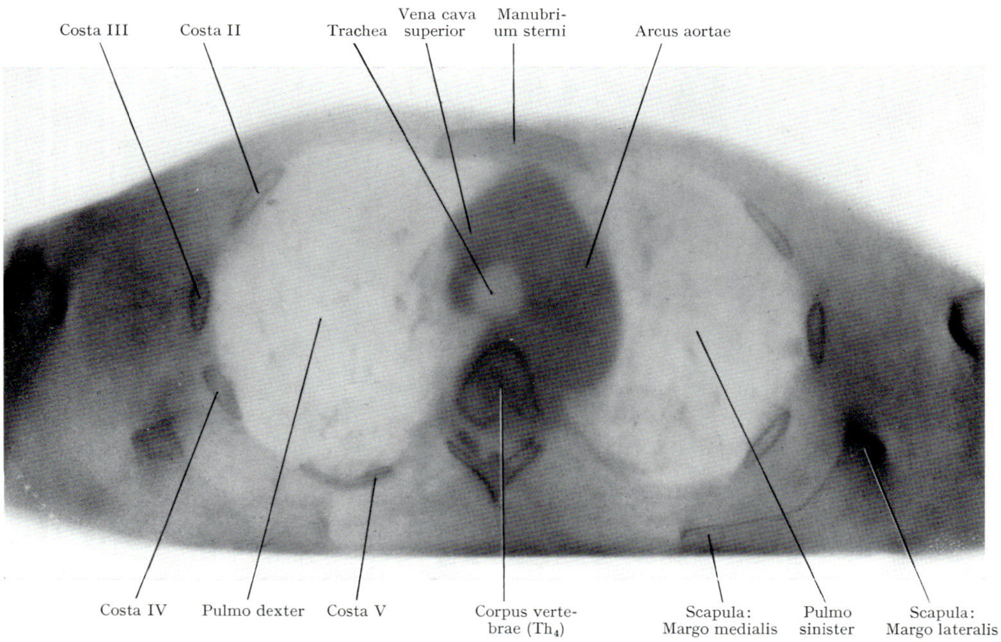

Fig. 189. Interpretation

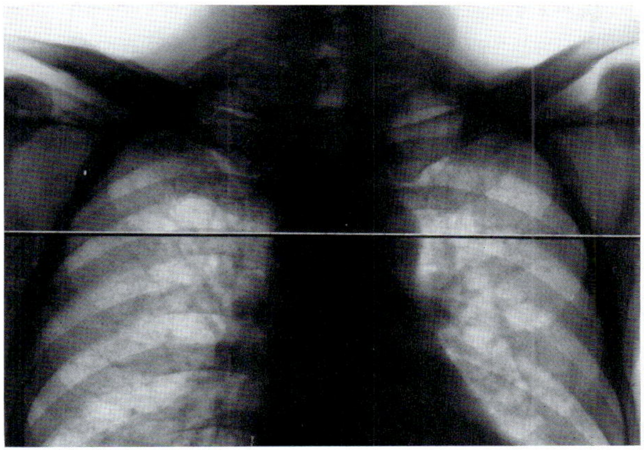

Fig. 190. Normal roentgenogram. Horizontal line showing the level tomographed

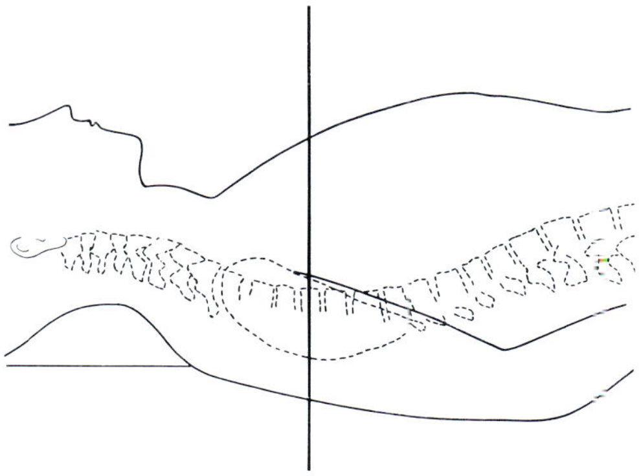

Fig. 191. Schematic drawing of the level tomographed. Subject supine with arms parallel to body axis

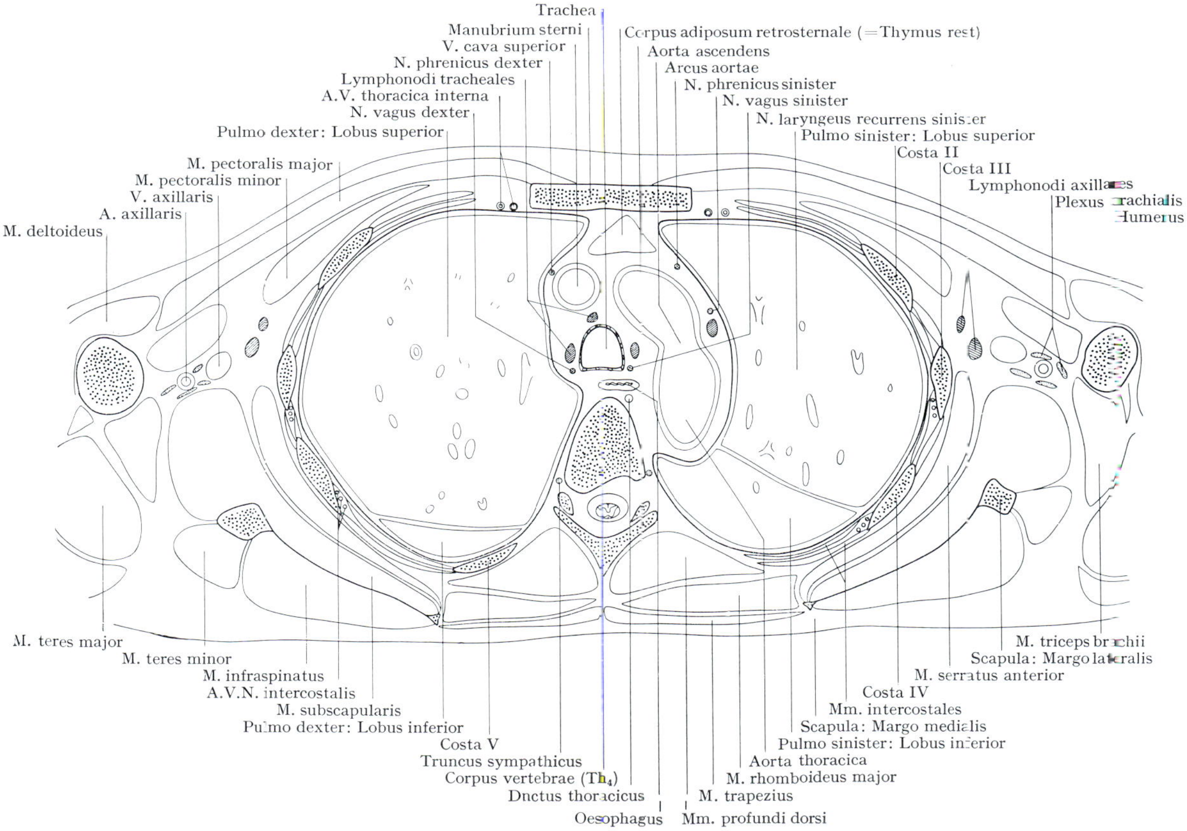

Fig. 192. Anatomical chart

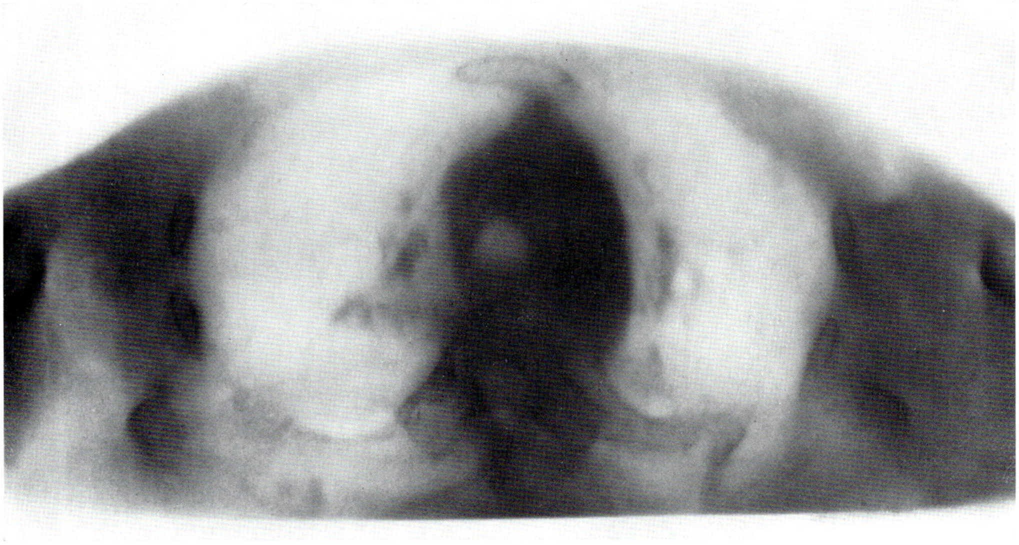

Fig. 193. Axial transverse tomogram

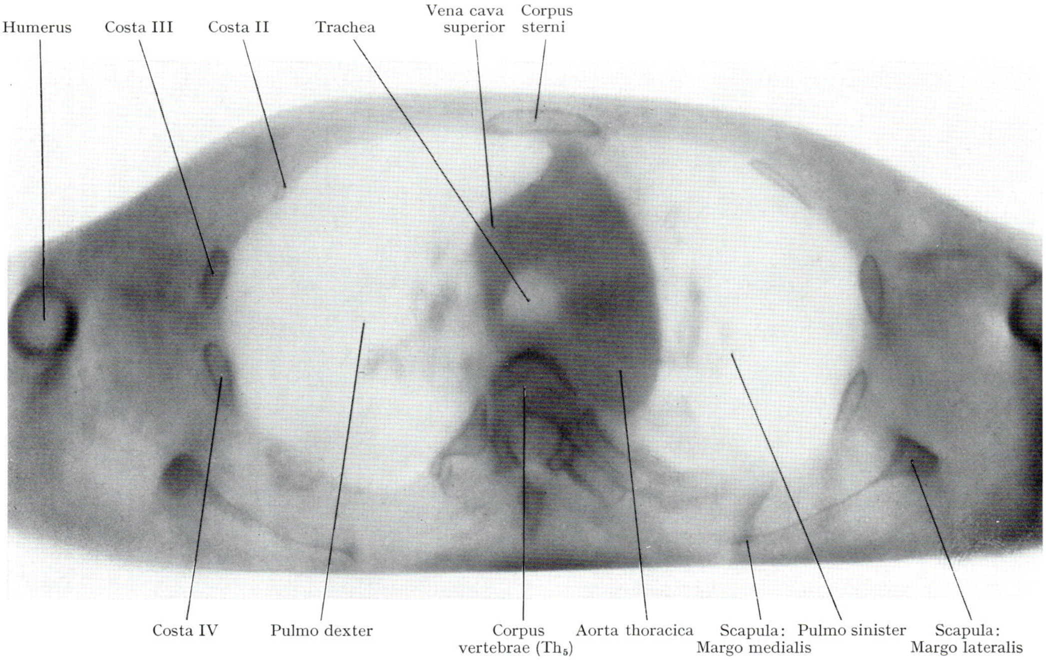

Fig. 194. Interpretation

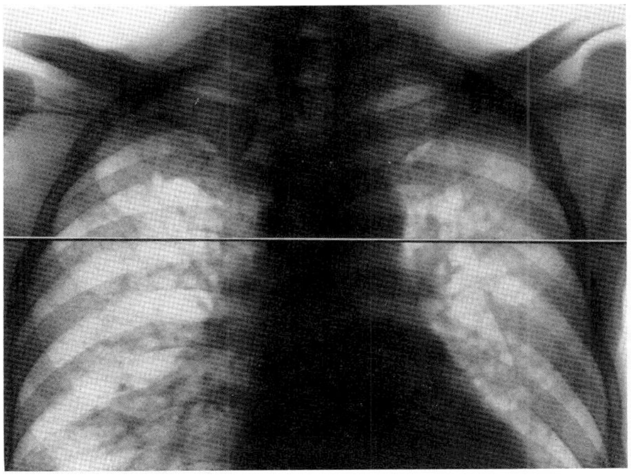

Fig. 195. Normal roentgenogram. Horizontal line showing the level tomographed

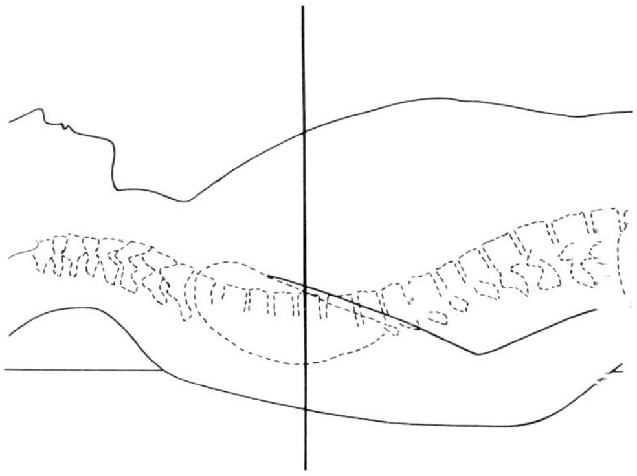

Fig. 196. Schematic drawing of the level tomographed. Subject supine with arms parallel to body axis

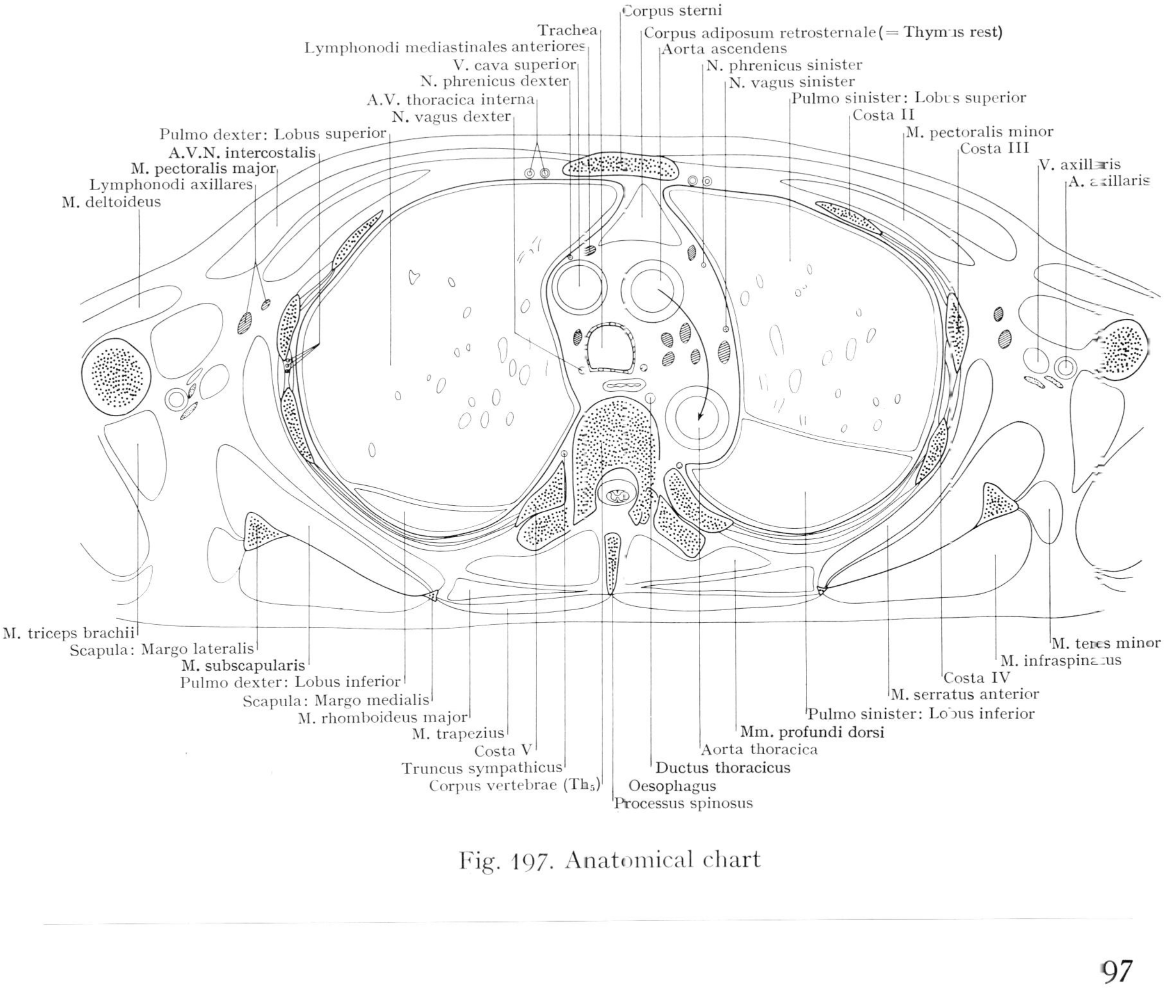

Fig. 197. Anatomical chart

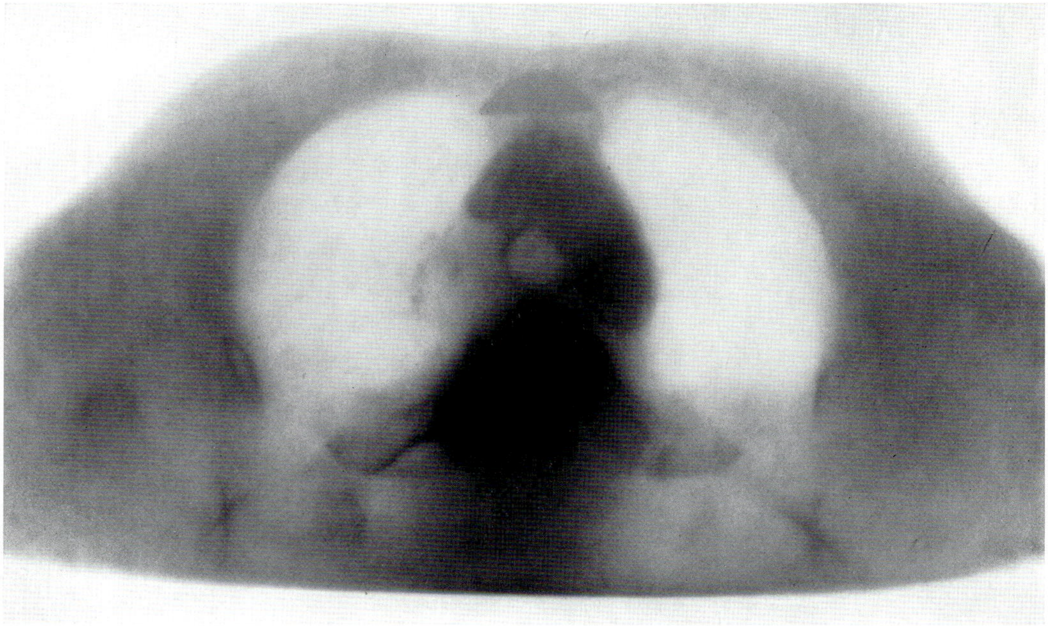

Fig. 198. Axial transverse tomogram

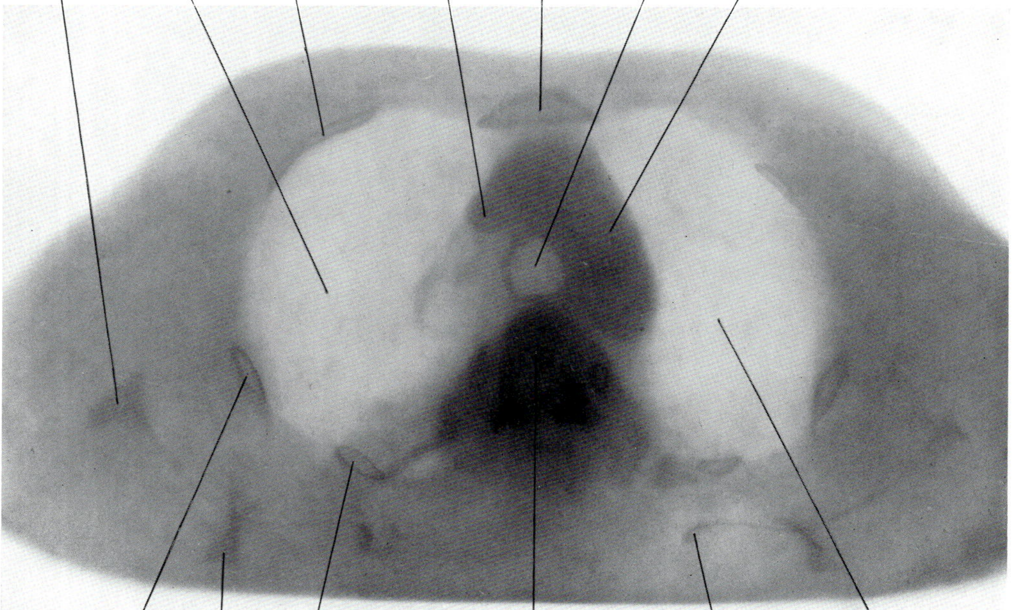

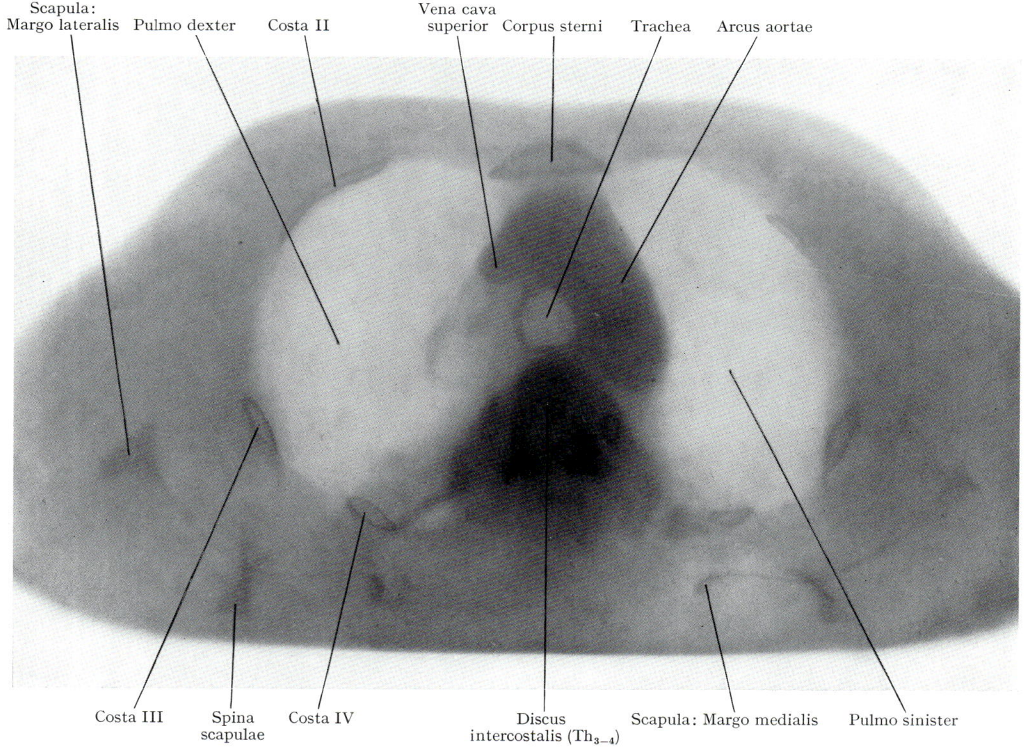

Fig. 199. Interpretation

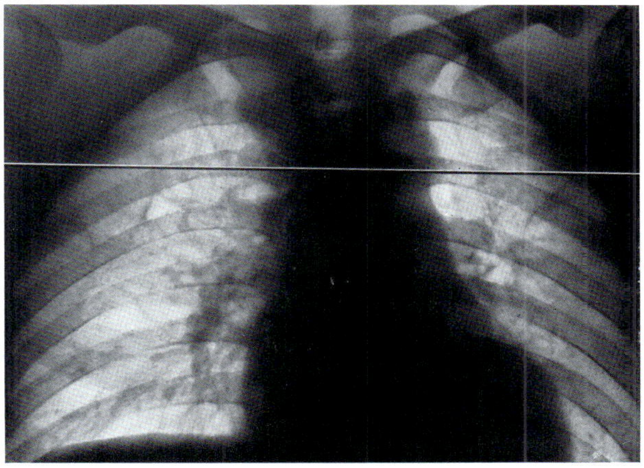

Fig. 200. Normal roentgenogram. Horizontal line showing the level tomographed

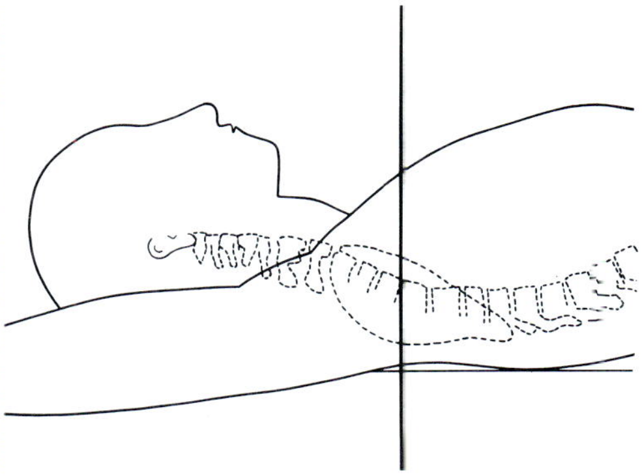

Fig. 201. Schematic drawing of the level tomographed. Subject supine with hands folded behind the head

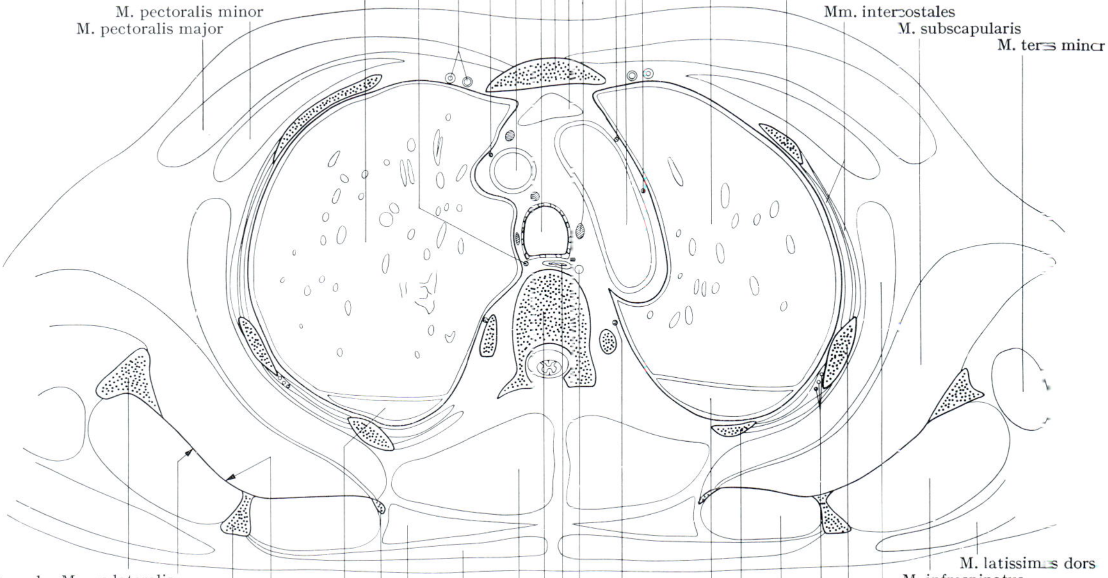

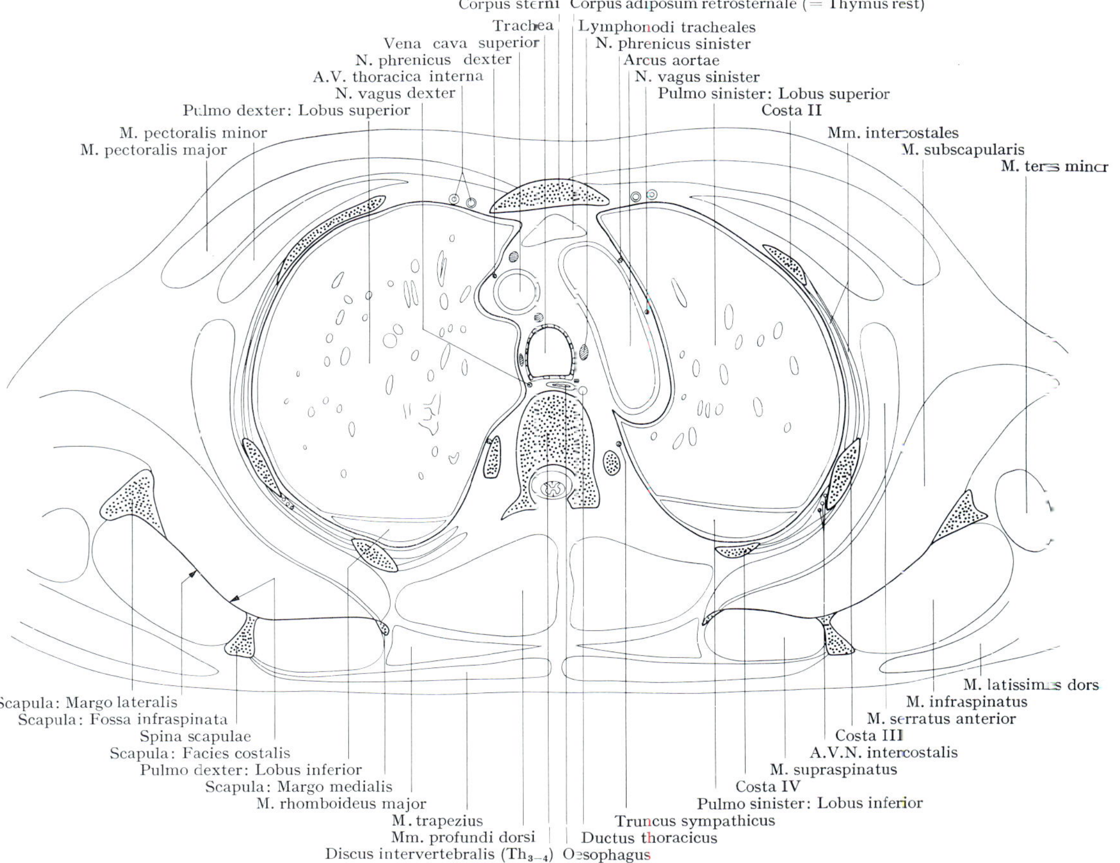

Fig. 202. Anatomical chart

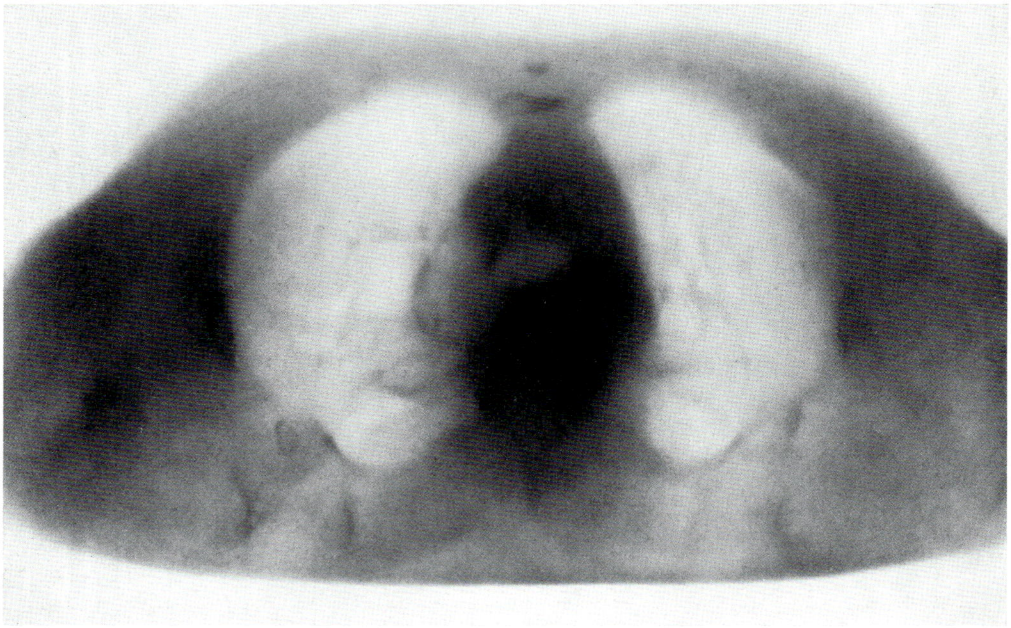

Fig. 203. Axial transverse tomogram

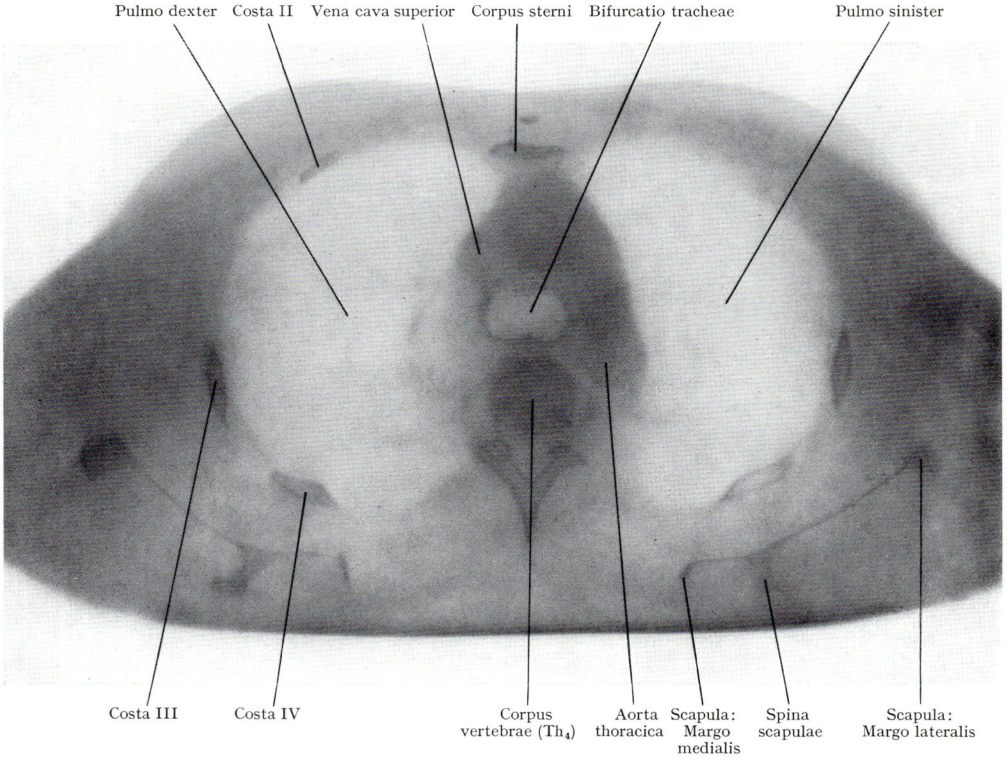

Fig. 204. Interpretation

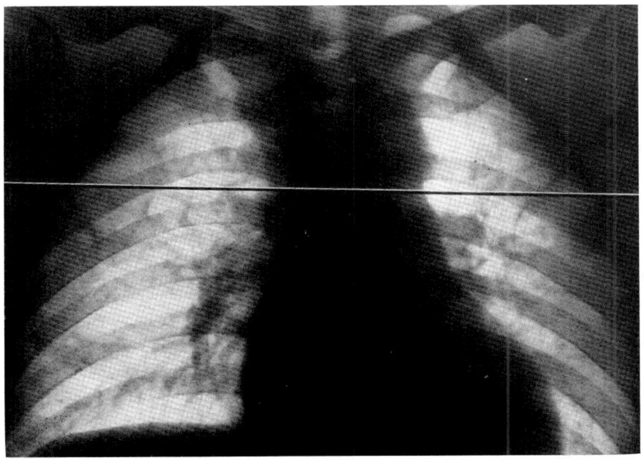

Fig. 205. Normal roentgenogram. Horizontal line showing the level tomographed

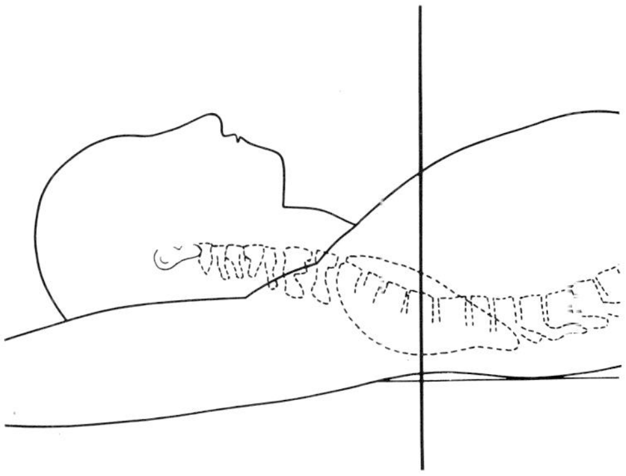

Fig. 206. Schematic drawing of the level tomographed. Subject supine with hands folded behind the head

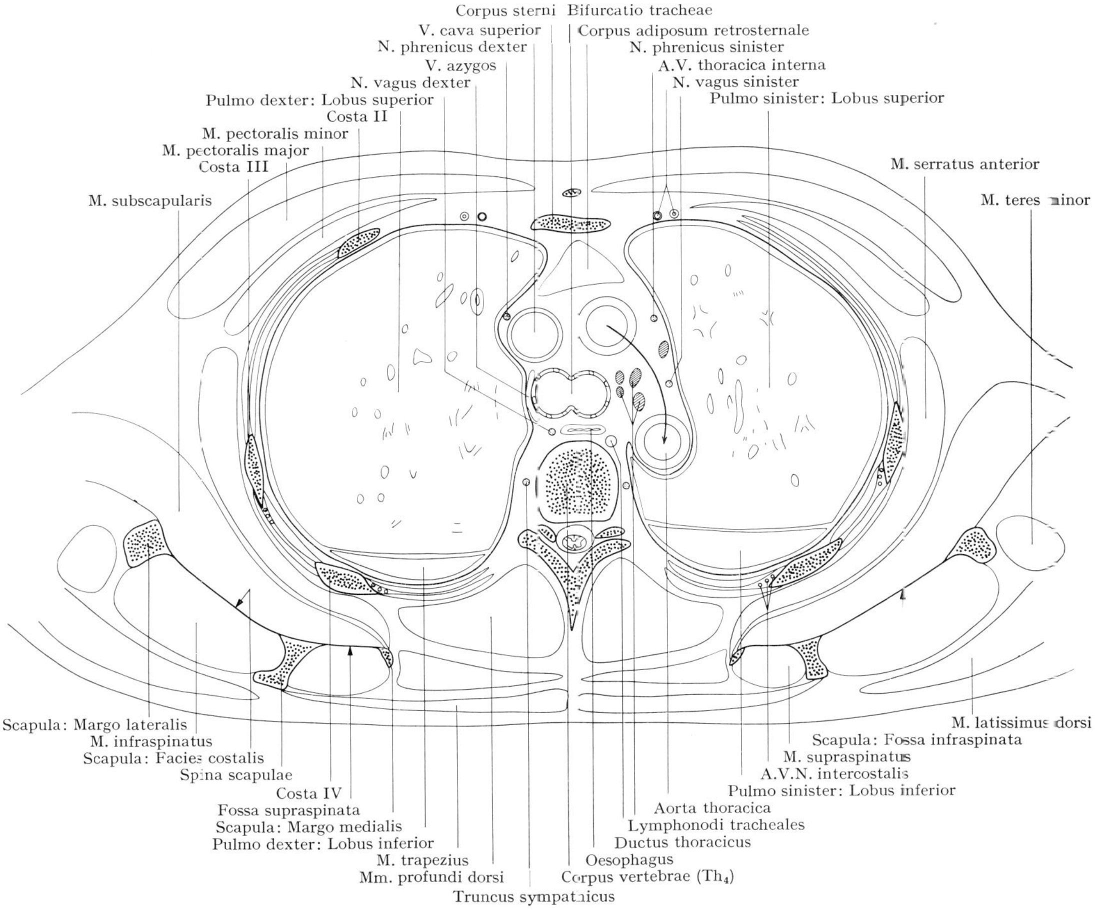

Fig. 207. Anatomical chart

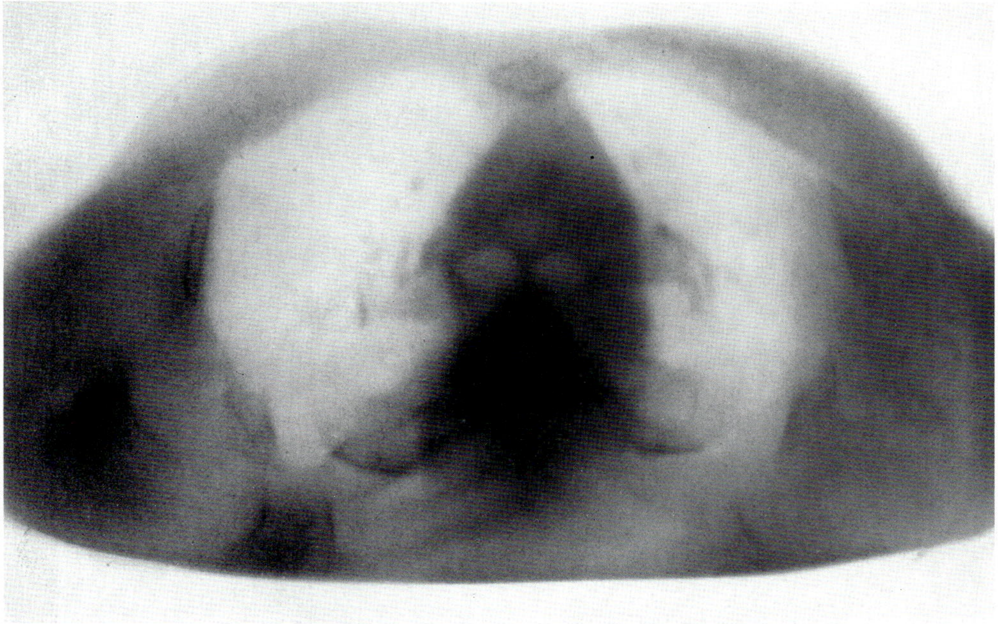

Fig. 208. Axial transverse tomogram

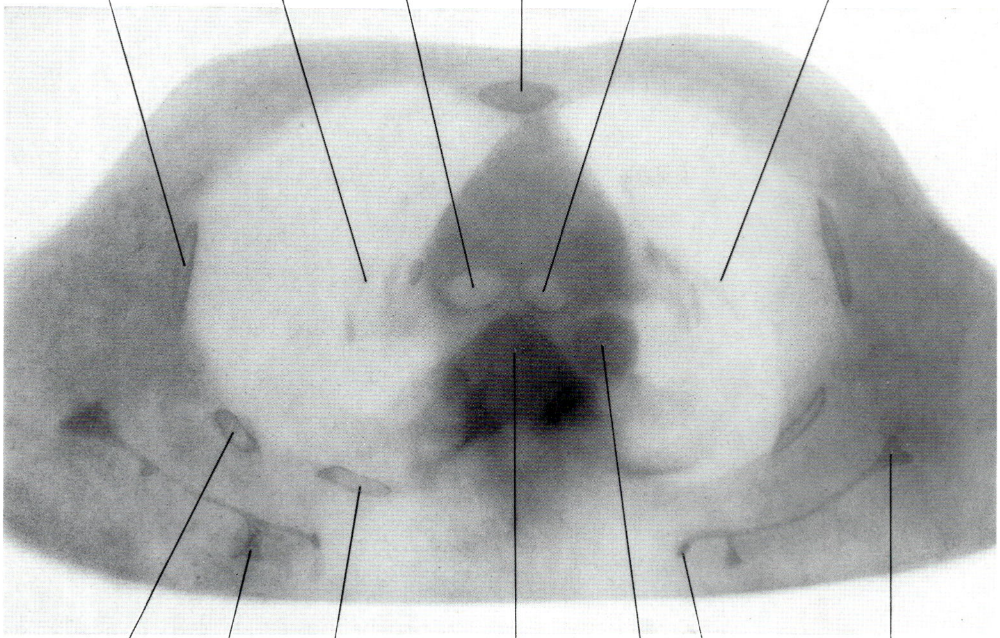

Fig. 209. Interpretation

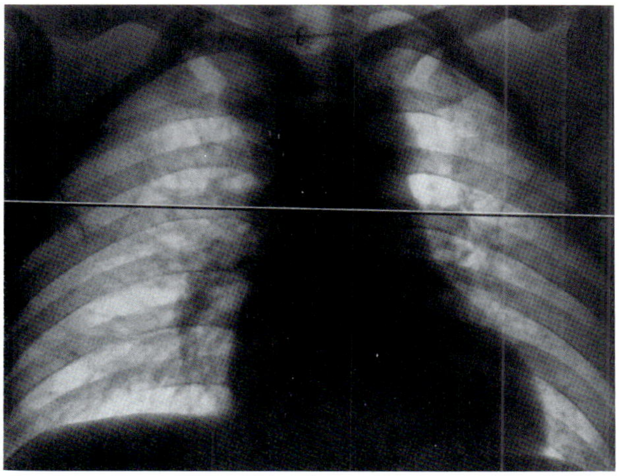

Fig. 210. Normal roentgenogram. Horizontal line showing the level tomographed

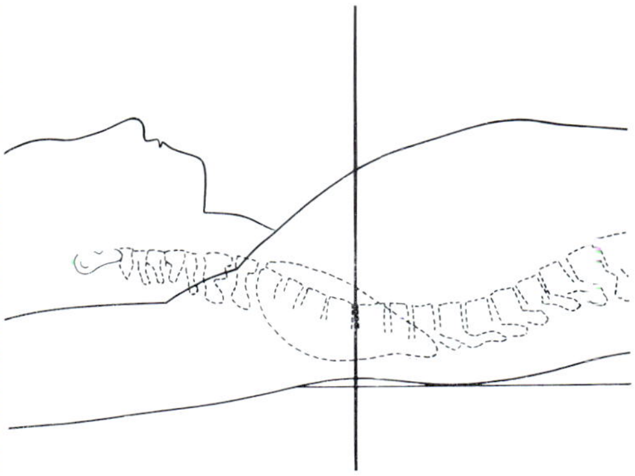

Fig. 211. Schematic drawing of the level tomographed. Subject supine with hands folded behind the head

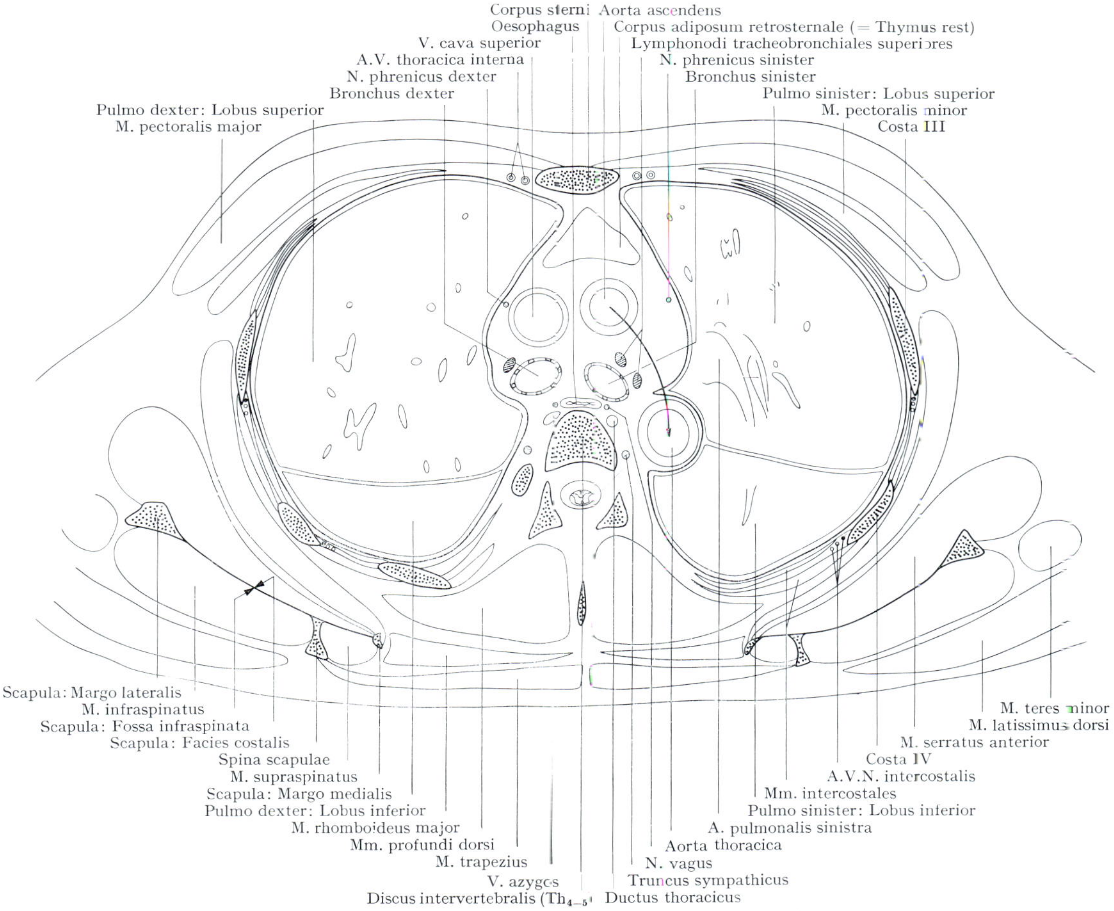

Fig. 212. Anatomical chart

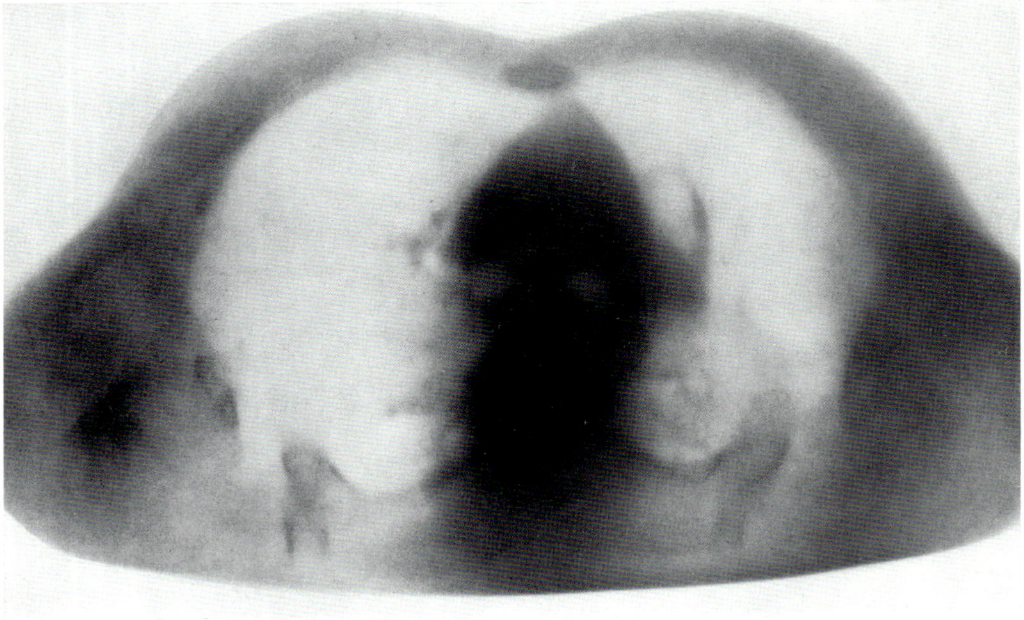

Fig. 213. Axial transverse tomogram

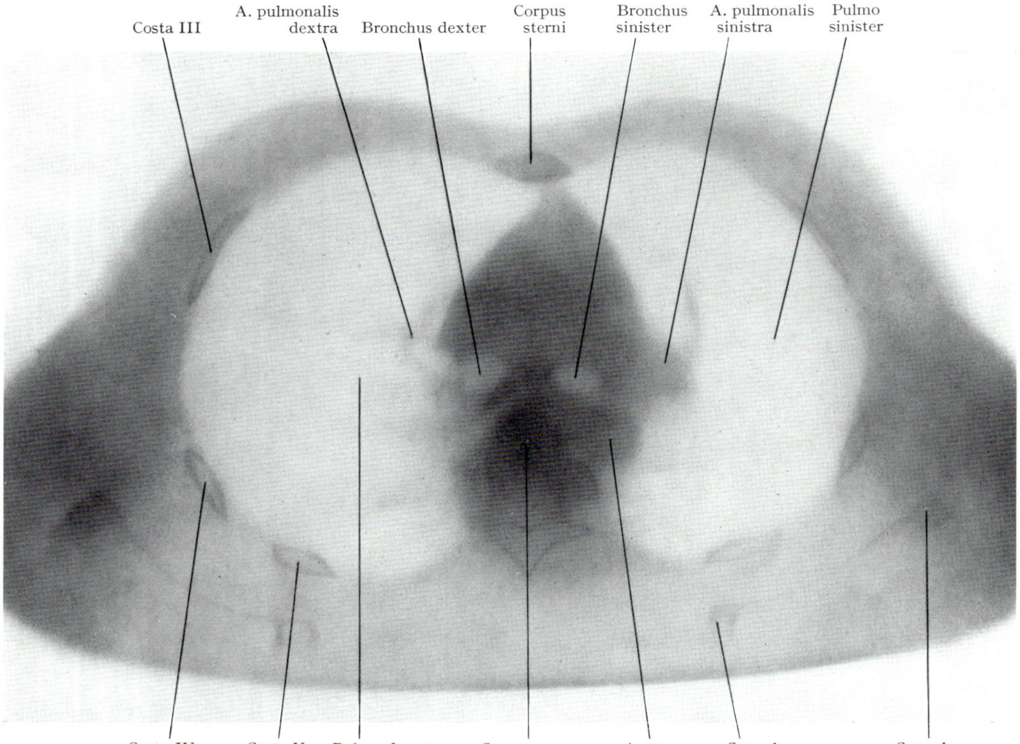

Fig. 214. Interpretation

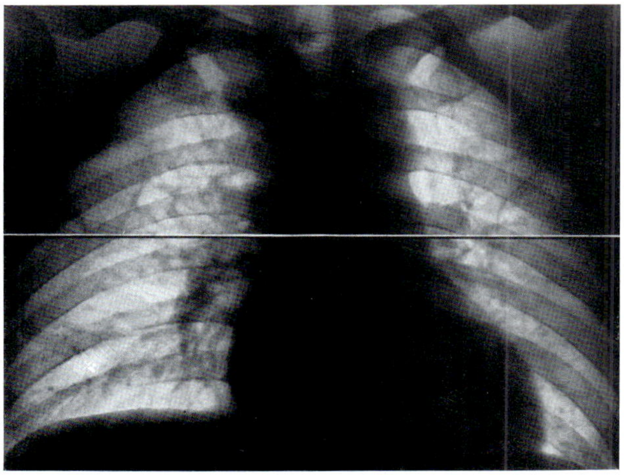

Fig. 215. Normal roentgenogram. Horizontal line showing the level tomographed

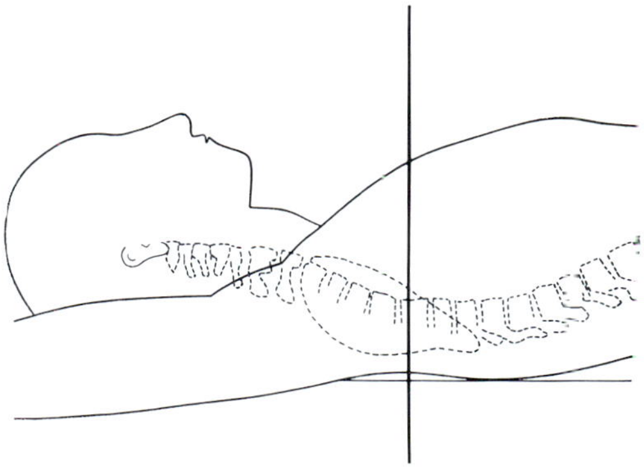

Fig. 216. Schematic drawing of the level tomographed. Subject supine with hands folded behind the head

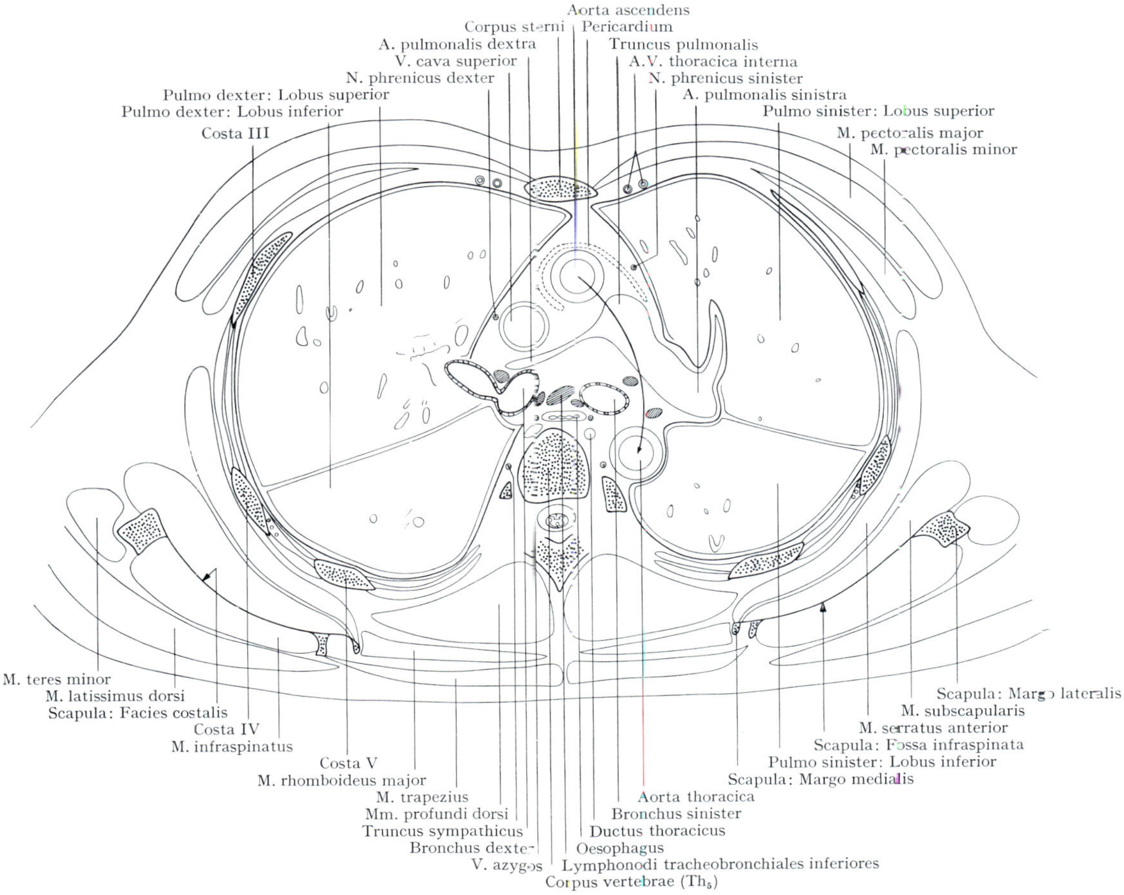

Fig. 217. Anatomical chart

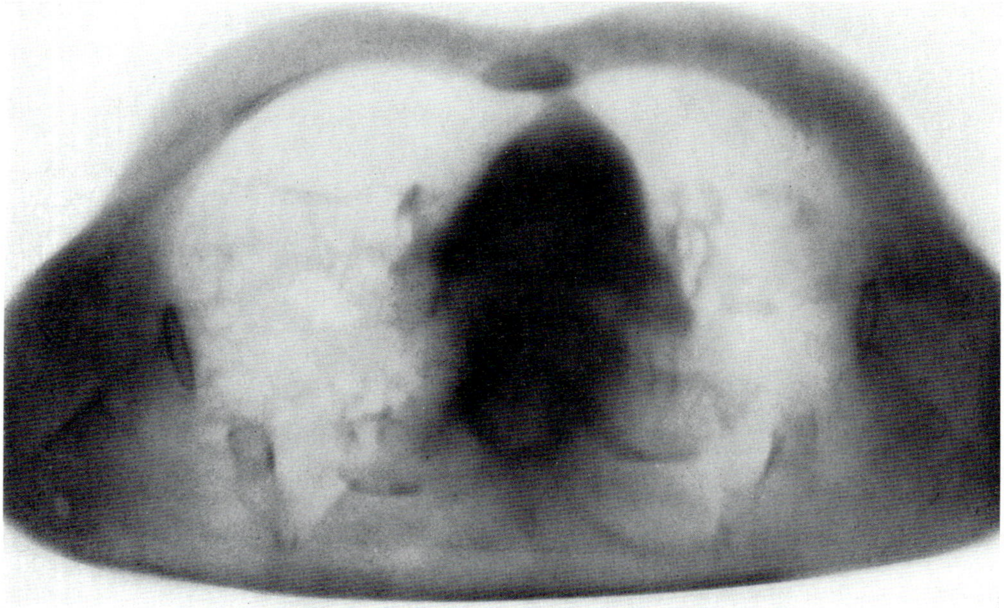

Fig. 218. Axial transverse tomogram

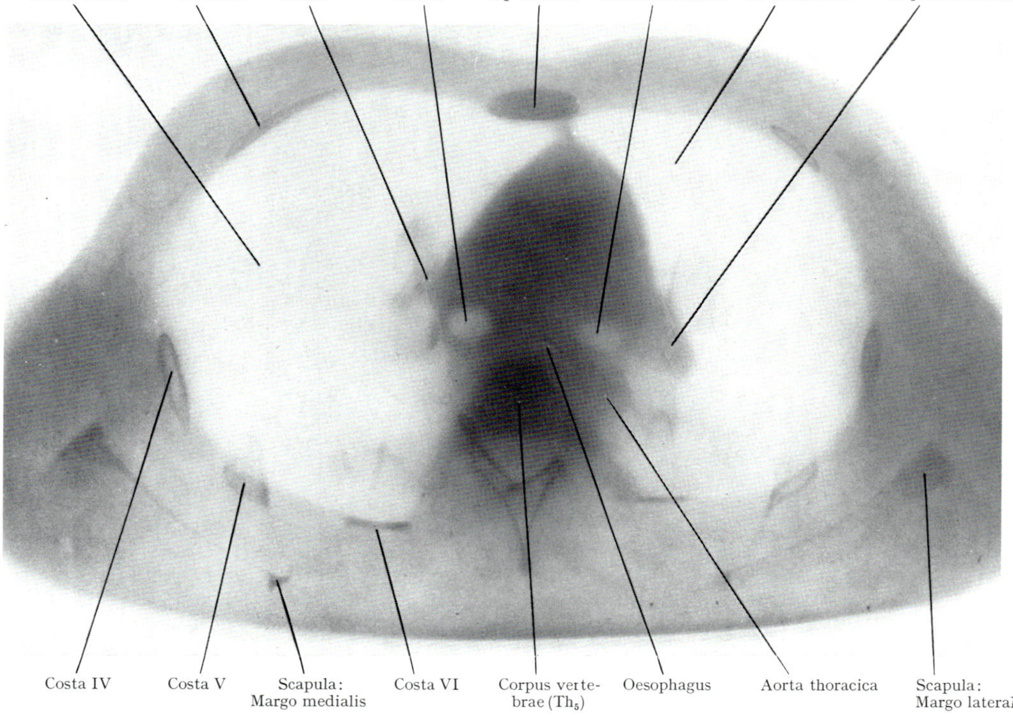

Fig. 219. Interpretation

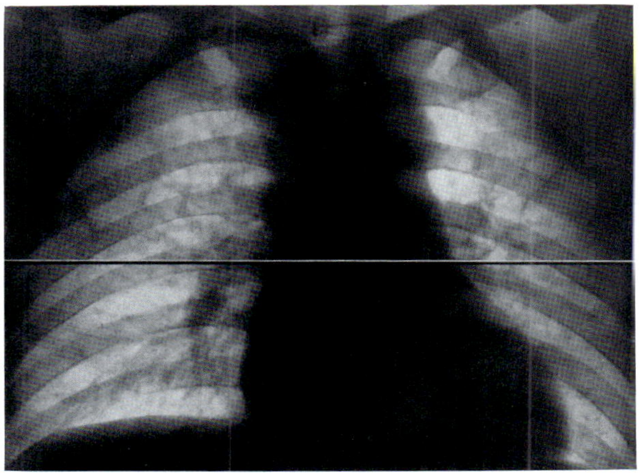

Fig. 220. Normal roentgenogram. Horizontal line showing the level tomographed

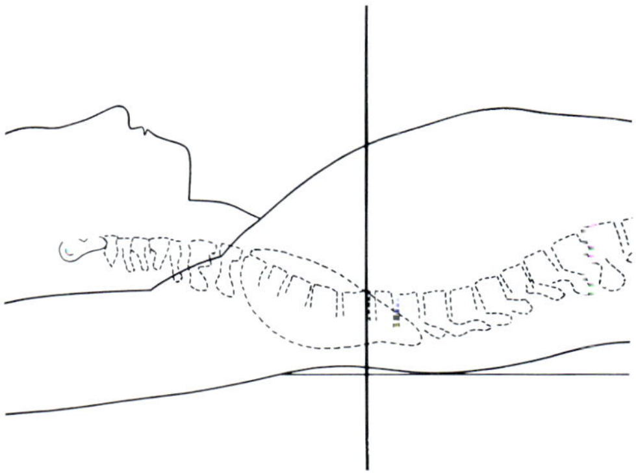

Fig. 221. Schematic drawing of the level tomographed. Subject supine with hands folded behind the head

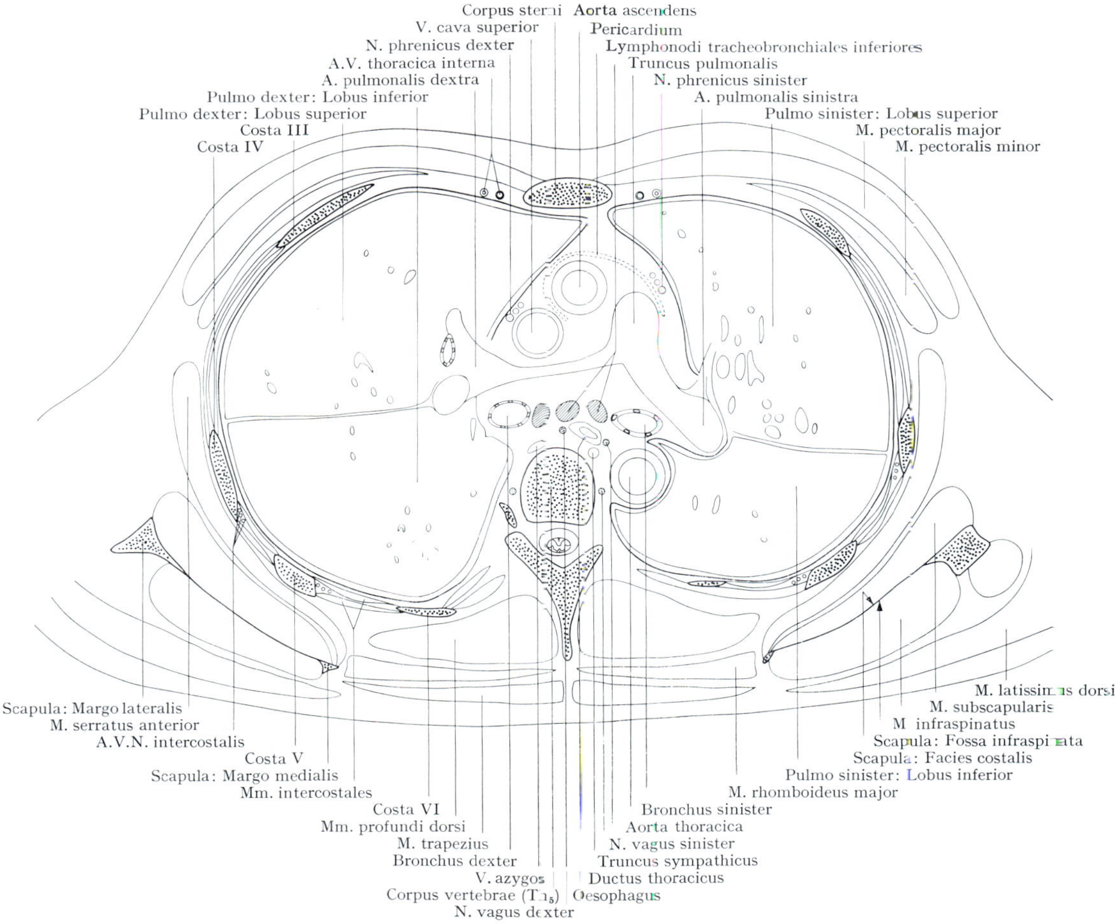

Fig. 222. Anatomical chart

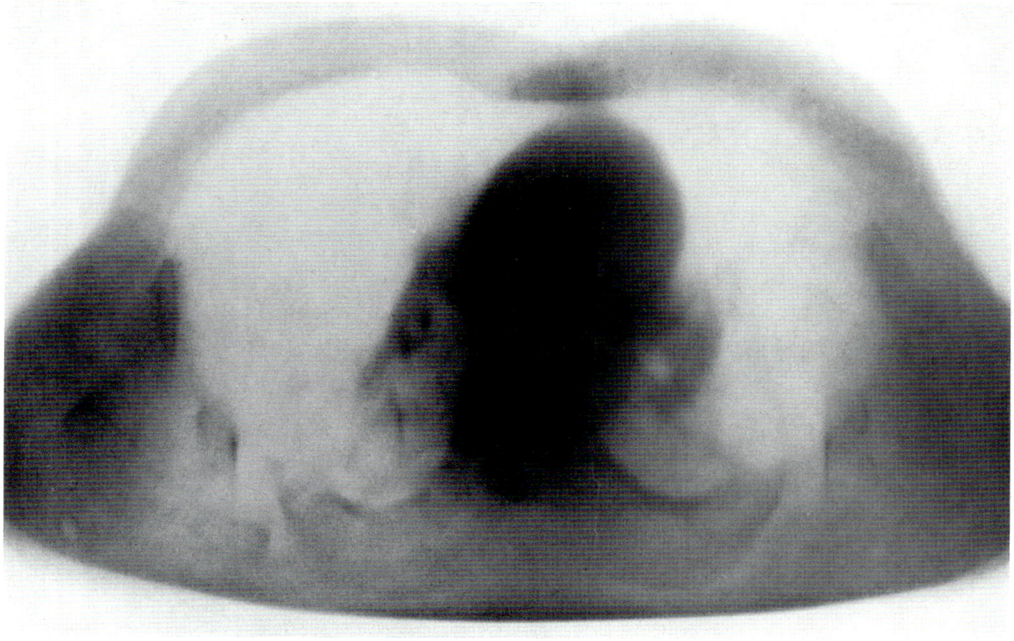

Fig. 223. Axial transverse tomogram

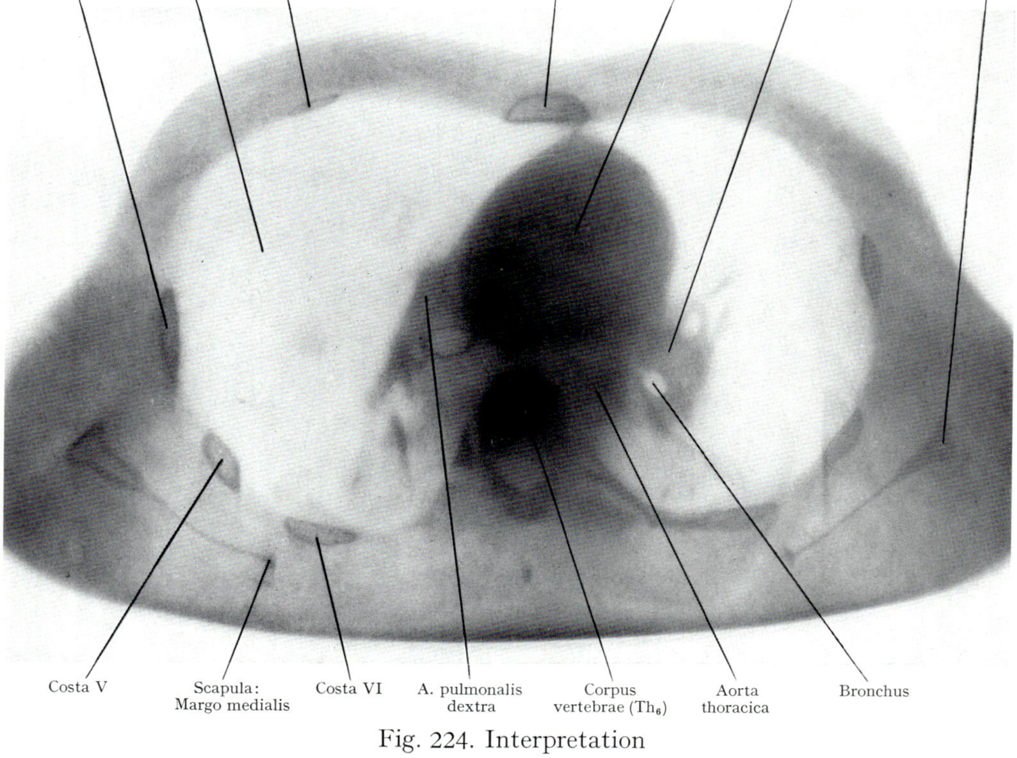

Fig. 224. Interpretation

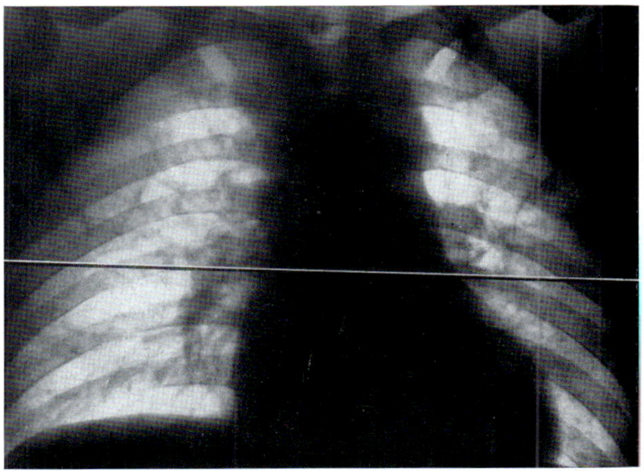

Fig. 225. Normal roentgenogram. Horizontal line showing the level tomographed

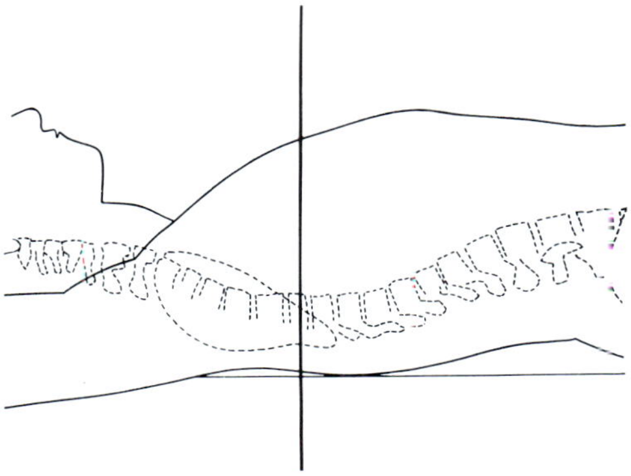

Fig. 226. Schematic drawing of the level tomographed. Subject supine with hands folded behind the head

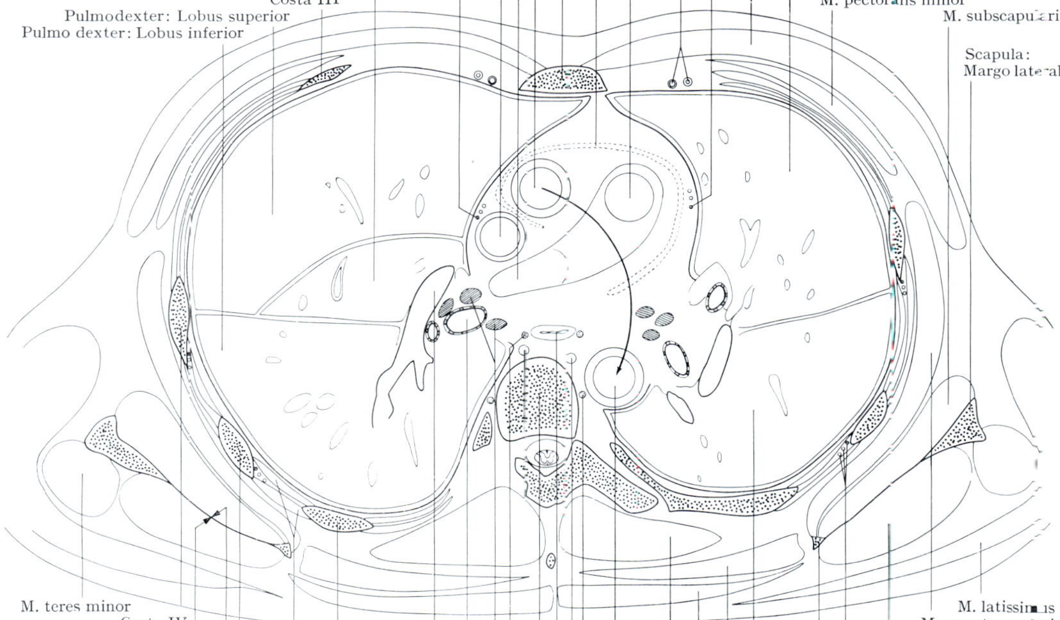

Fig. 227. Anatomical chart

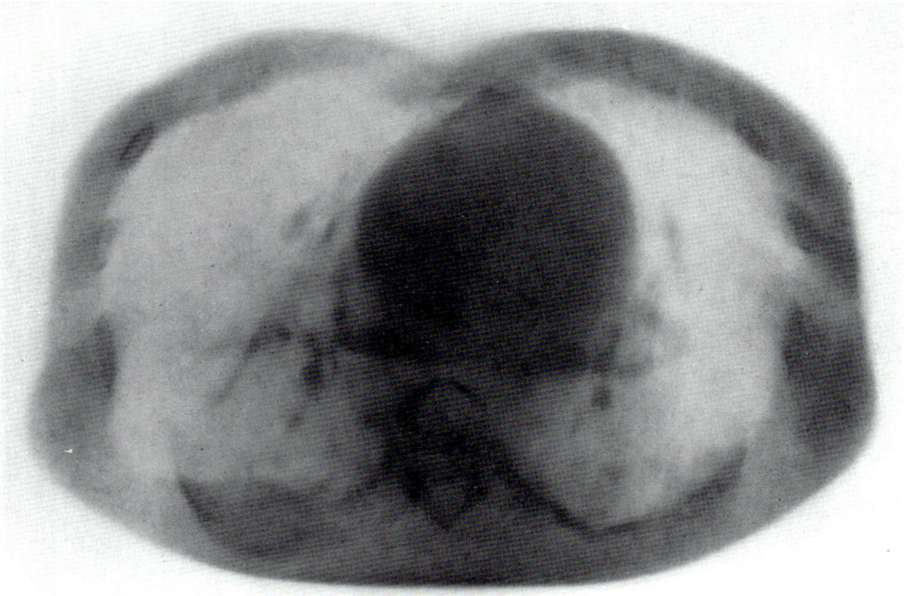

Fig. 228. Axial transverse tomogram

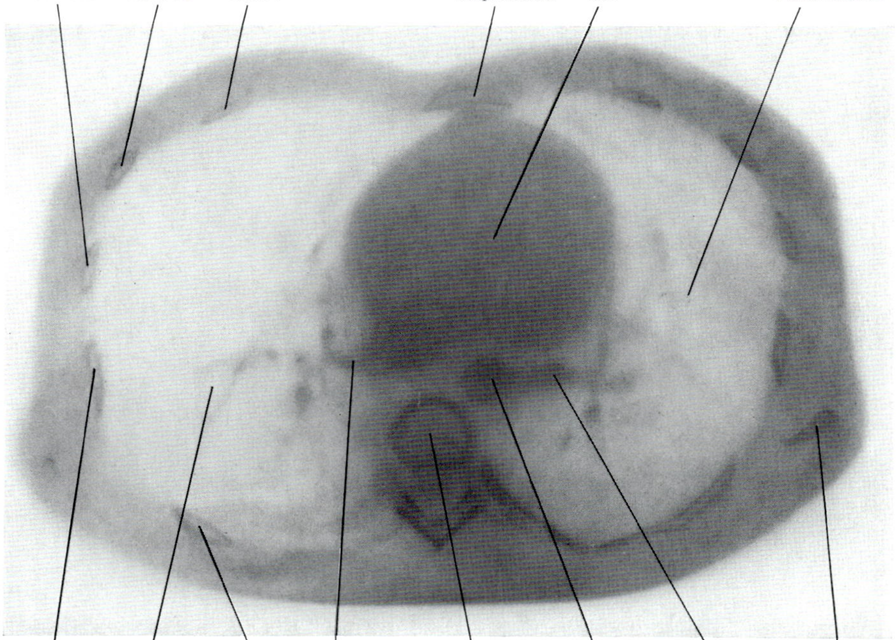

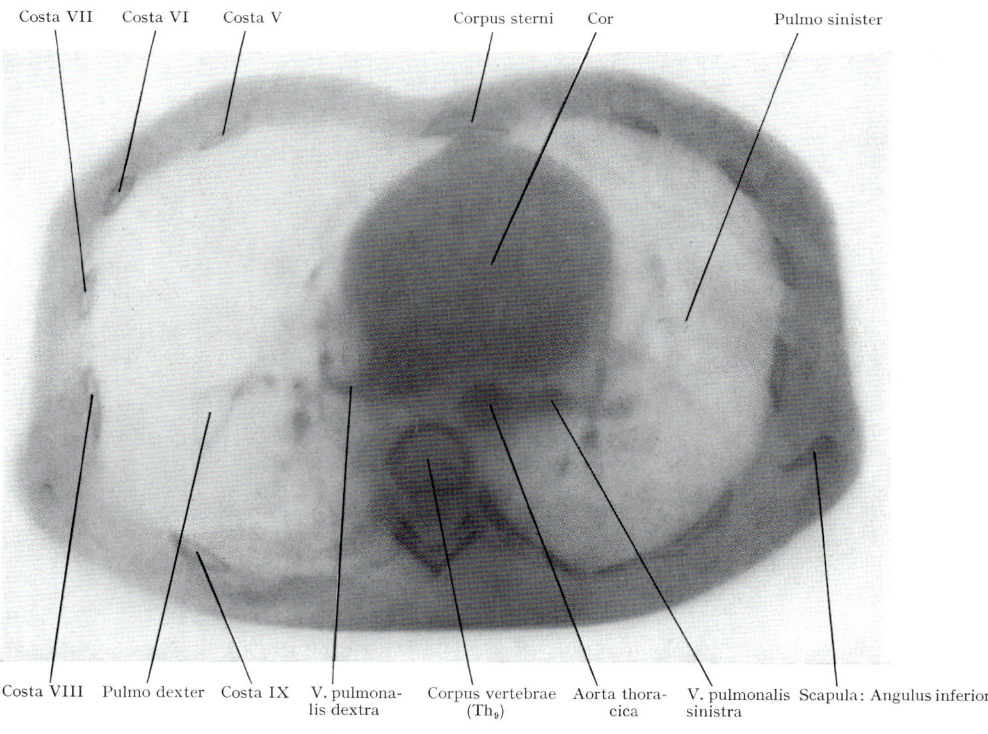

Fig. 229. Interpretation

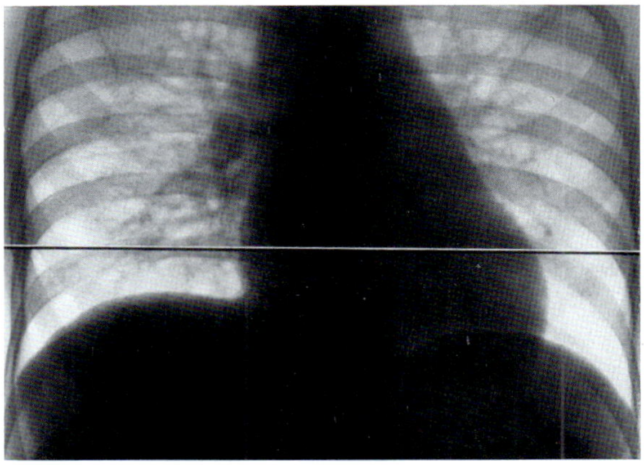

Fig. 230. Normal roentgenogram. Horizontal line showing the level tomographed

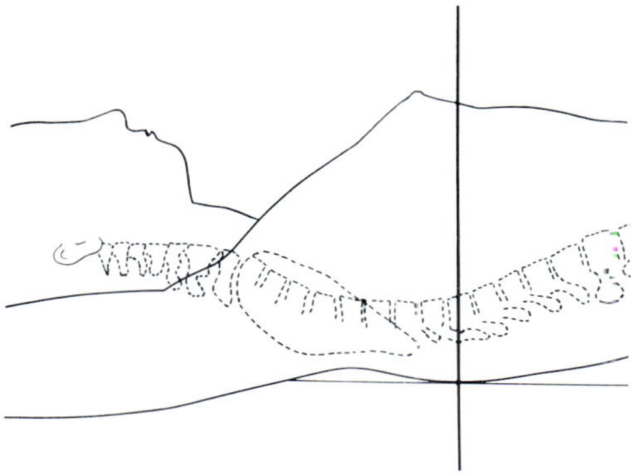

Fig. 231. Schematic drawing of the level tomographed. Subject supine with hands folded behind the head

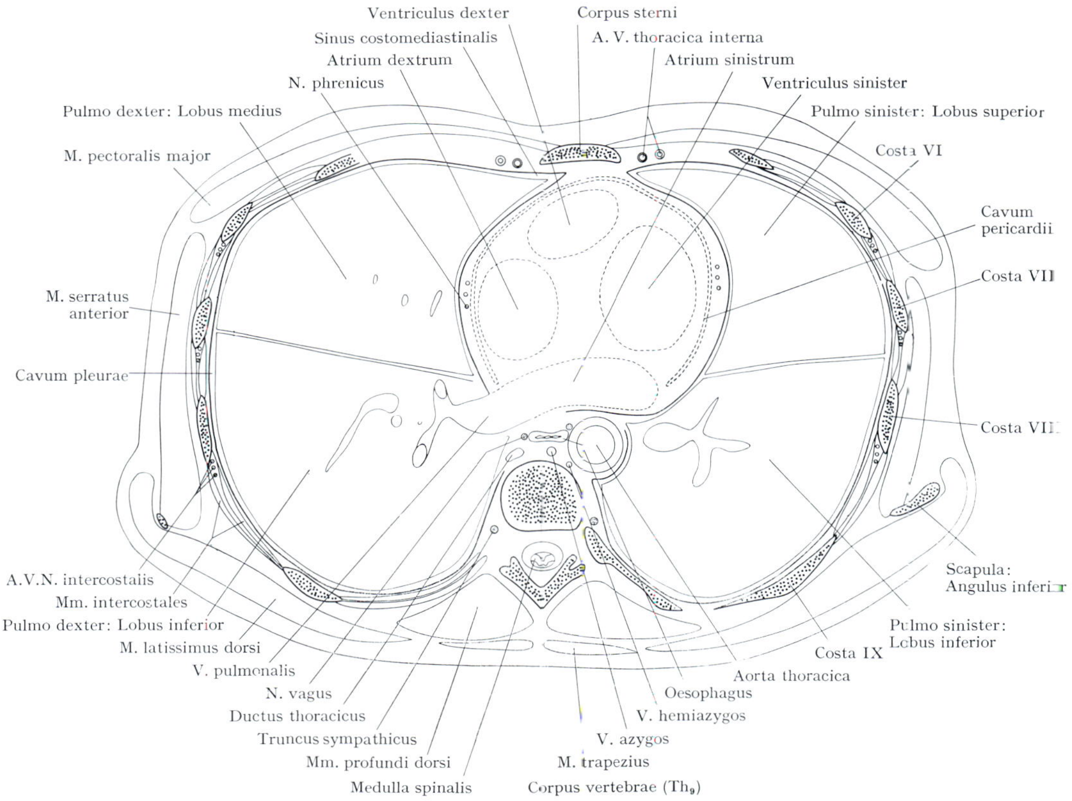

Fig. 232. Anatomical chart

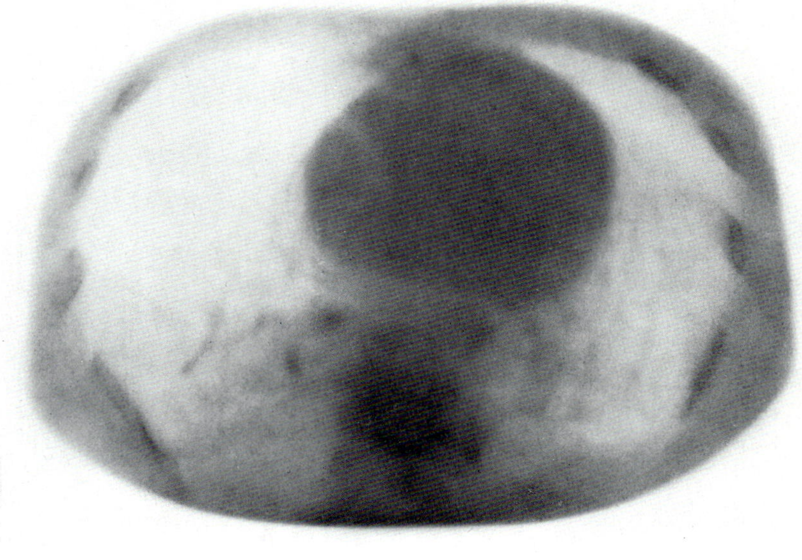

Fig. 233. Axial transverse tomogram

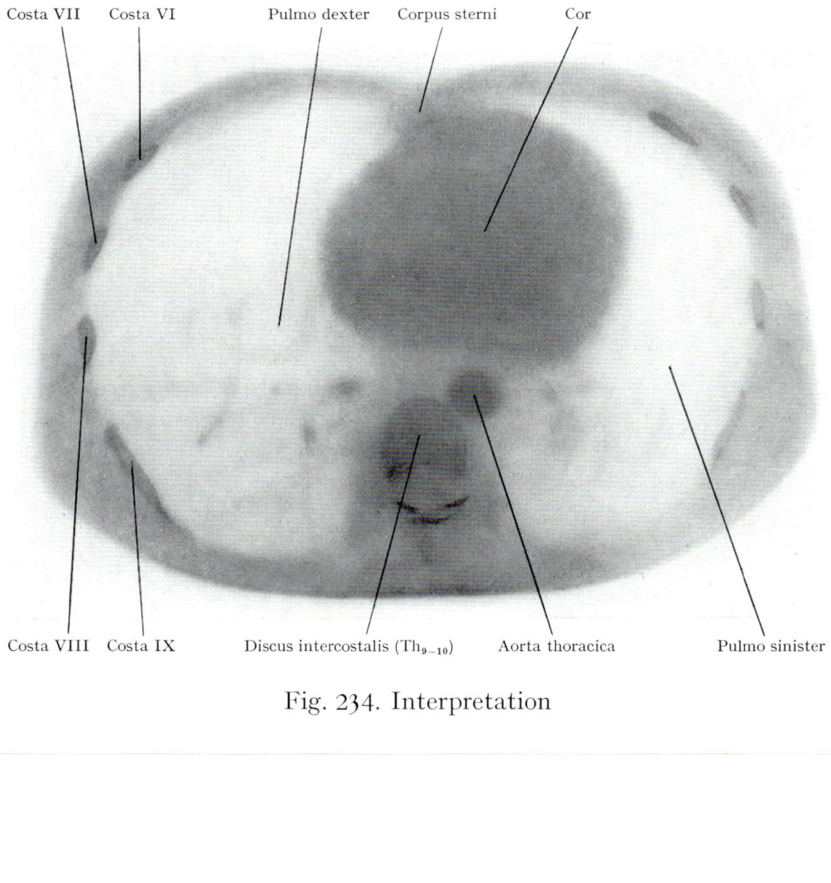

Fig. 234. Interpretation

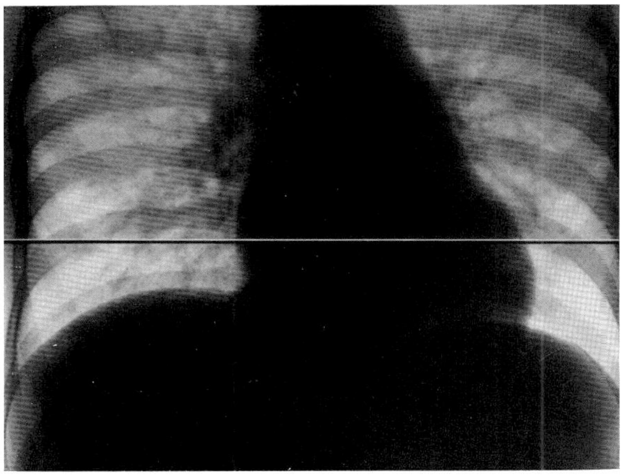

Fig. 235. Normal roentgenogram. Horizontal line showing the level tomographed

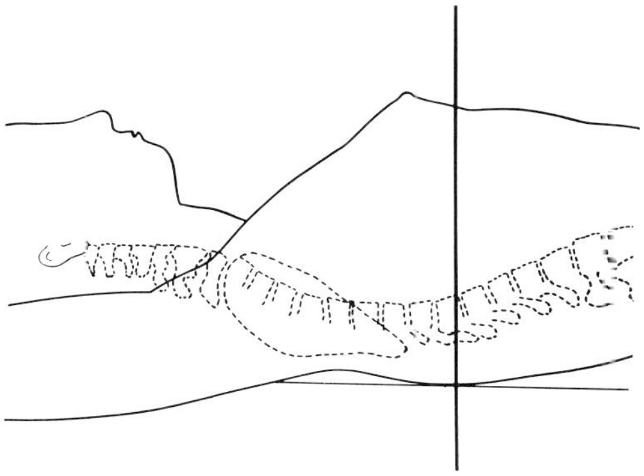

Fig. 236. Schematic drawing of the level tomographed. Subject supine with hands folded behind the head

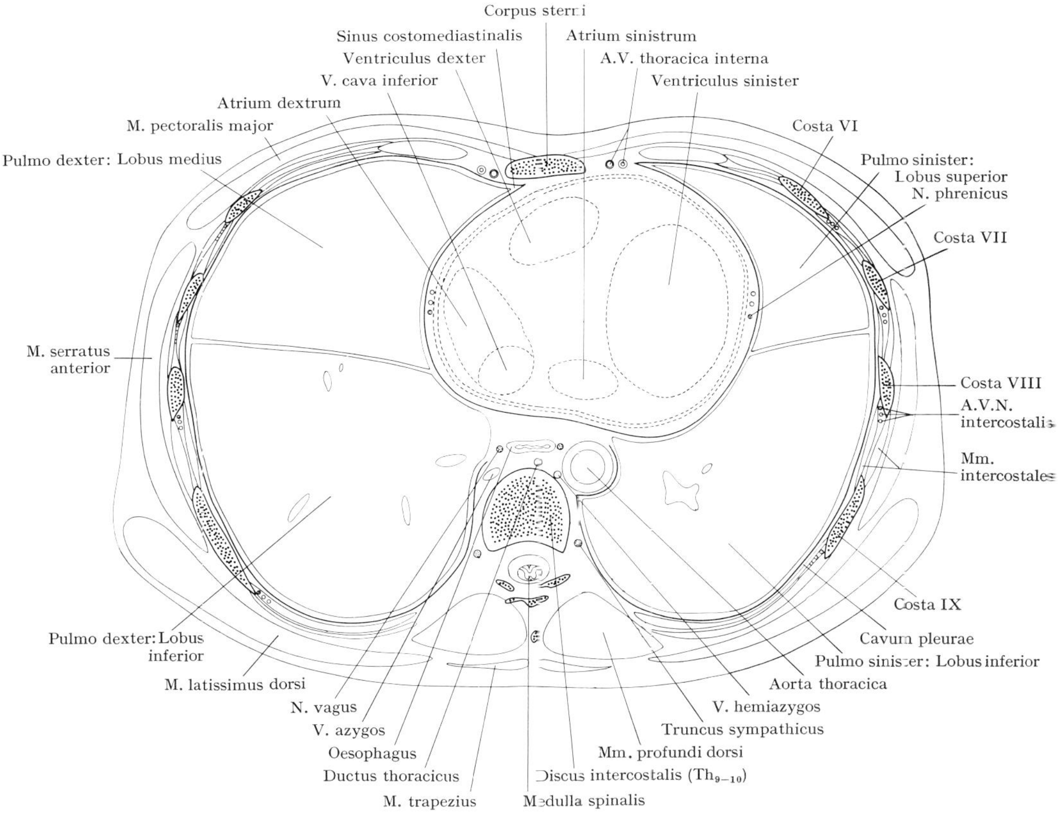

Fig. 237. Anatomical chart

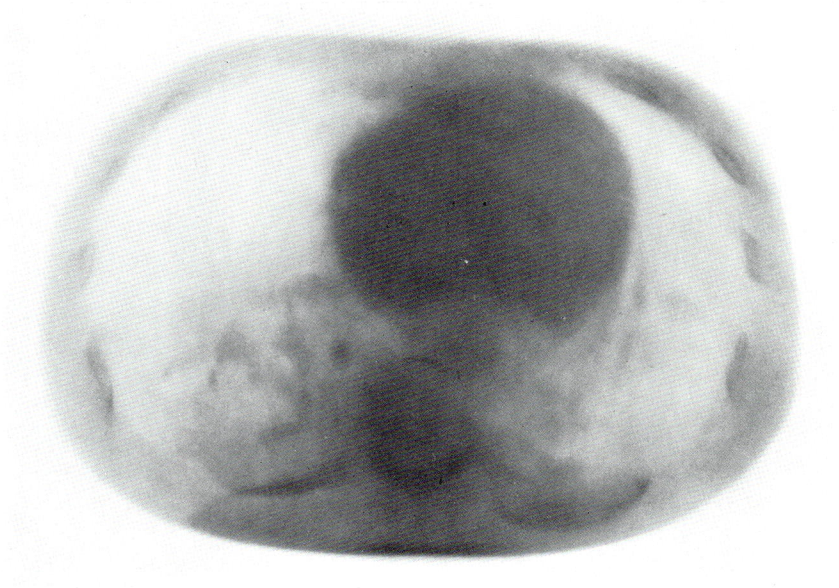

Fig. 238. Axial transverse tomogram

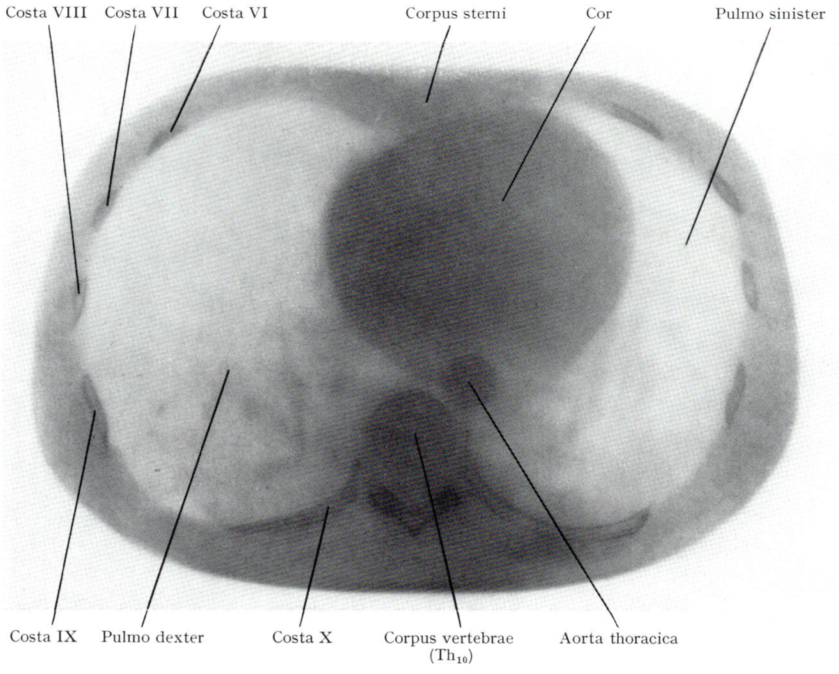

Fig. 239. Interpretation

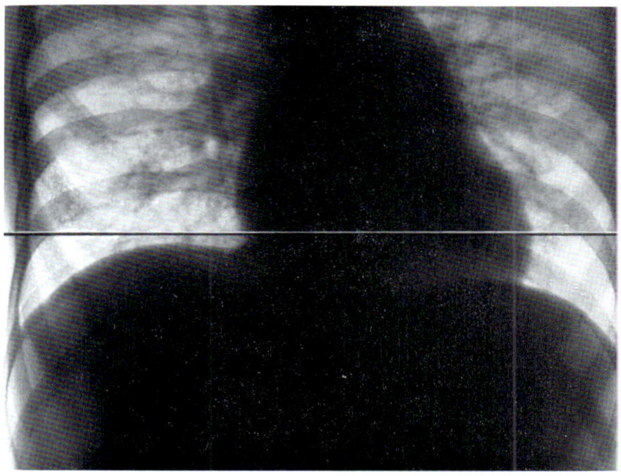

Fig. 240. Normal roentgenogram. Horizontal line showing the level tomographed

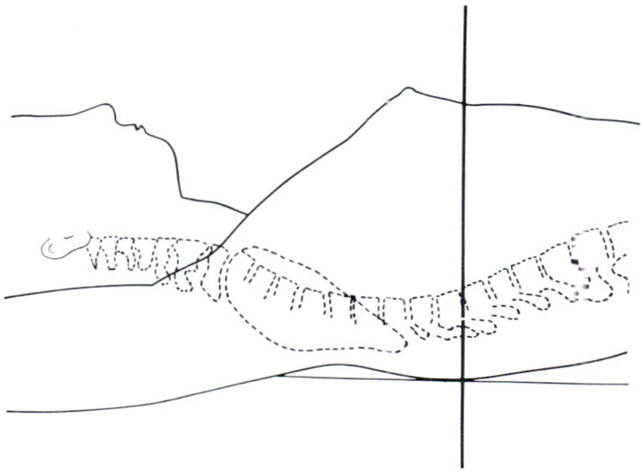

Fig. 241. Schematic drawing of the level tomographed. Subject supine with hands folded behind the head

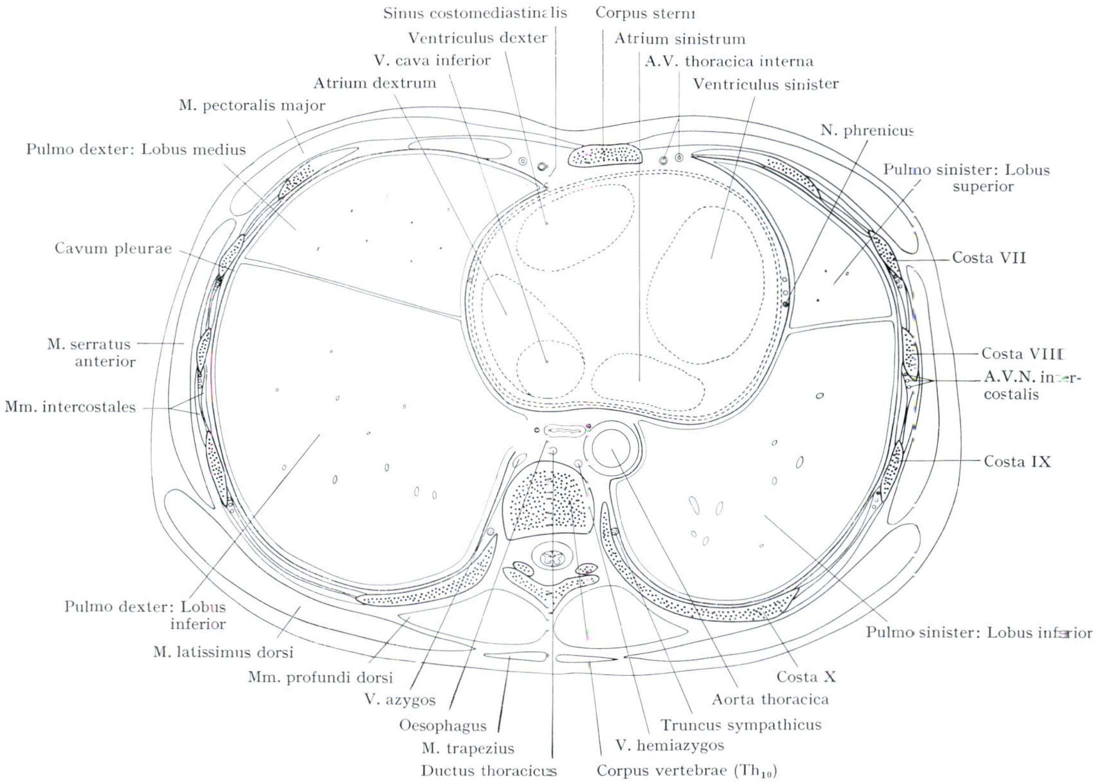

Fig. 242. Anatomical chart

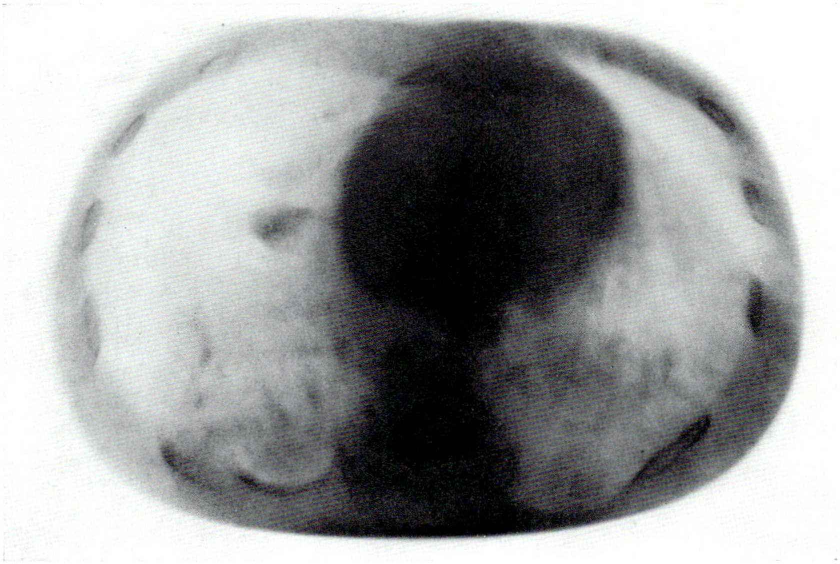

Fig. 243. Axial transverse tomogram

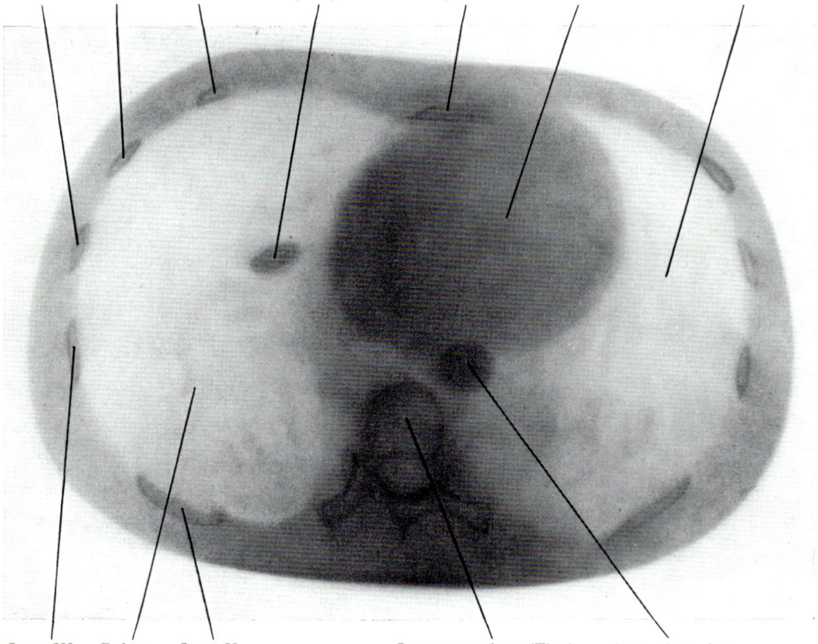

Fig. 244. Interpretation

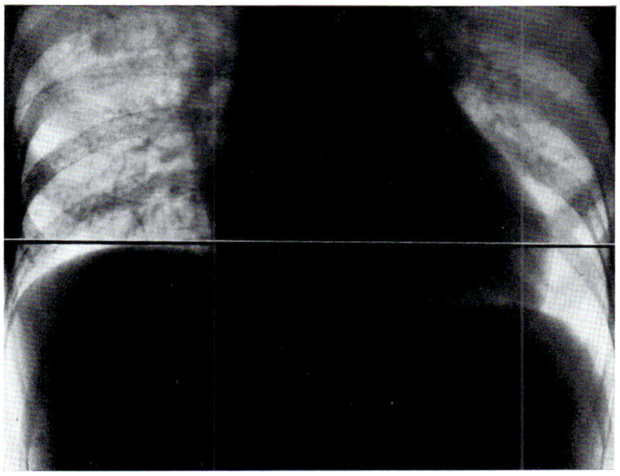

Fig. 245. Normal roentgenogram. Horizontal line showing the level tomographed

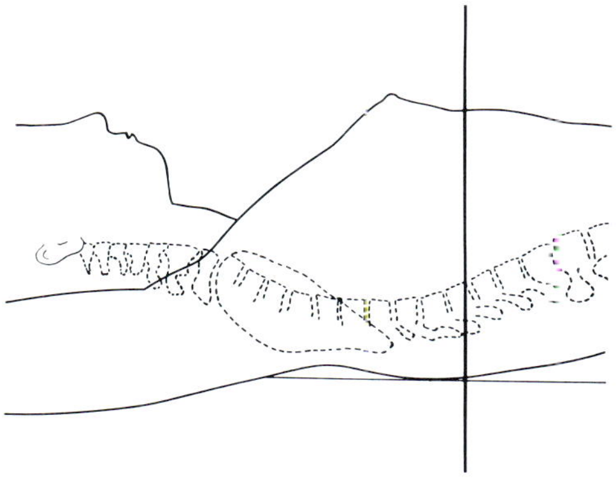

Fig. 246. Schematic drawing of the level tomographed. Subject supine with hands folded behind the head

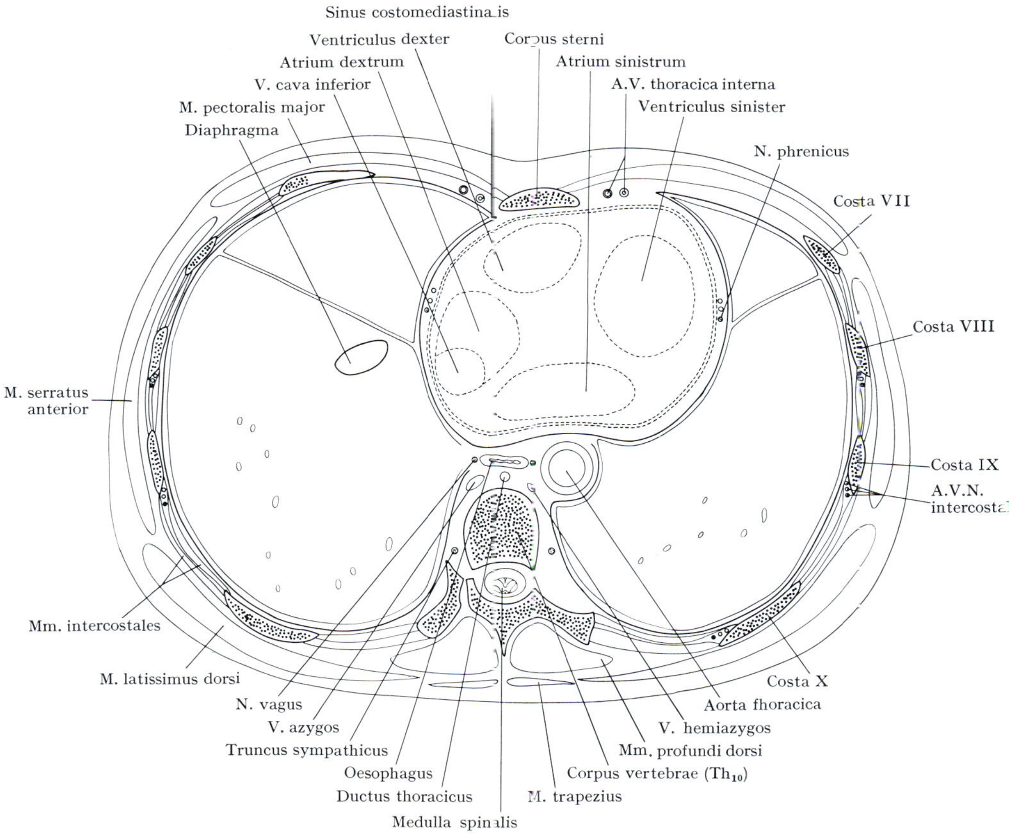

Fig. 247. Anatomical chart

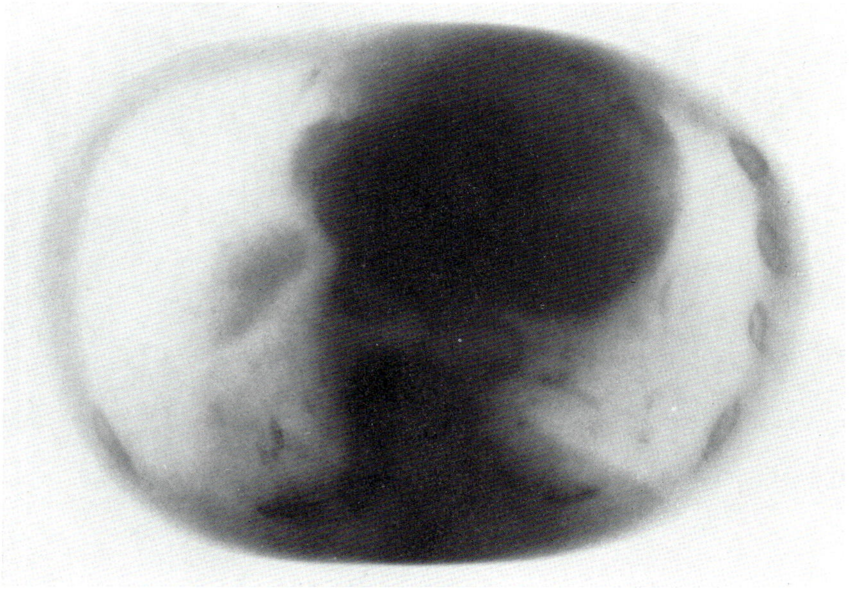

Fig. 248. Axial transverse tomogram

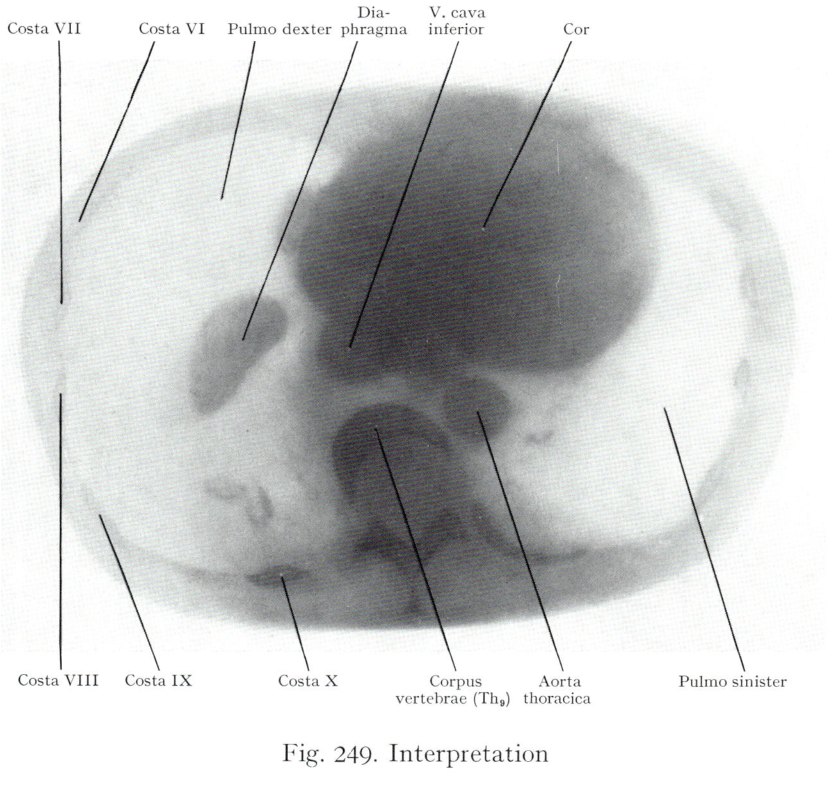

Fig. 249. Interpretation

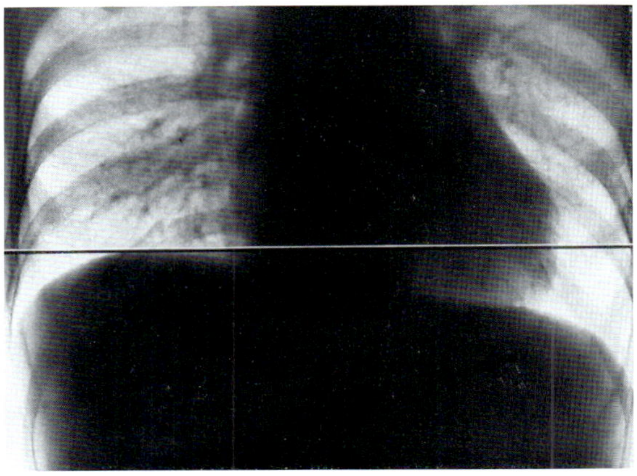

Fig. 250. Normal roentgenogram. Horizontal line showing the level tomographed

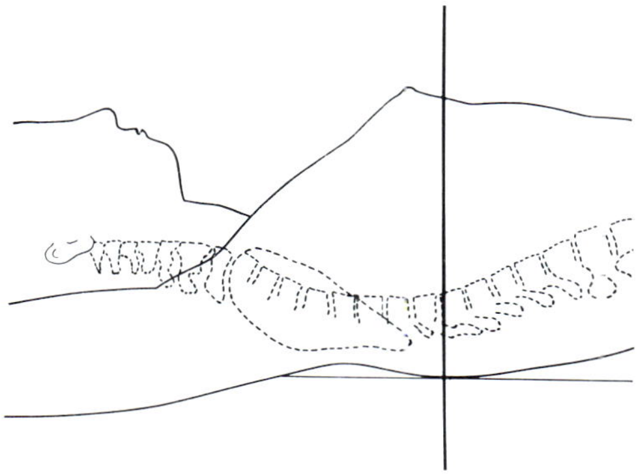

Fig. 251. Schematic drawing of the level tomographed. Subject supine with hands folded behind the head

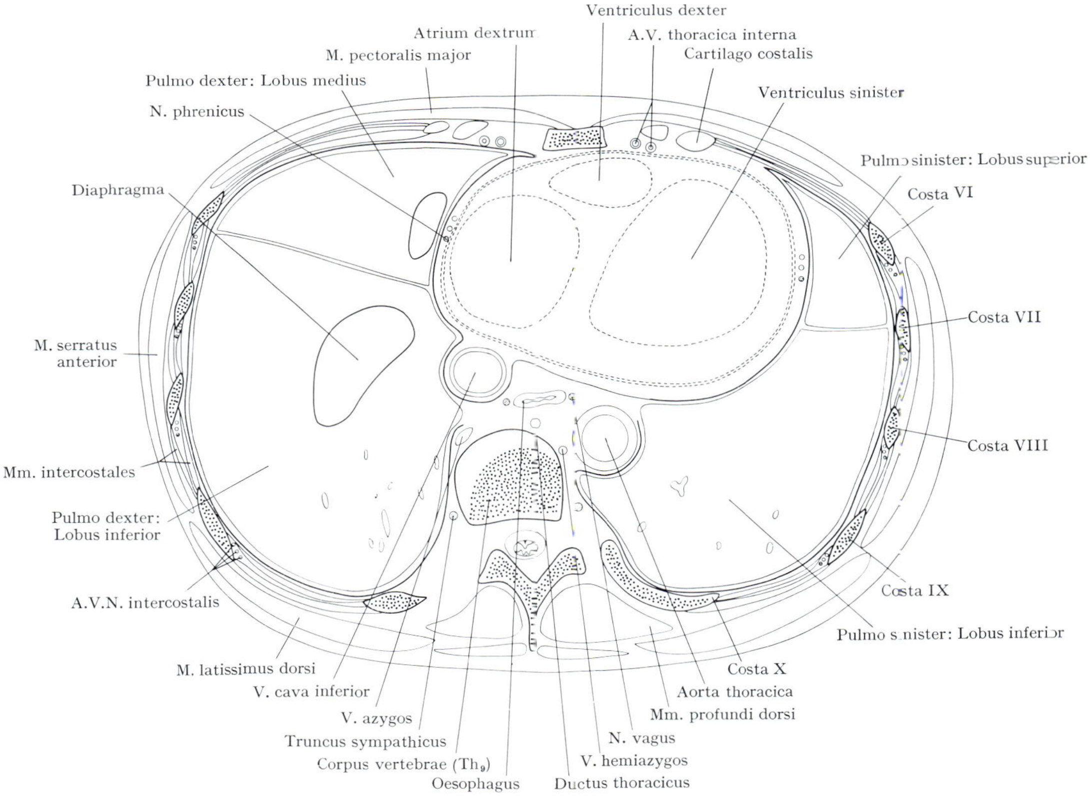

Fig. 252. Anatomical chart

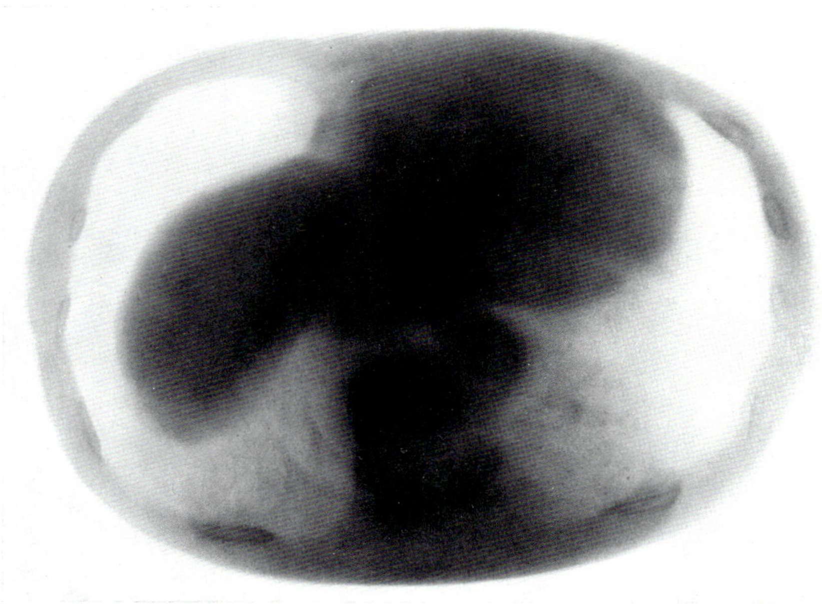

Fig. 253. Axial transverse tomogram

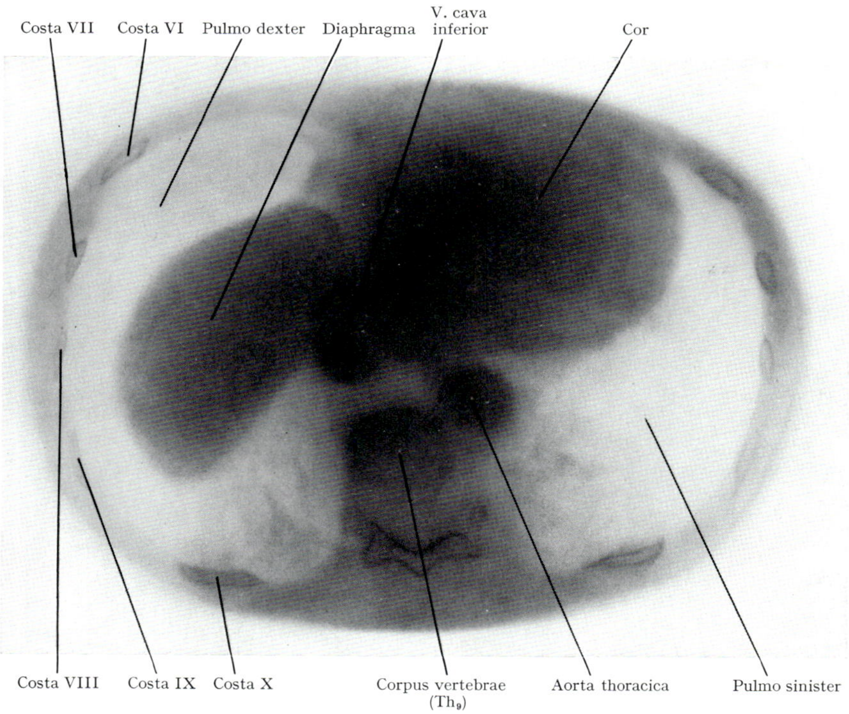

Fig. 254. Interpretation

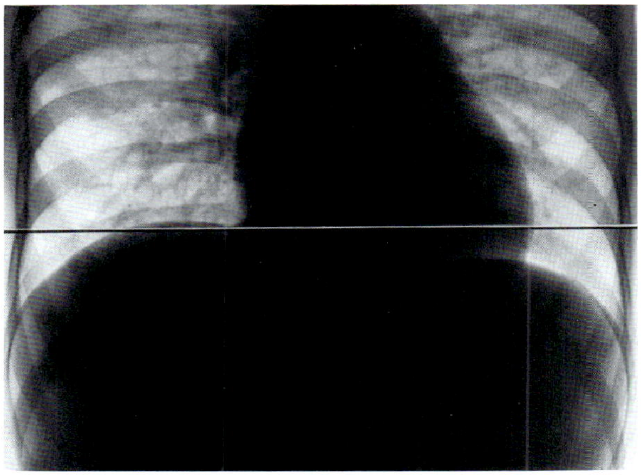

Fig. 255. Normal roentgenogram. Horizontal line showing the level tomographed

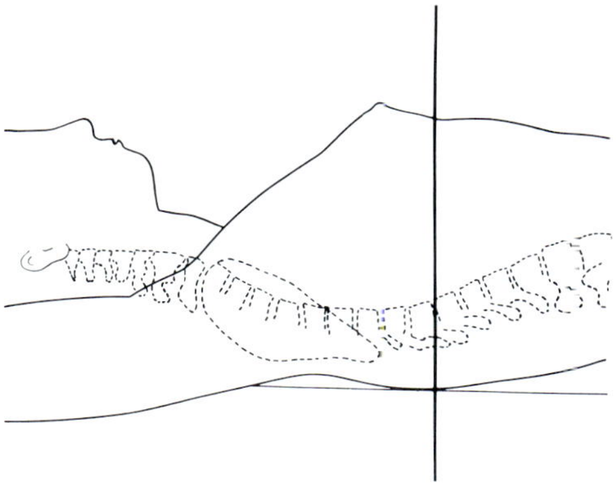

Fig. 256. Schematic drawing of the level tomographed. Subject supine with hands folded behind the head

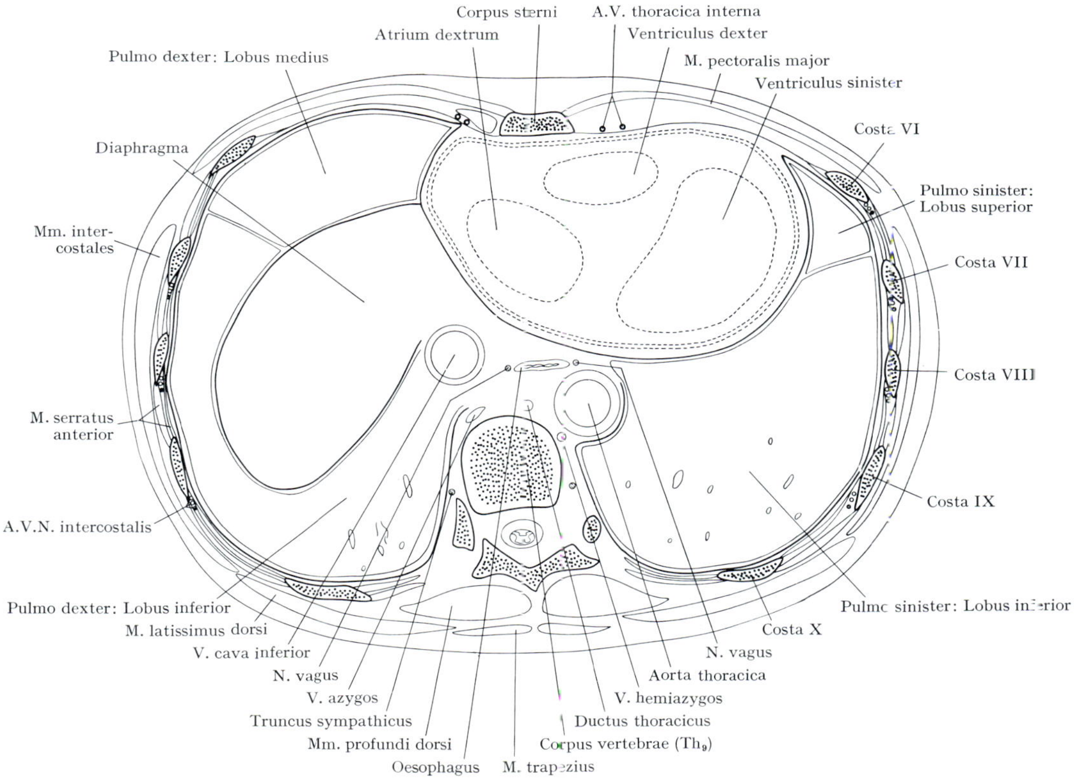

Fig. 257. Anatomical chart

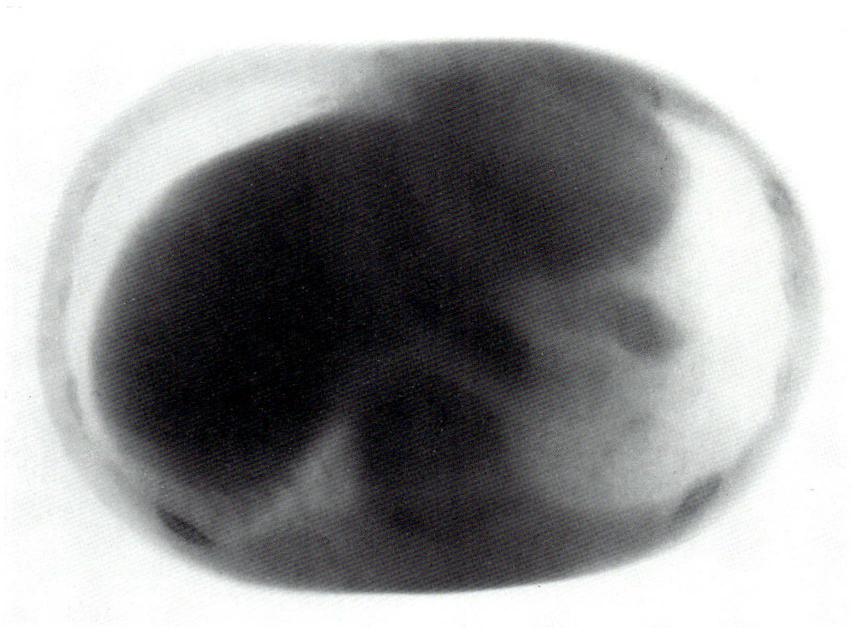

Fig. 258. Axial transverse tomogram

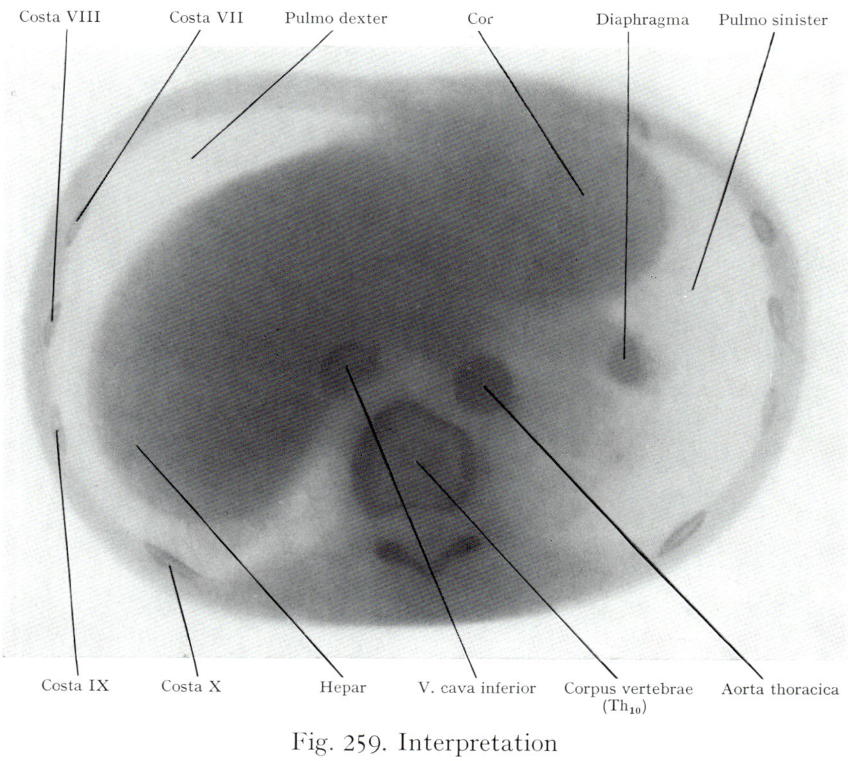

Fig. 259. Interpretation

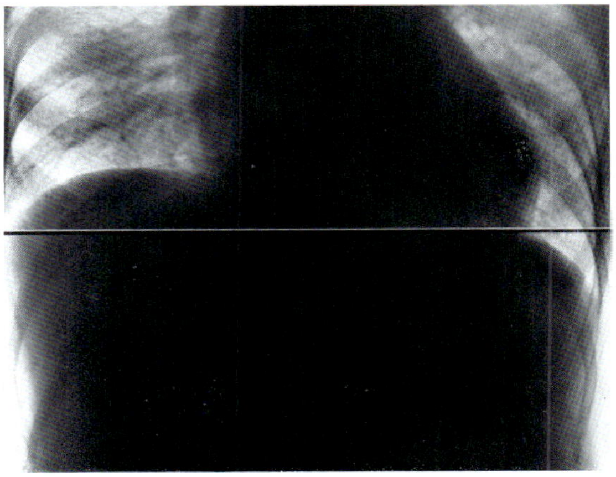

Fig. 260. Normal roentgenogram. Horizontal line showing the level tomographed

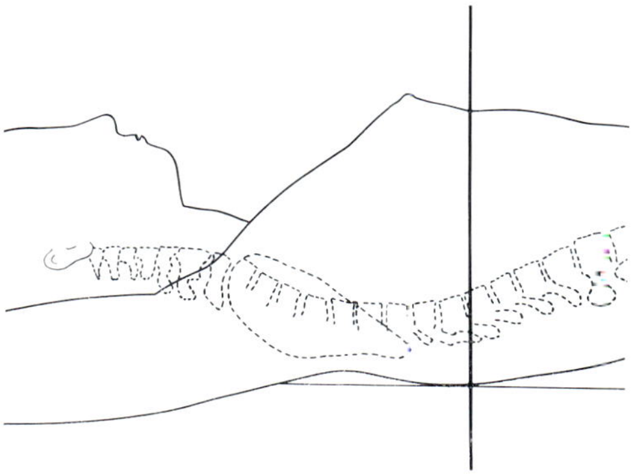

Fig. 261. Schematic drawing of the level tomographed. Subject supine with hands folded behind the head

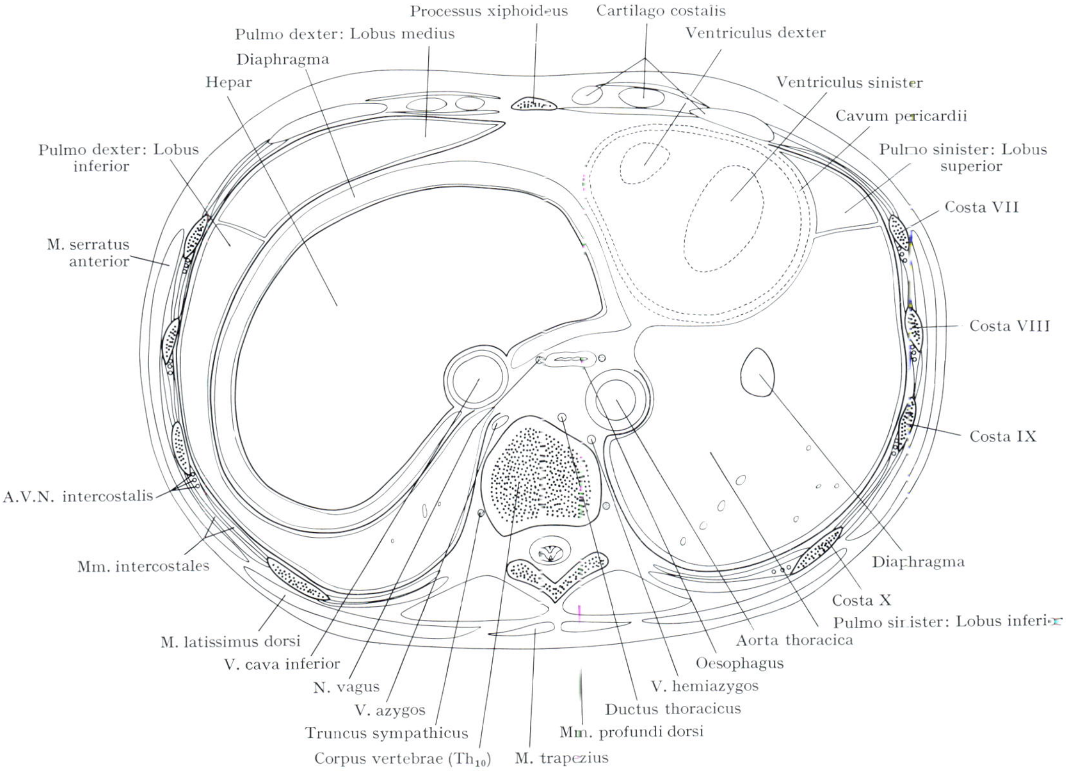

Fig. 262. Anatomical chart

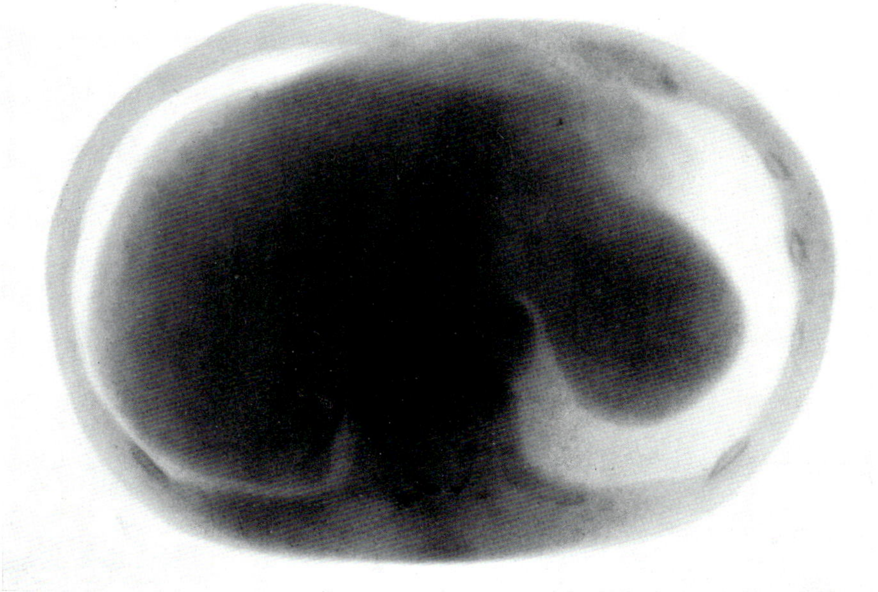

Fig. 263. Axial transverse tomogram

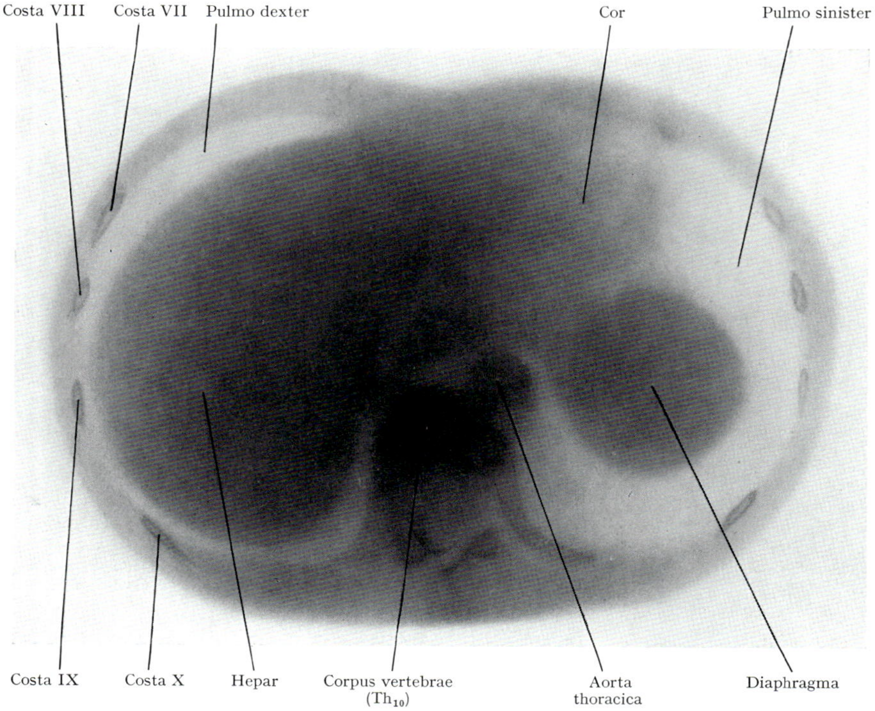

Fig. 264. Interpretation

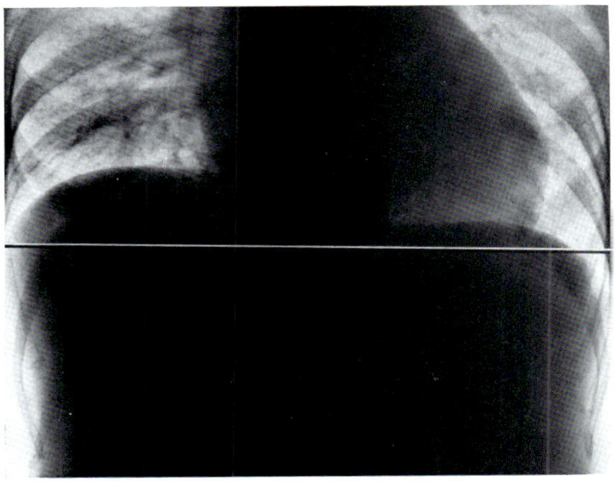

Fig. 265. Normal roentgenogram. Horizontal line showing the level tomographed

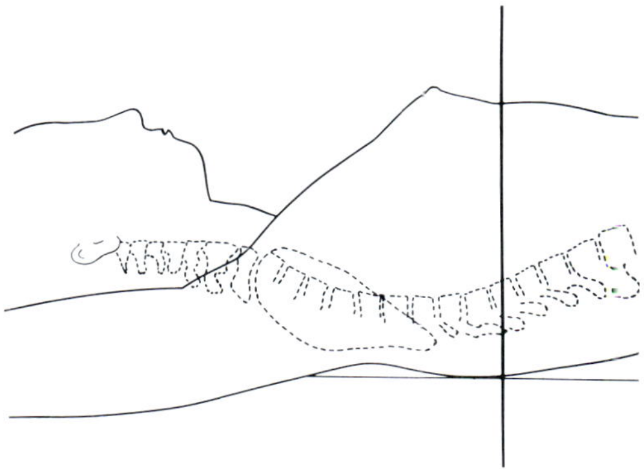

Fig. 266. Schematic drawing of the level tomographed. Subject supine with hands folded behind the head

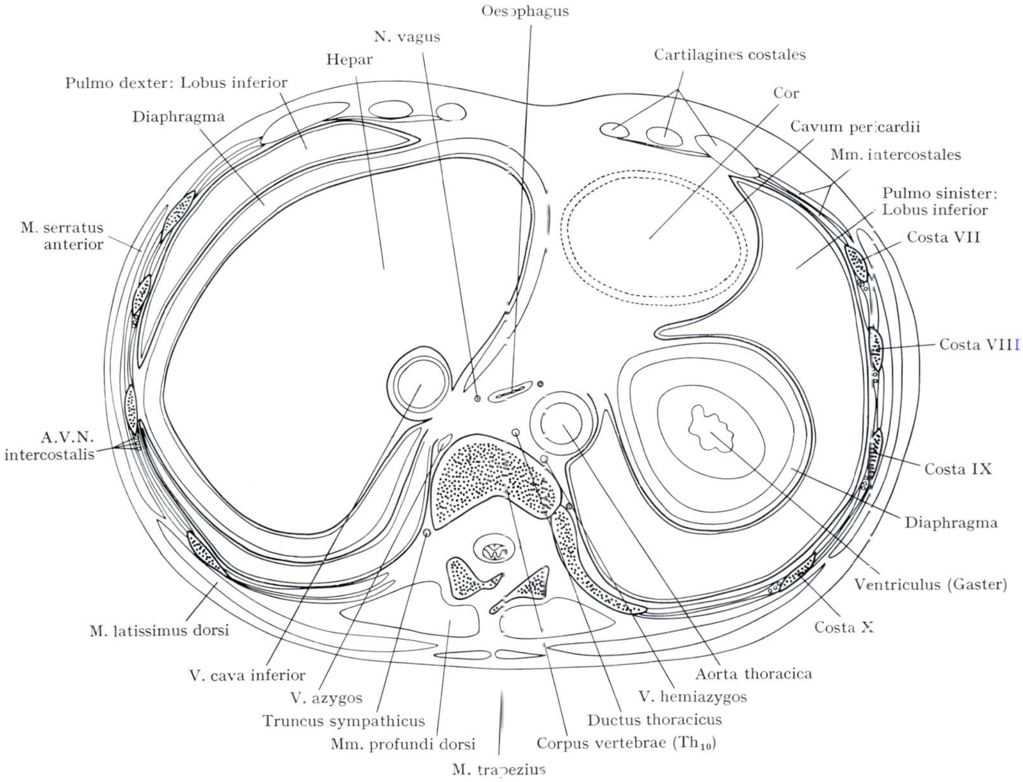

Fig. 267. Anatomical chart

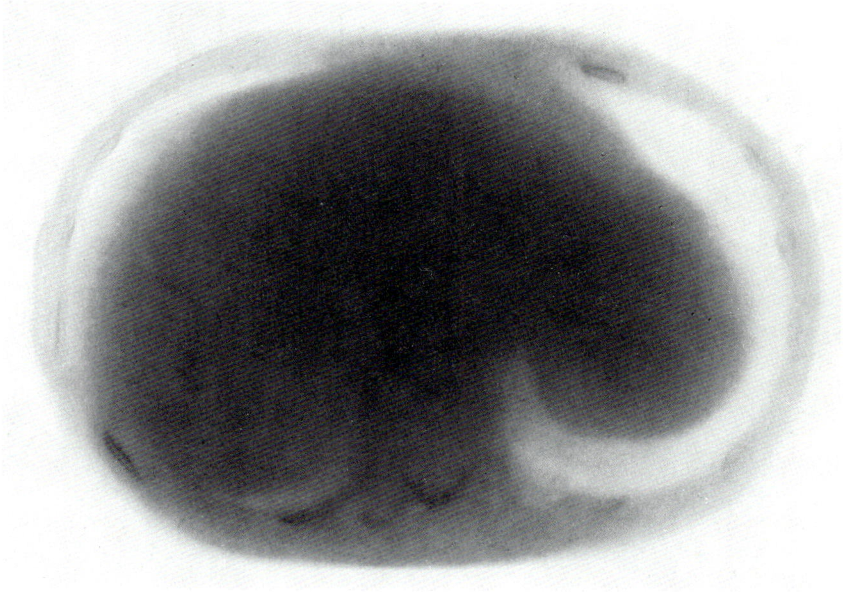

Fig. 268. Axial transverse tomogram

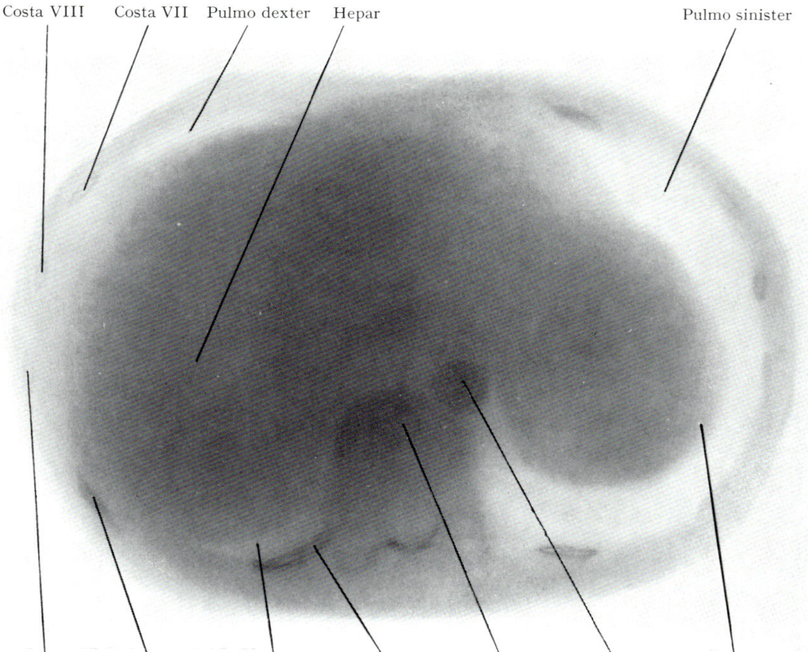

Fig. 269. Interpretation

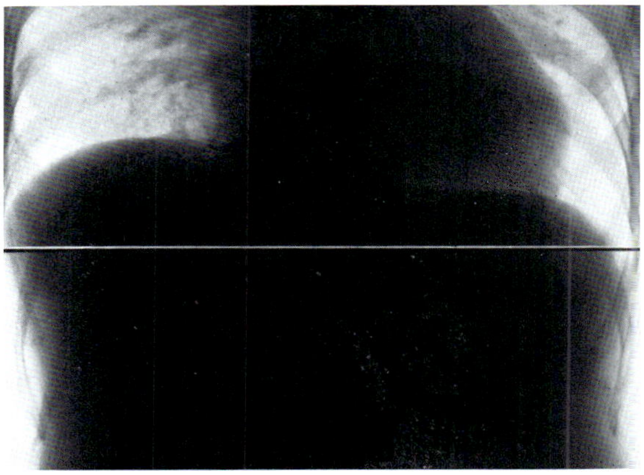

Fig. 270. Normal roentgenogram. Horizontal line showing the level tomographed

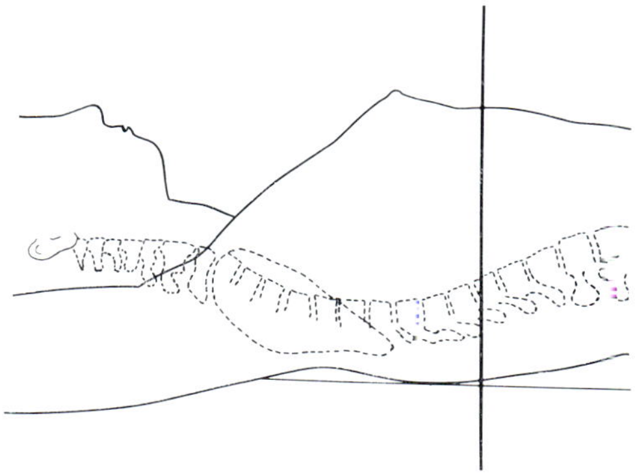

Fig. 271. Schematic drawing of the level tomographed. Subject supine with hands folded behind the head

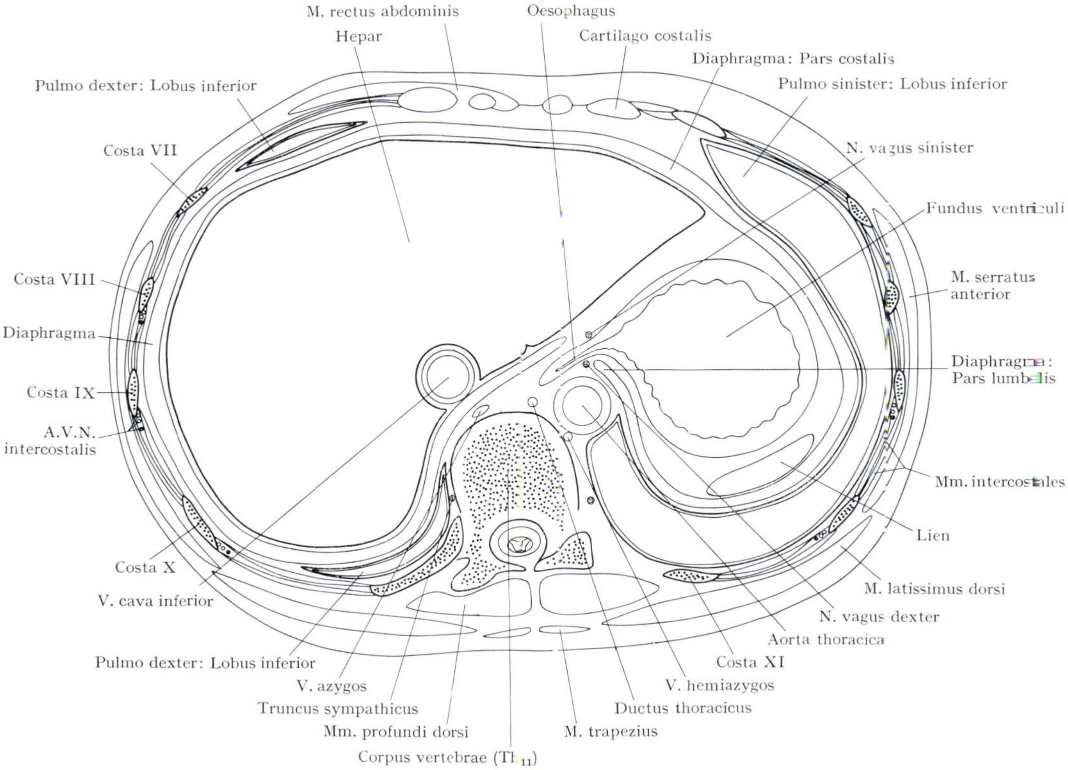

Fig. 272. Anatomical chart

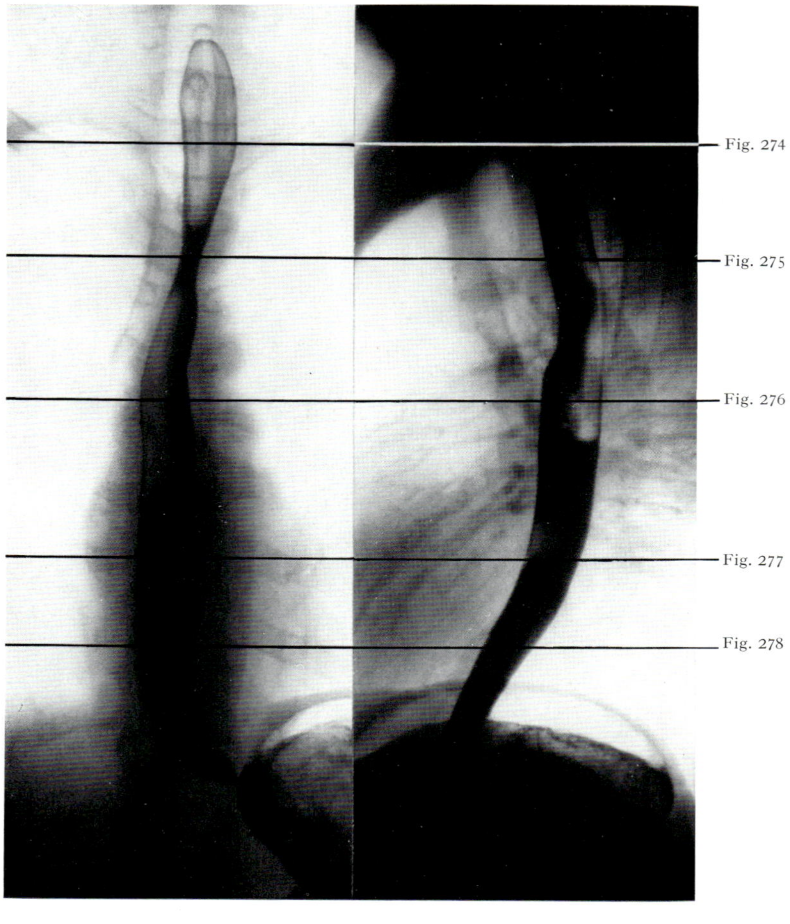

Fig. 273. Normal roentgenograms of the esophagus in the a.p. view and in the lateral view. Horizontal lines showing the level tomographed

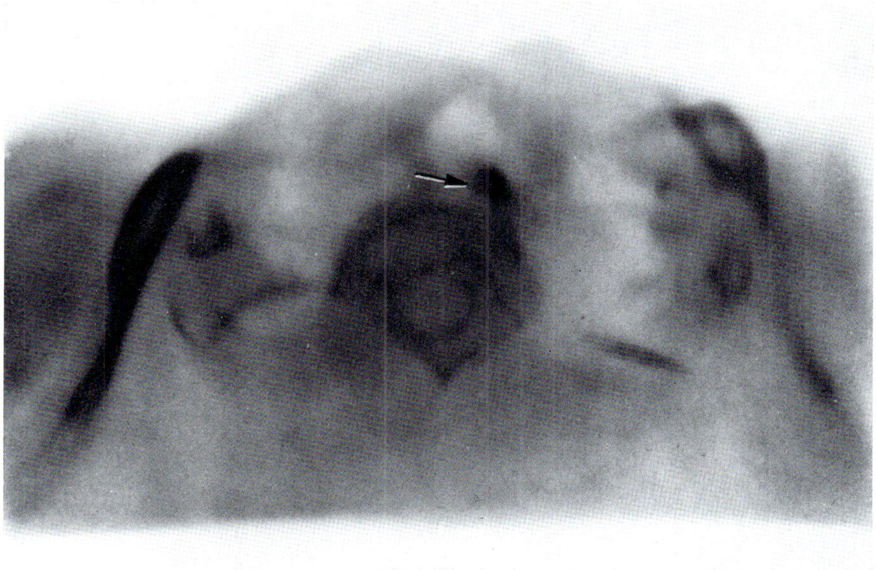

Fig. 274. Axial transverse tomogram of the esophagus (↗) (see Figs. 158—162)

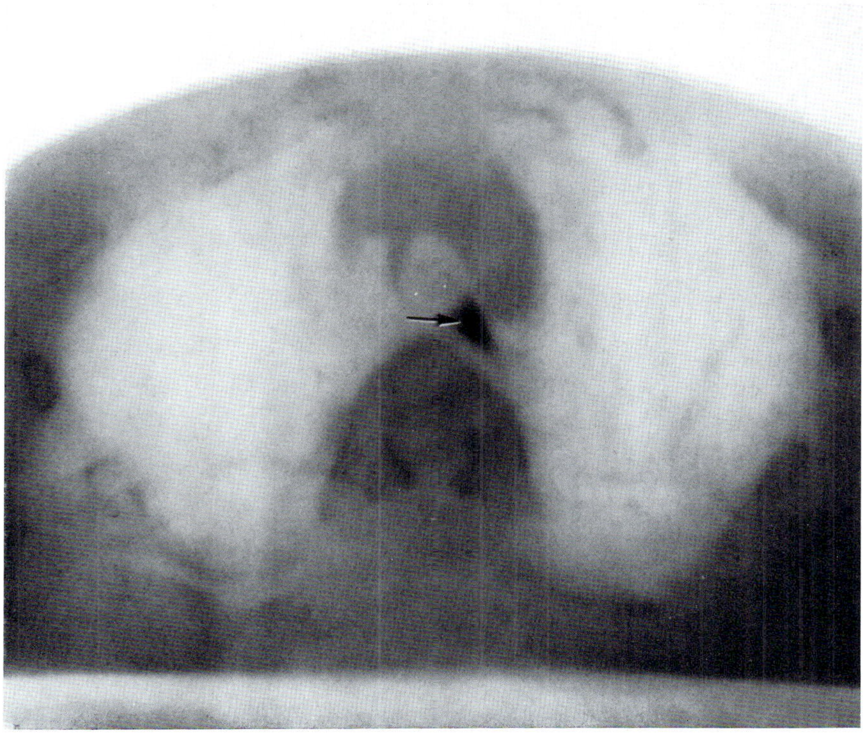

Fig. 275. Axial transverse tomogram of the esophagus (↗) (see Figs. 178—182)

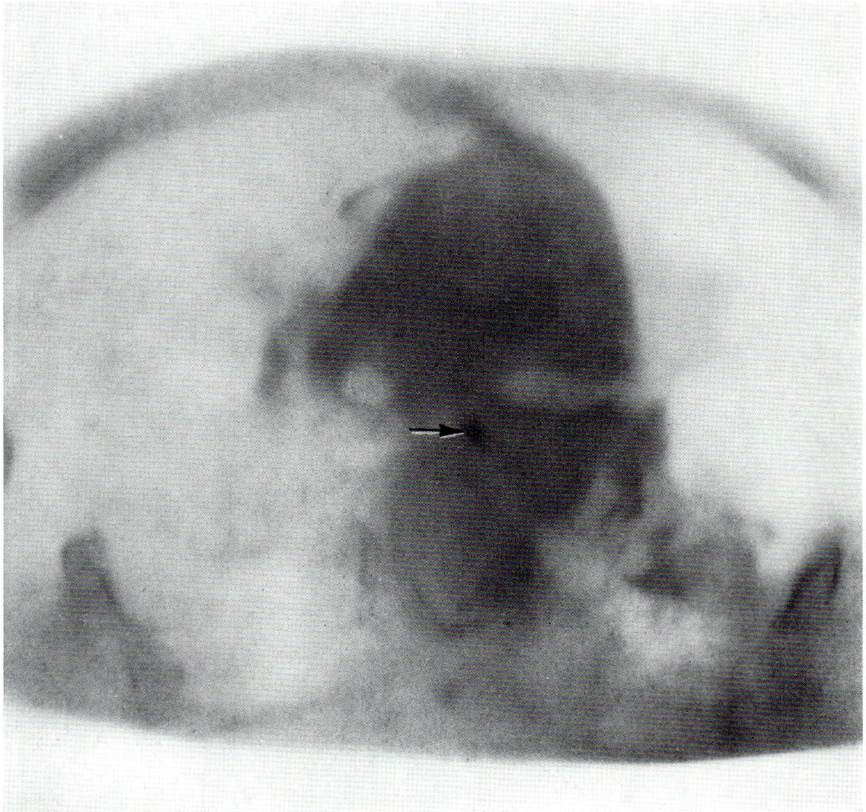

Fig. 276. Axial transverse tomogram of the esophagus (↗) (see Figs. 218—222)

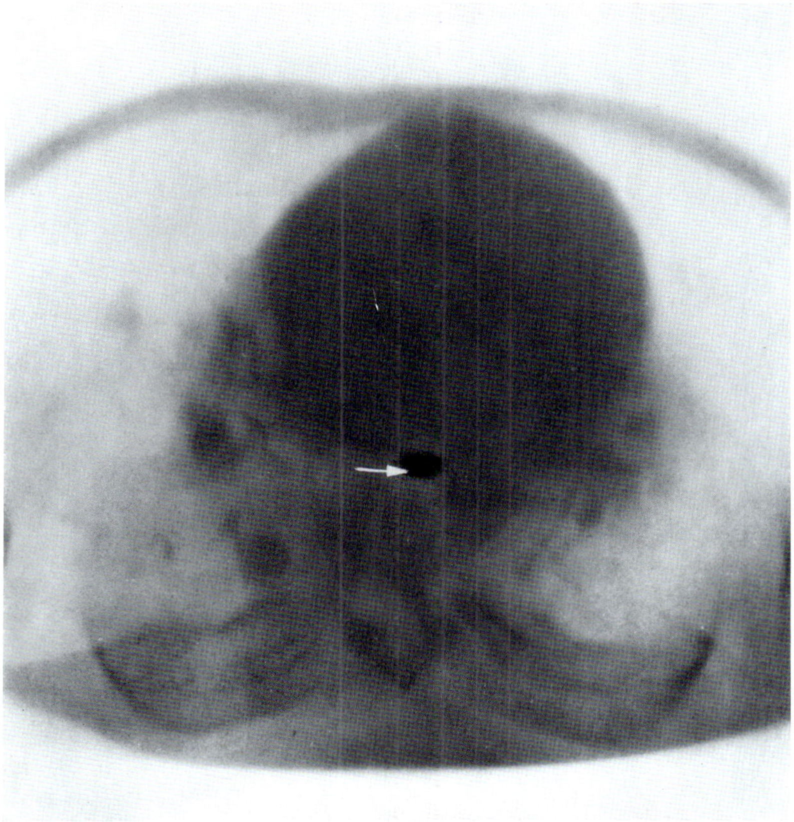

Fig. 277. Axial transverse tomogram of the esophagus (↗) (see Figs. 228—232)

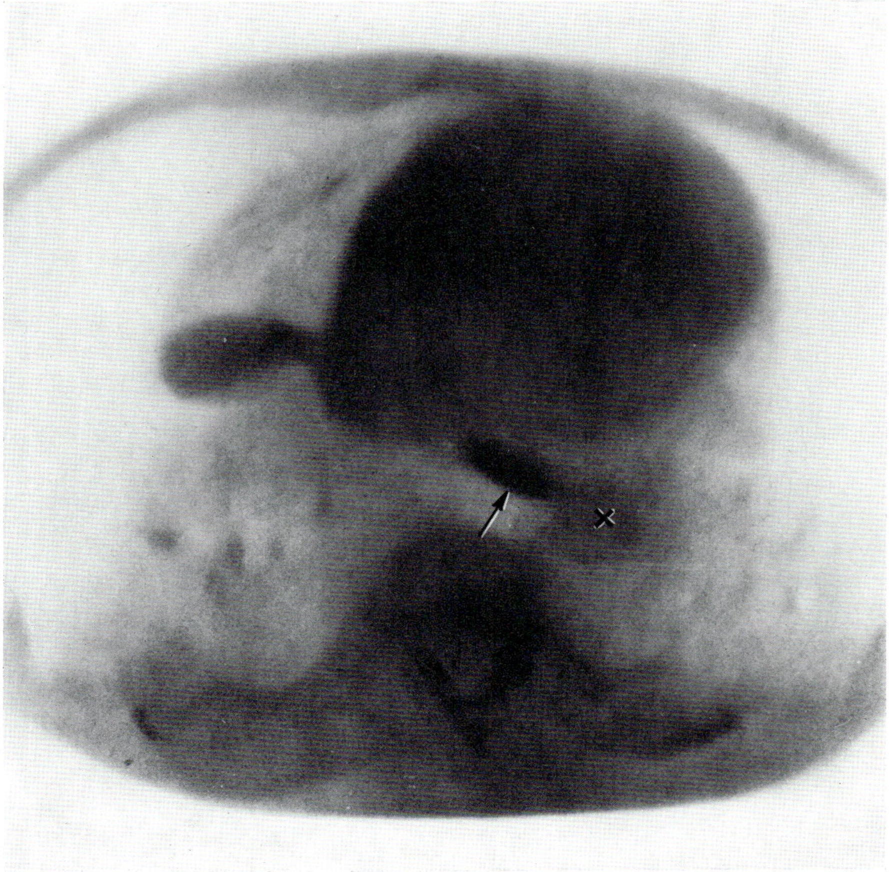

Fig. 278. Axial transverse tomogram of the esophagus (↗) (see Figs. 243—247). Thoracic aorta (×)

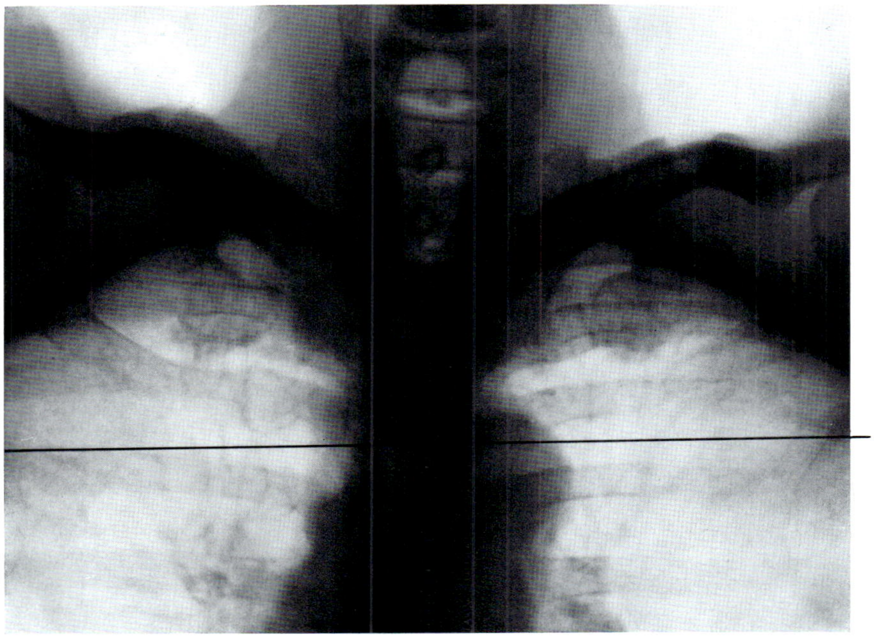

Fig. 279. Normal roentgenogram of the thoracic duct. Horizontal line showing the level tomographed

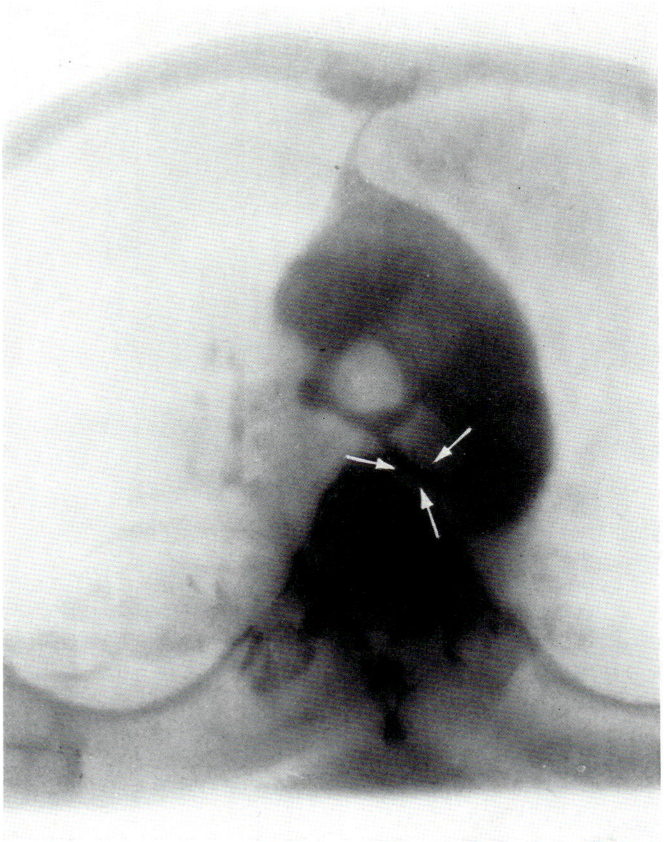

Fig. 280. Axial transverse tomogram of the thoracic duct (↗) (see Figs. 188—192)

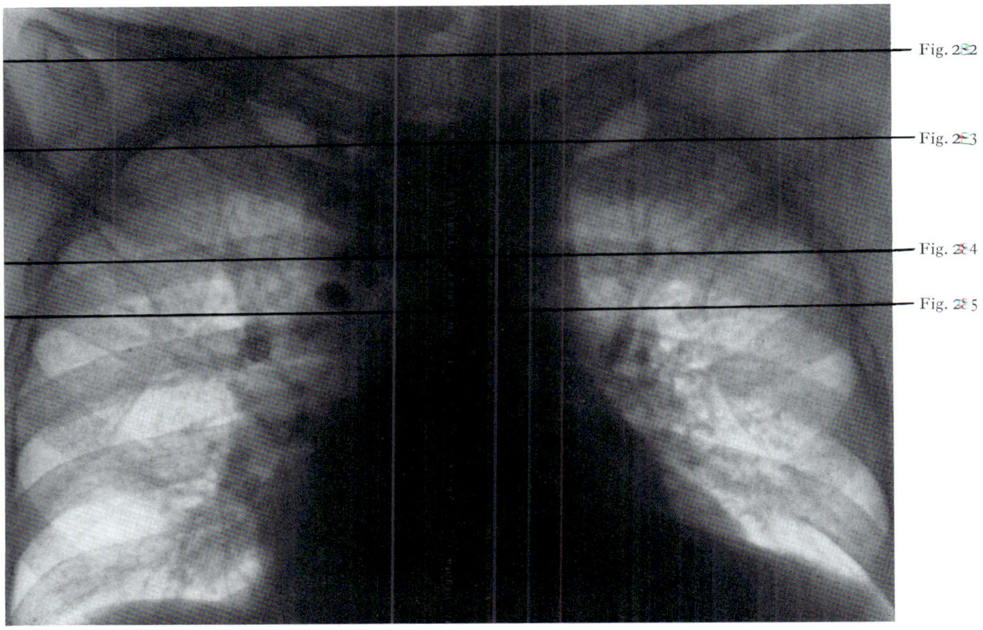

Fig. 281. Normal roentgenogram of the intrathoracic lymph nodes. Horizontal lines showing the level tomographed

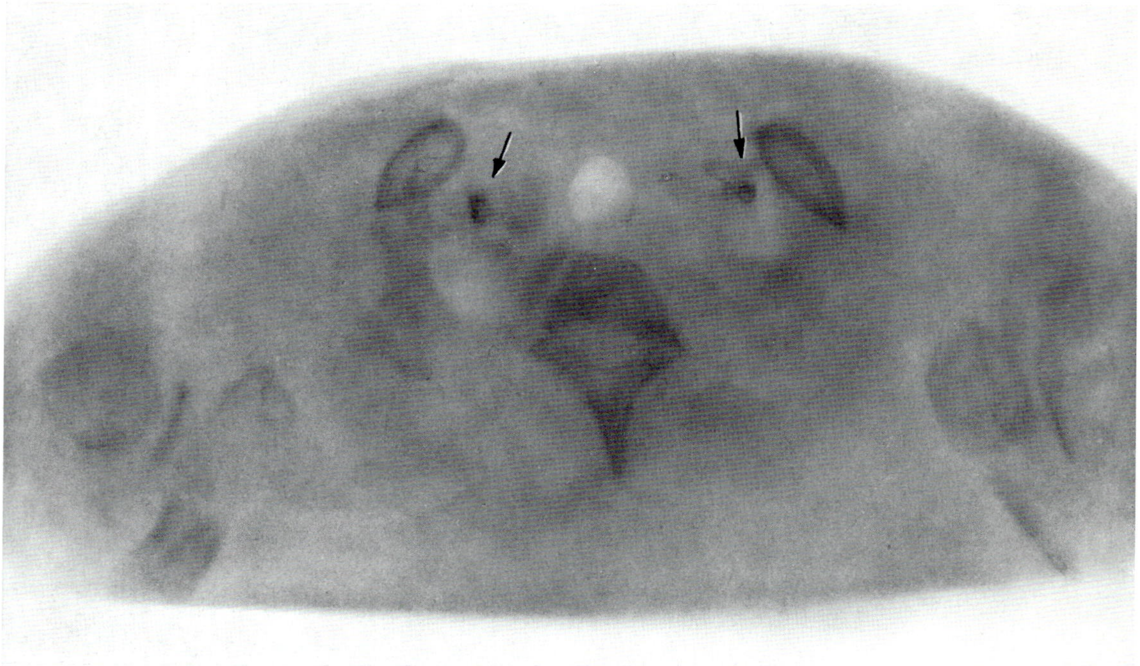

Fig. 282. Axial transverse tomogram of the infraclavicular lymph nodes (↗) (see Figs. 158—162)

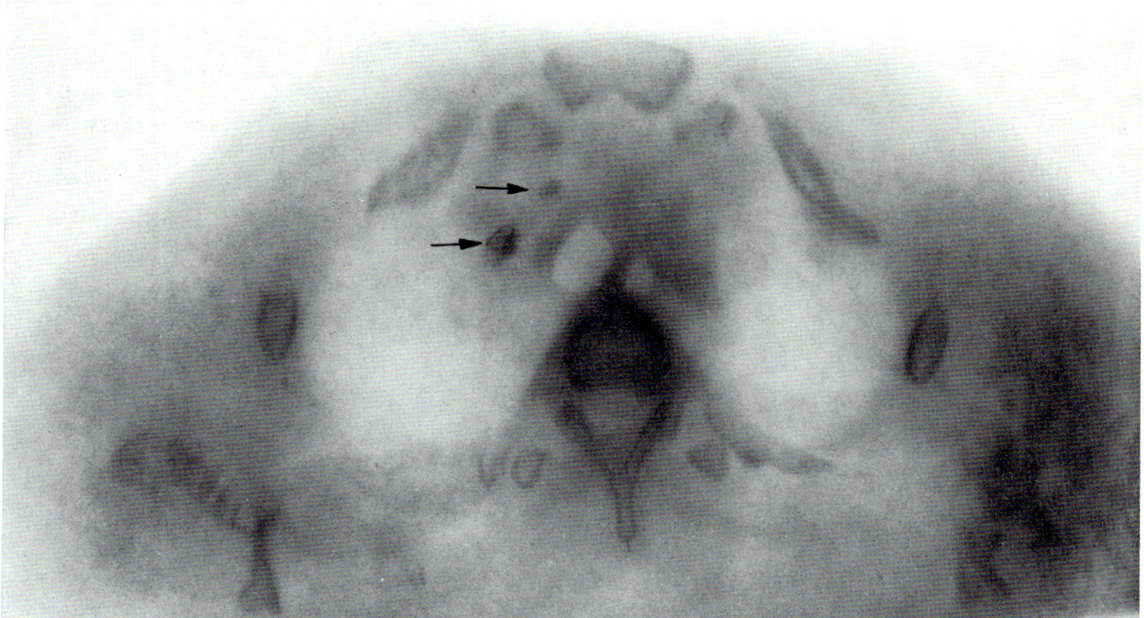

Fig. 283. Axial transverse tomogram of the tracheal lymph nodes (↗) (see Figs. 173—177)

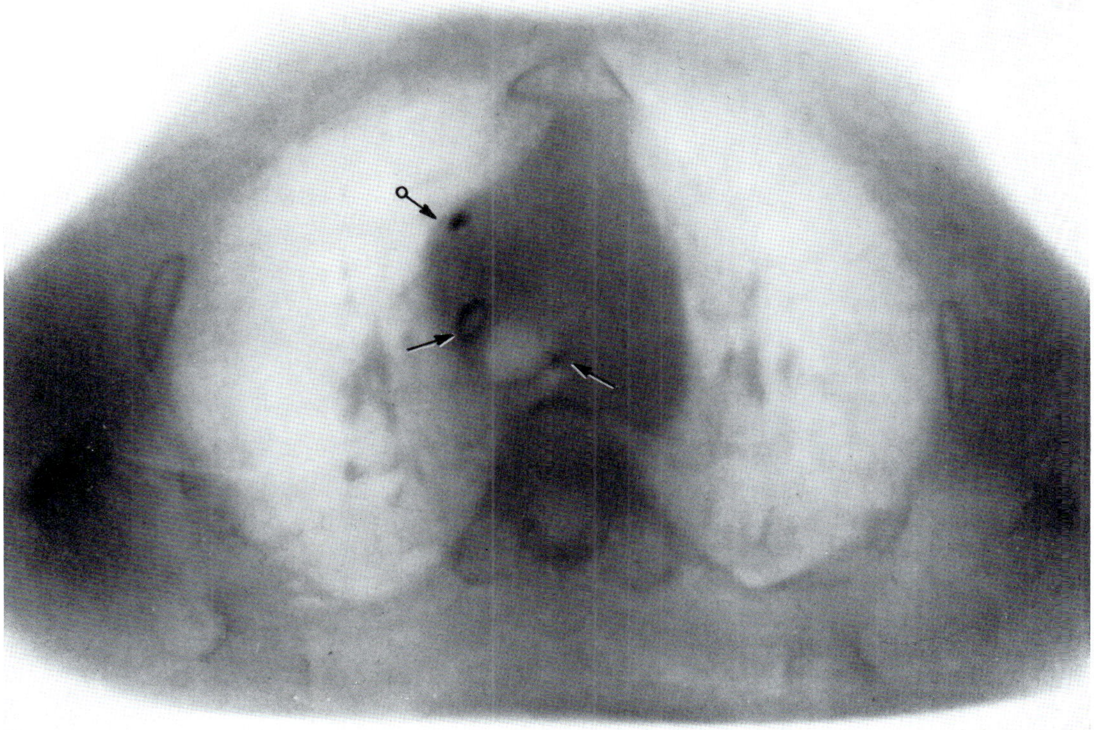

Fig. 284. Axial transverse tomogram of the tracheal lymph nodes (↗) and anterior mediastinal lymph nodes (o↗) (see Figs. 193—222)

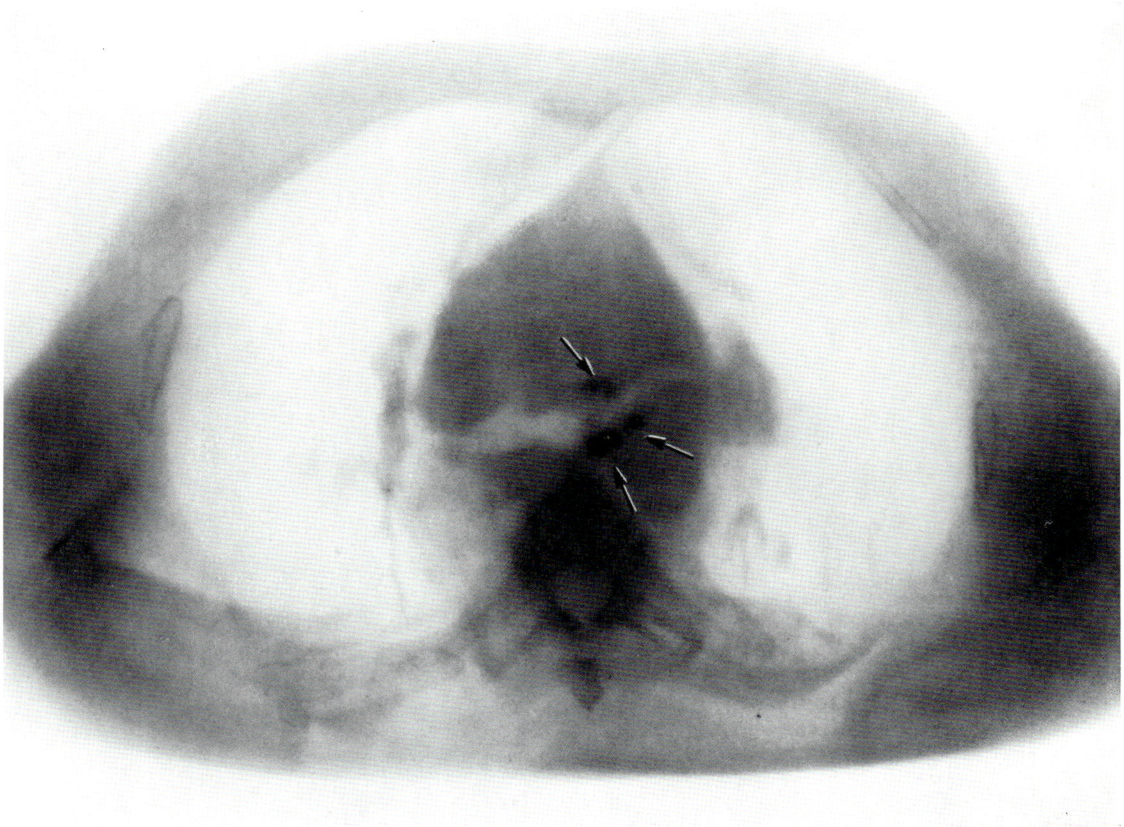

Fig. 285. Axial transverse tomogram of the superior tracheobronchial lymph nodes (↗) (see Figs. 213—217)

Upper Abdomen

Seventeen axial transverse tomograms of the subject with air insufflated into the retroperitoneal space.

Appendices:

1. Axial transverse tomograms of the duodenal loop with duodenal tube introduced.
2. Axial transverse tomogram of the stomach, the duodenum, the gall bladder and the renal pelvis.

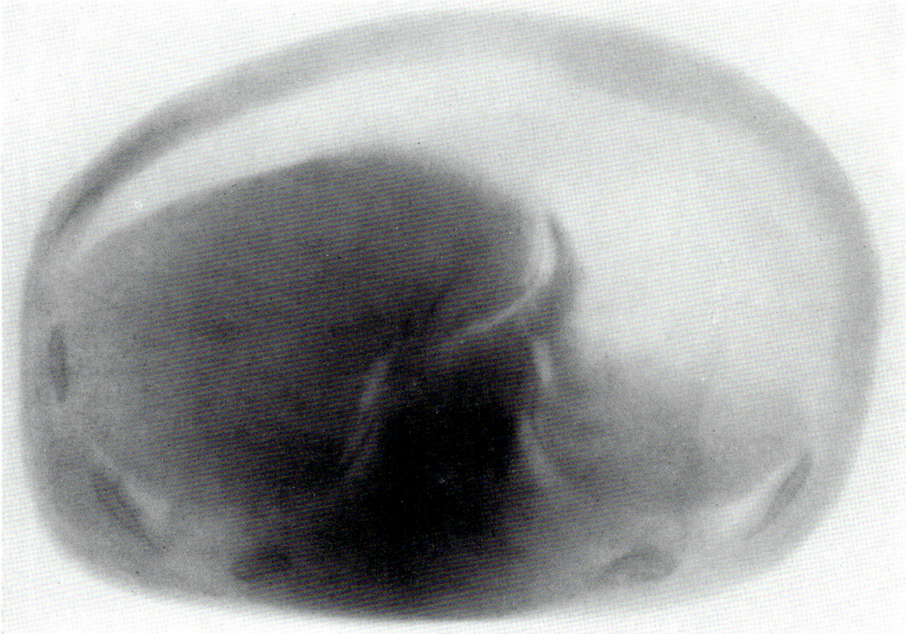

Fig. 286. Axial transverse tomogram

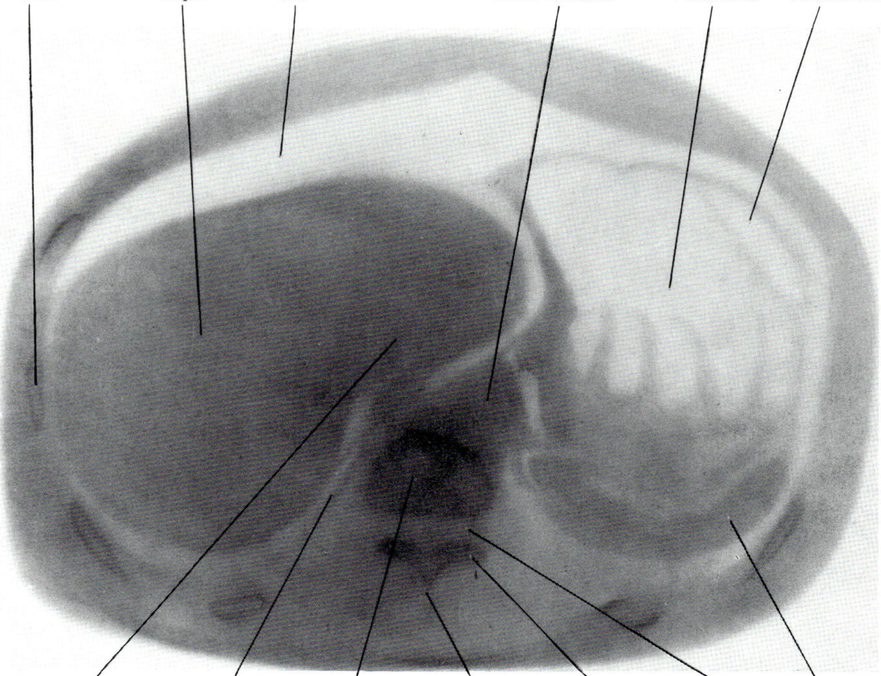

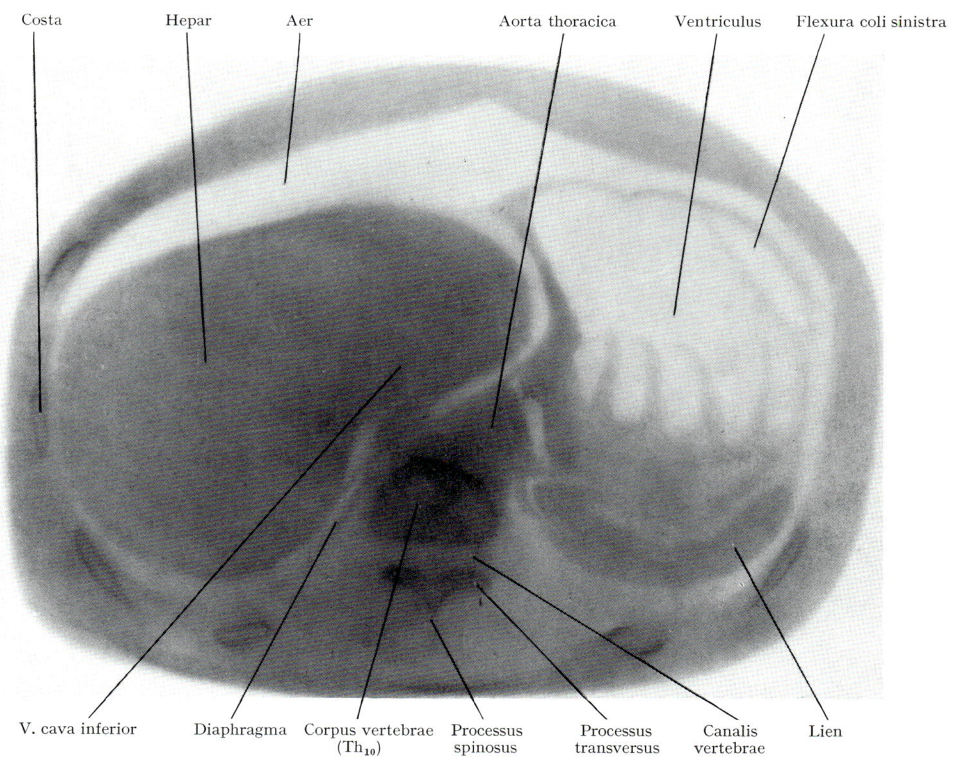

Fig. 287. Interpretation

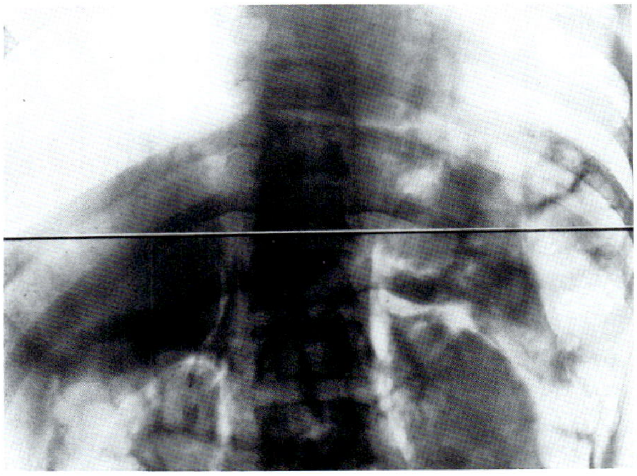

Fig. 288. Normal roentgenogram. Horizontal line showing the level tomographed

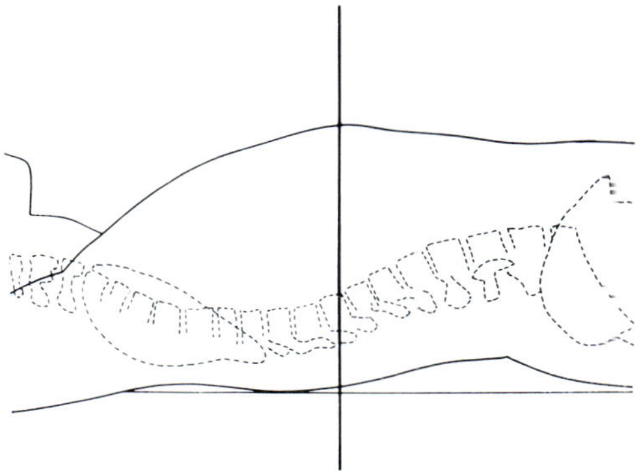

Fig. 289. Schematic drawing of the level tomographed

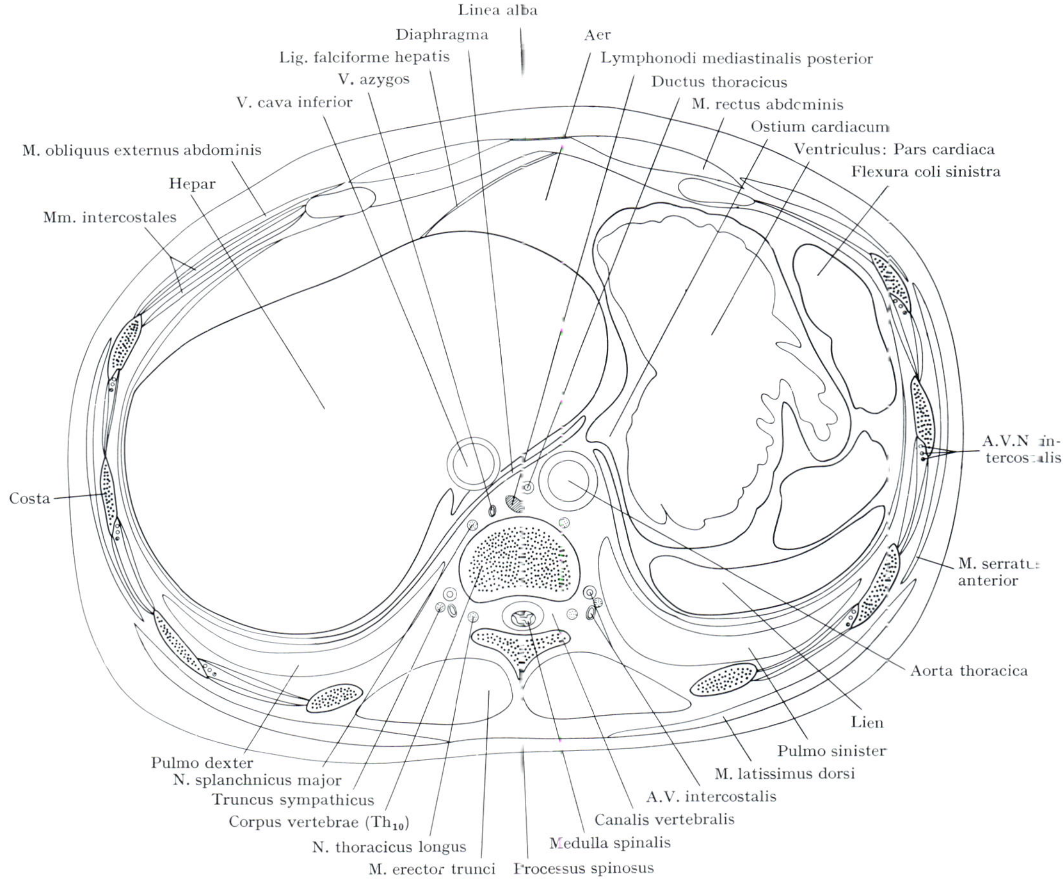

Fig. 290. Anatomical chart

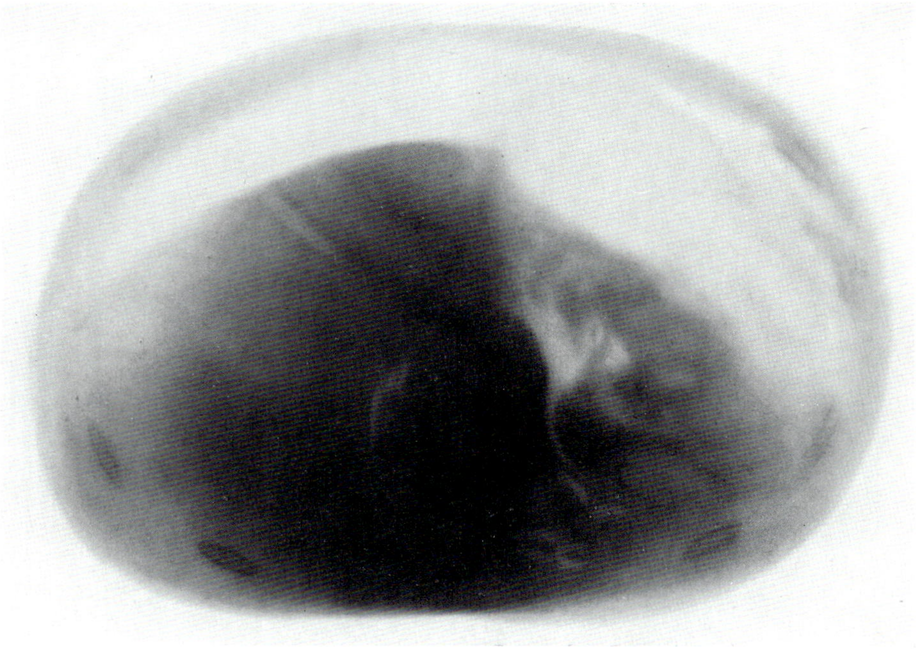

Fig. 291. Axial transverse tomogram

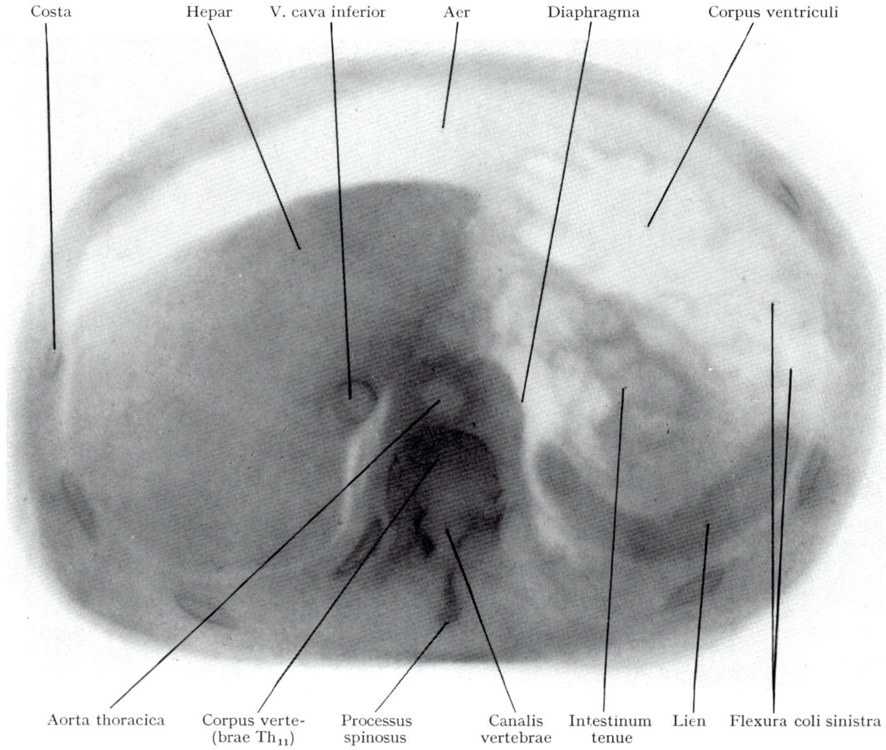

Fig. 292. Interpretation

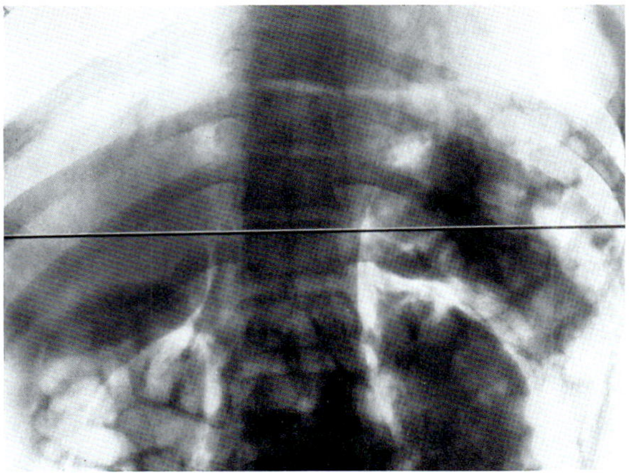

Fig. 293. Normal roentgenogram. Horizontal line showing the level tomographed

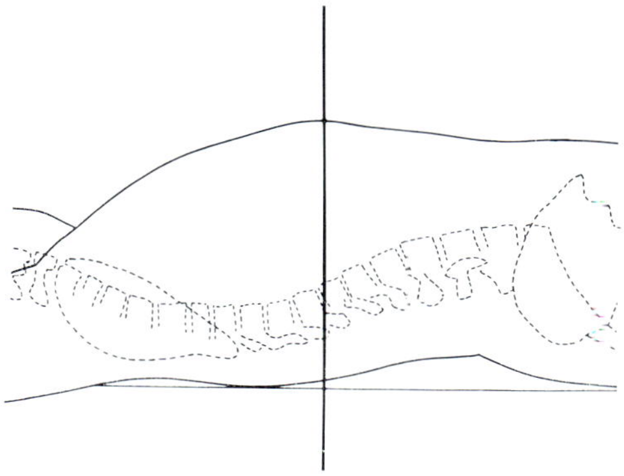

Fig. 294. Schematic drawing of the level tomographed

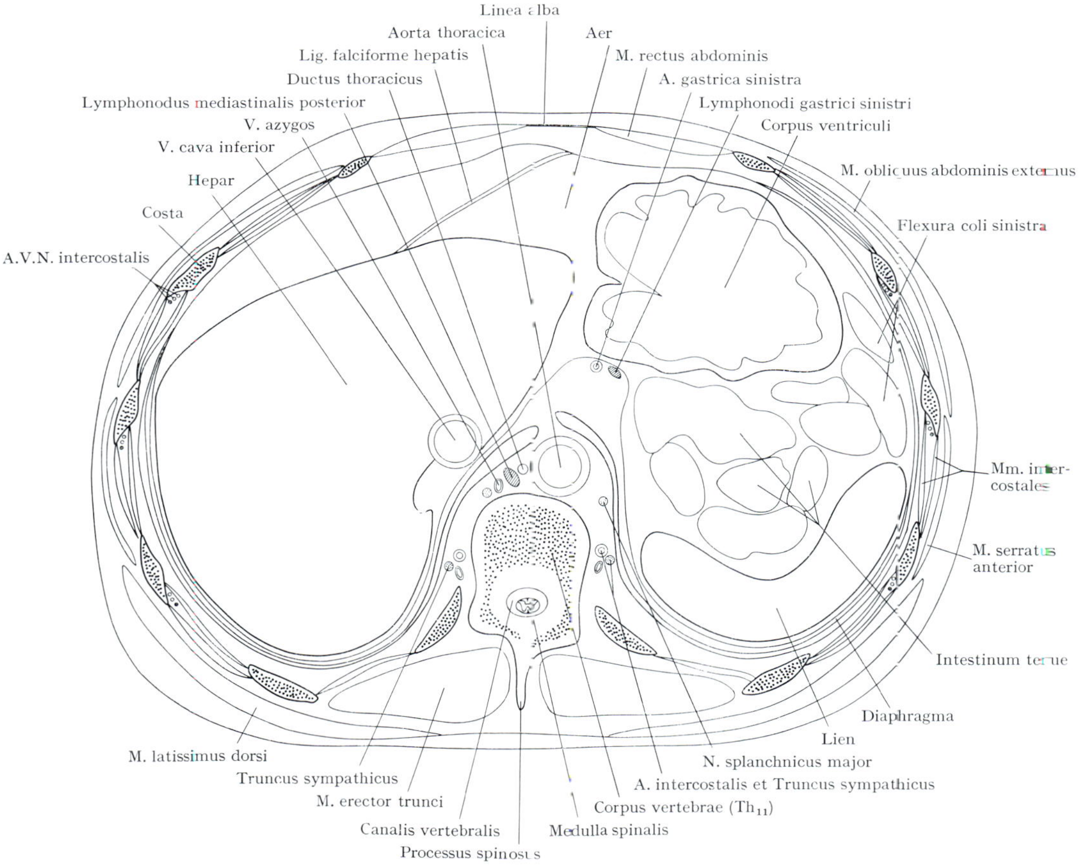

Fig. 295. Anatomical chart

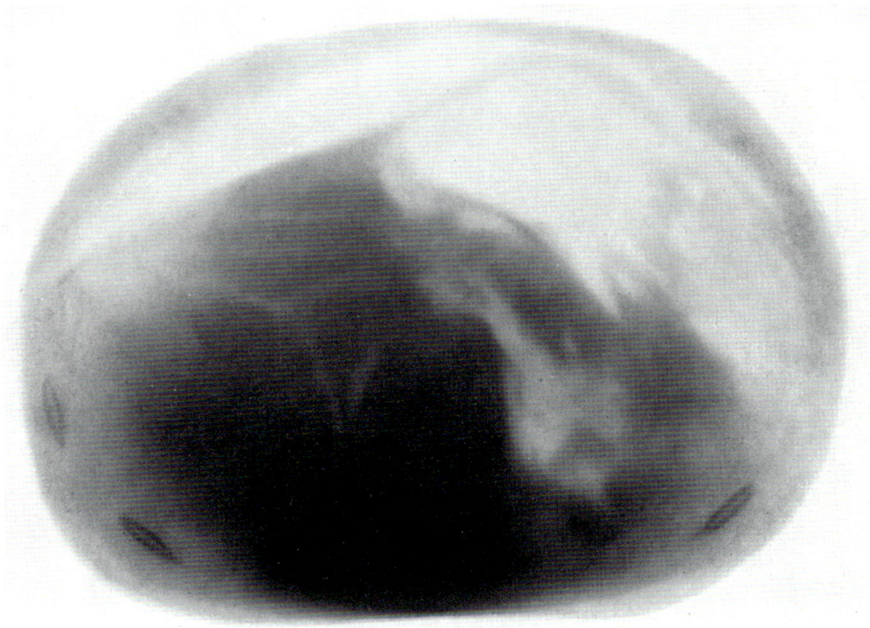

Fig. 296. Axial transverse tomogram

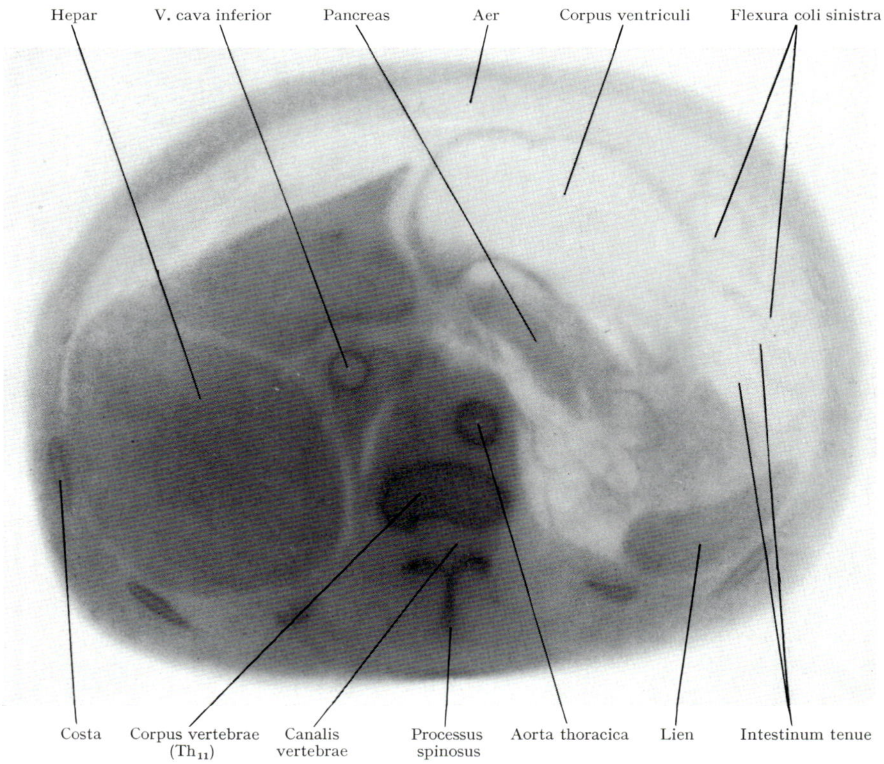

Fig. 297. Interpretation

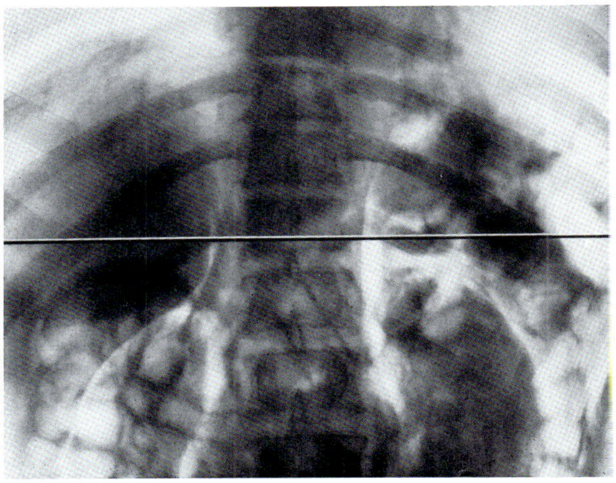

Fig. 298. Normal roentgenogram. Horizontal line showing the level tomographed

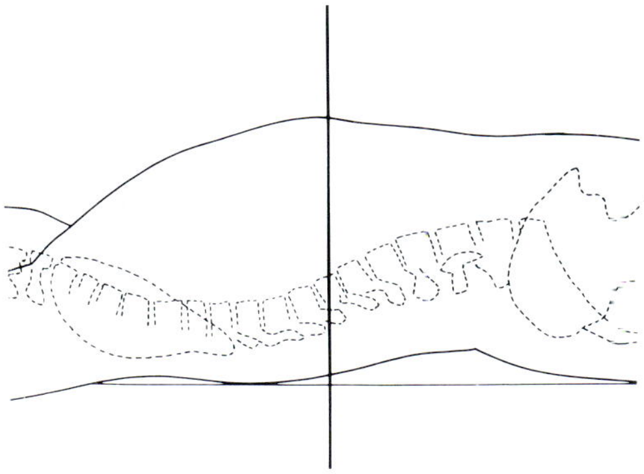

Fig. 299. Schematic drawing of the level tomographed

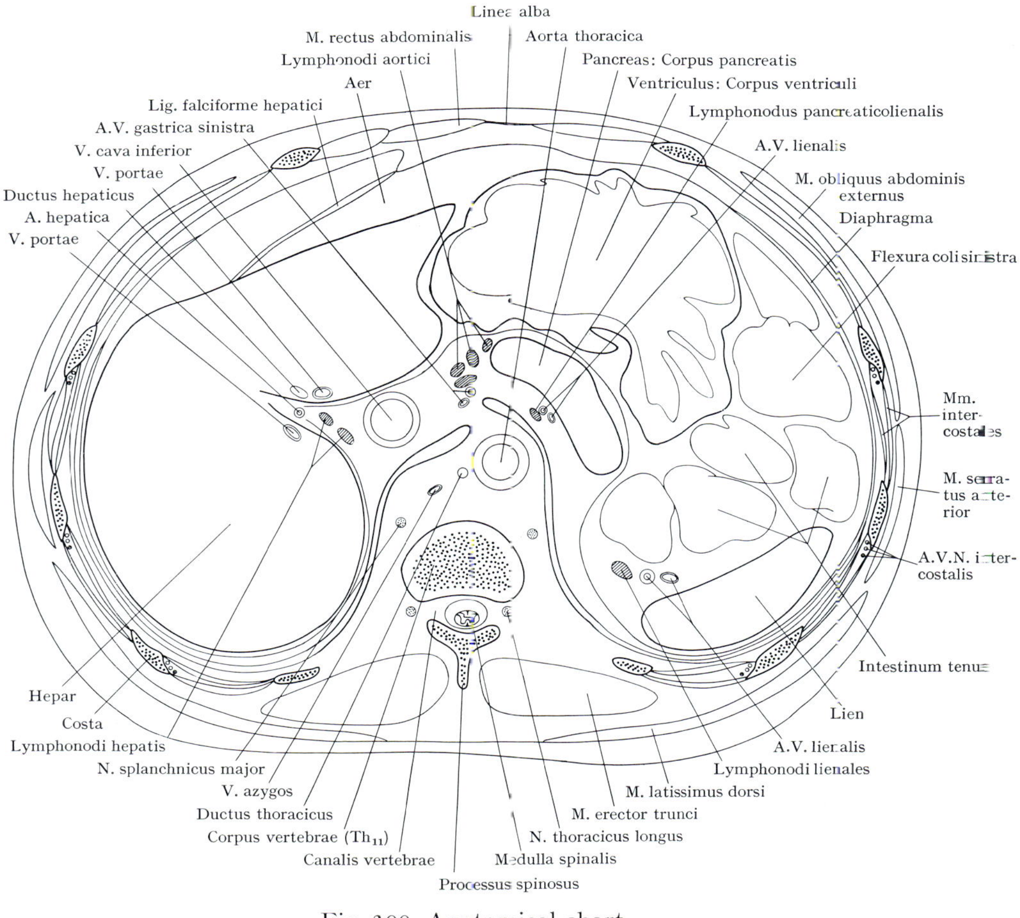

Fig. 300. Anatomical chart

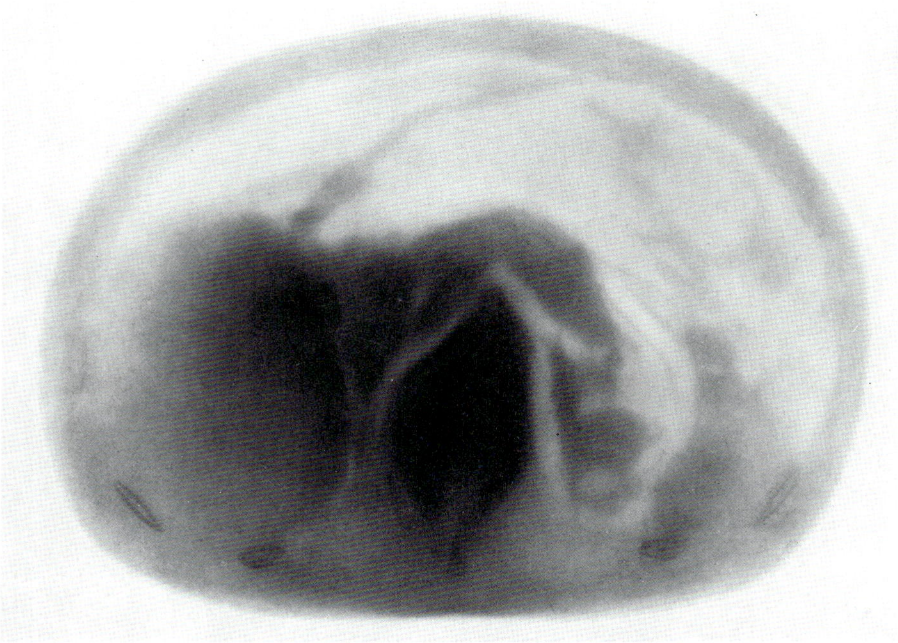

Fig. 301. Axial transverse tomogram

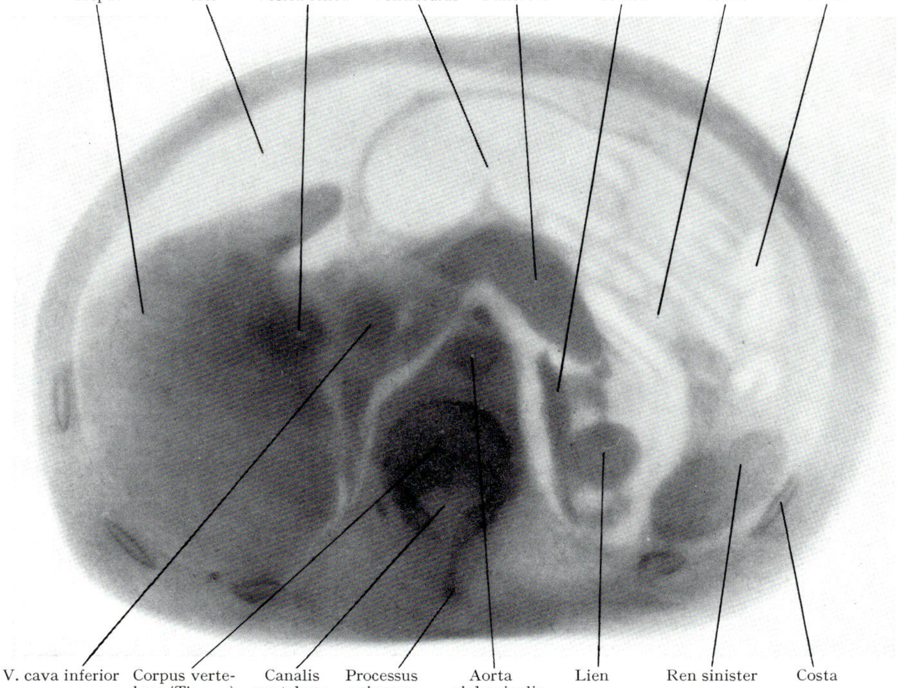

Fig. 302. Interpretation

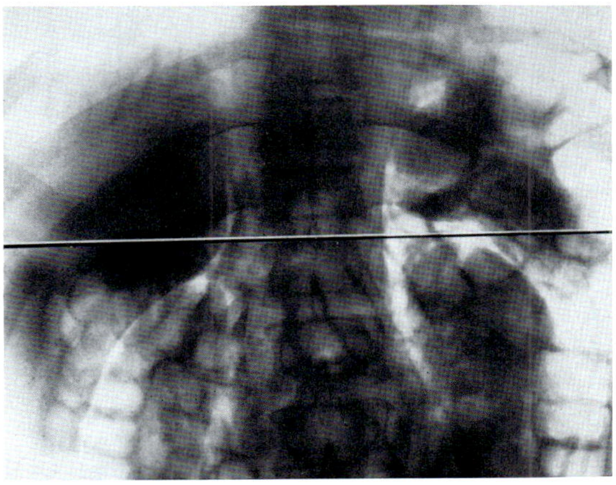

Fig. 303. Normal roentgenogram. Horizontal line showing the level tomographed

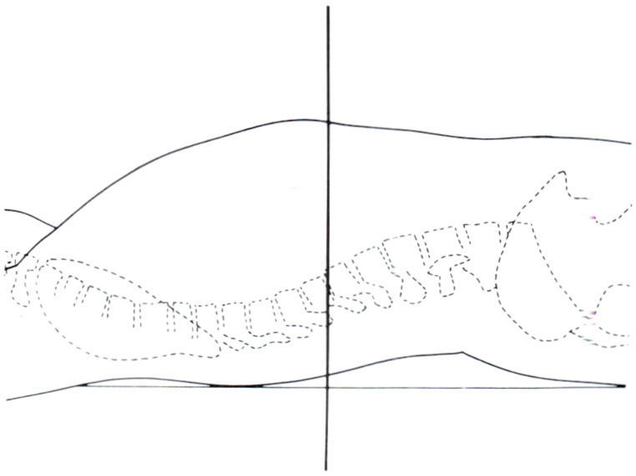

Fig. 304. Schematic drawing of the level tomographed

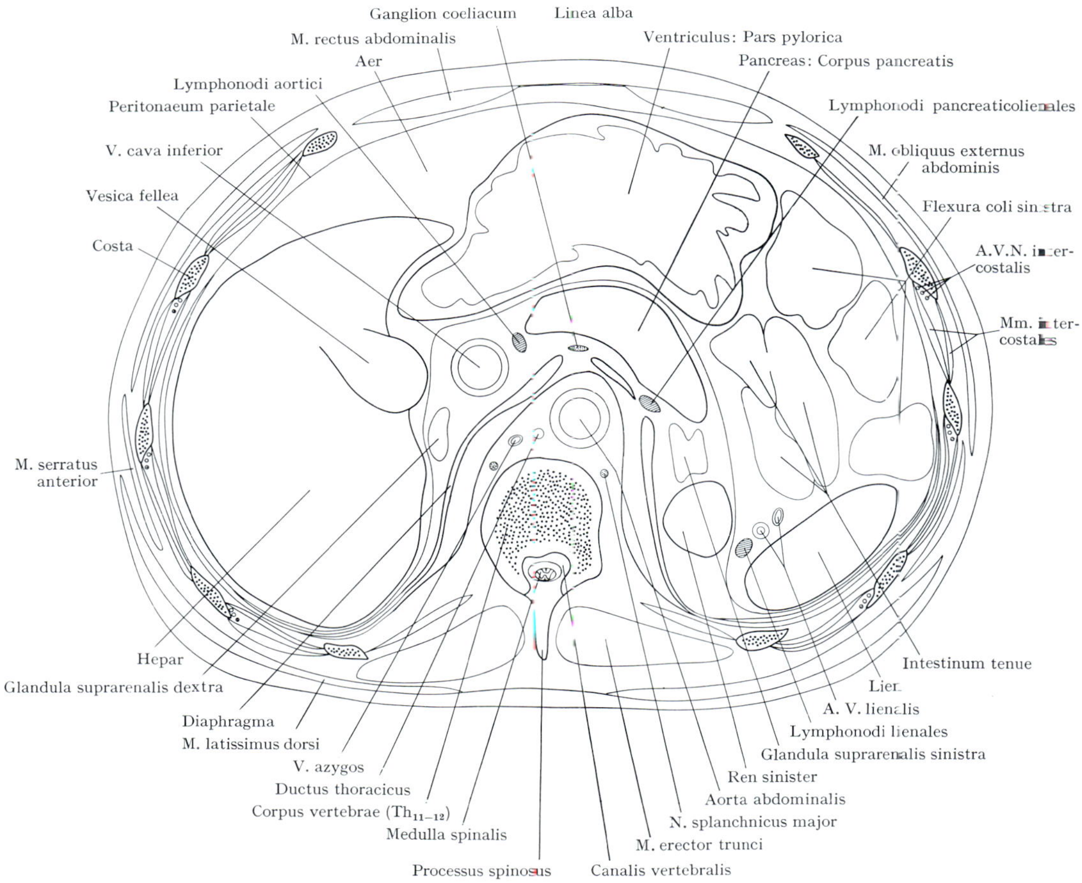

Fig. 305. Anatomical chart

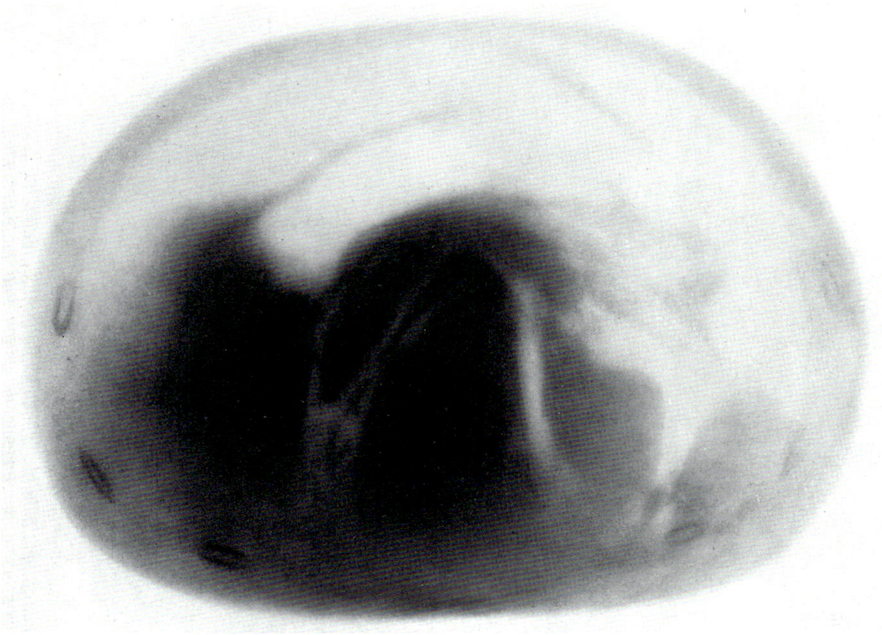

Fig. 306. Axial transverse tomogram

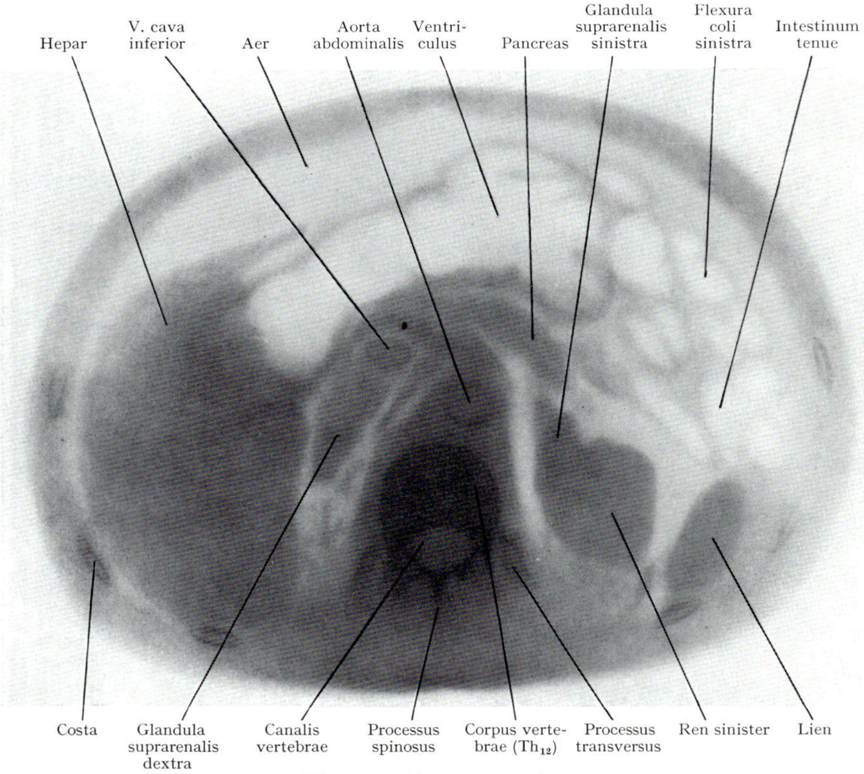

Fig. 307. Interpretation

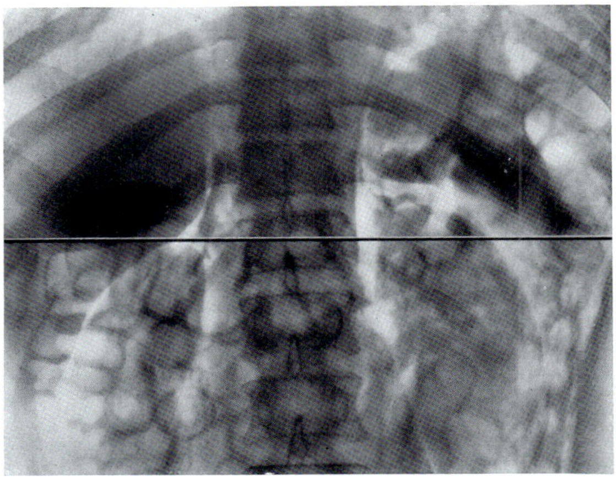

Fig. 308. Normal roentgenogram. Horizontal line showing the level tomographed

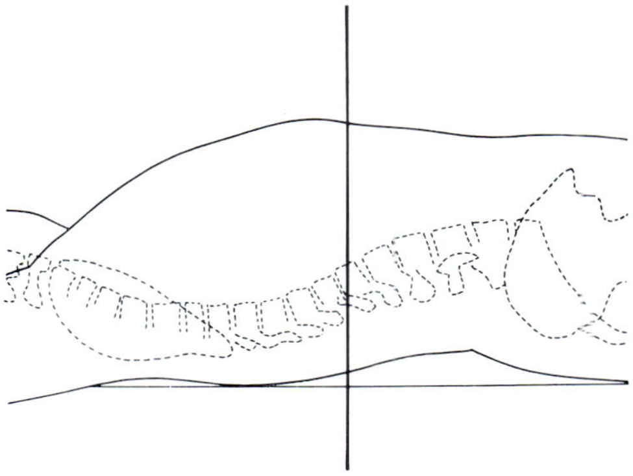

Fig. 309. Schematic drawing of the level tomographed

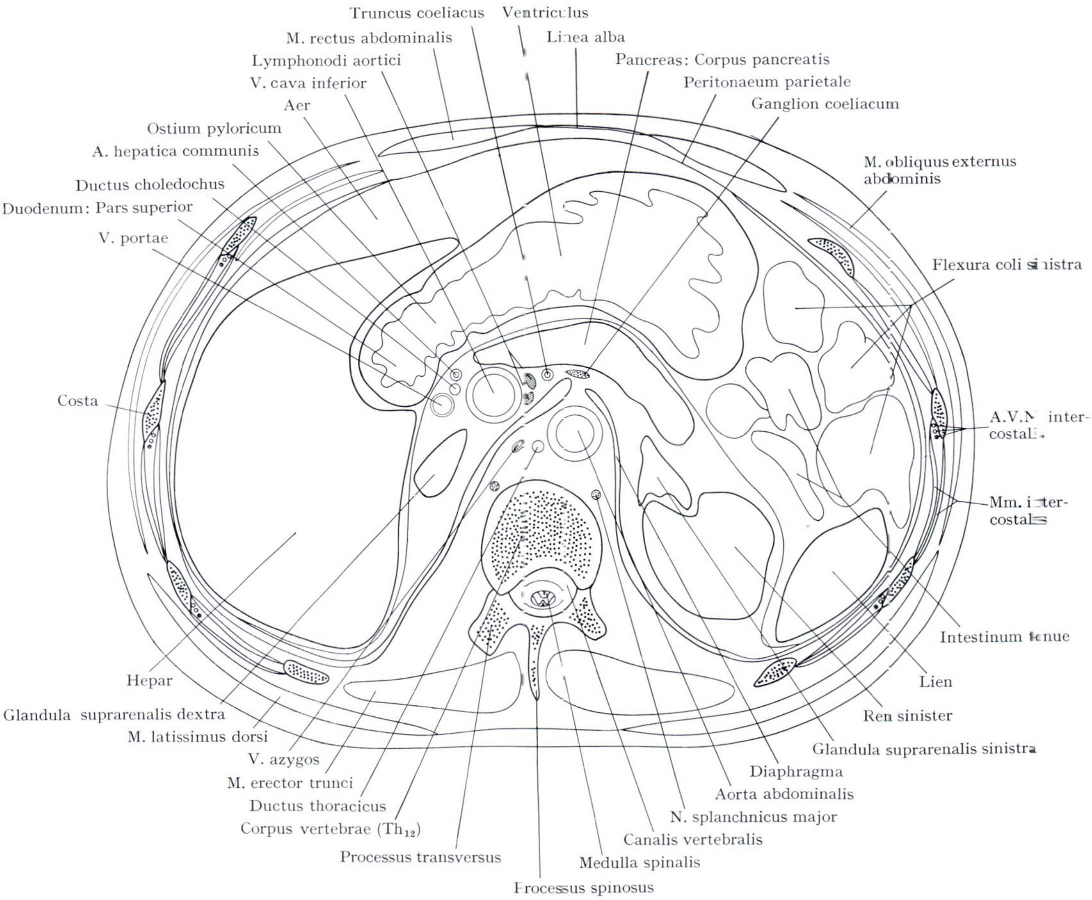

Fig. 310. Anatomical chart

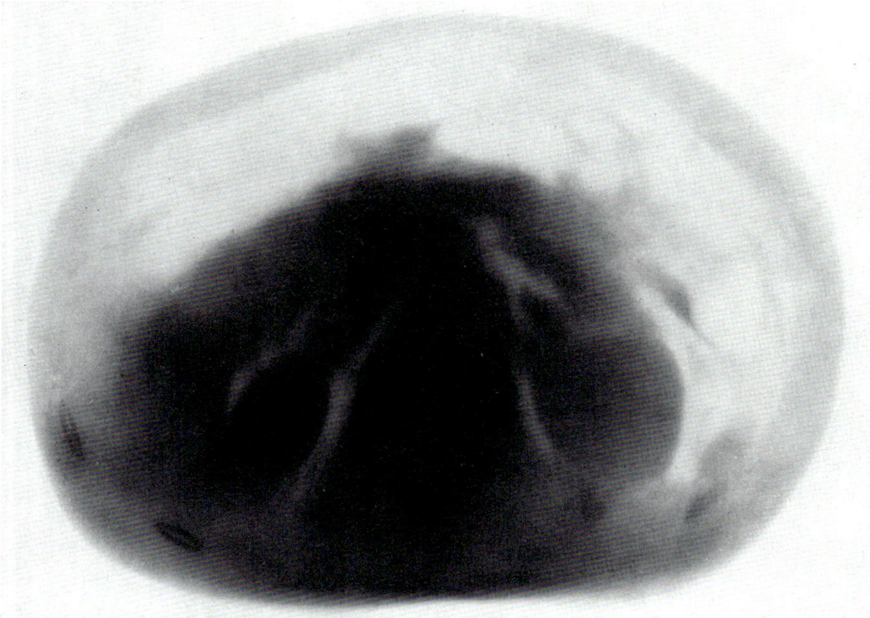

Fig. 311. Axial transverse tomogram

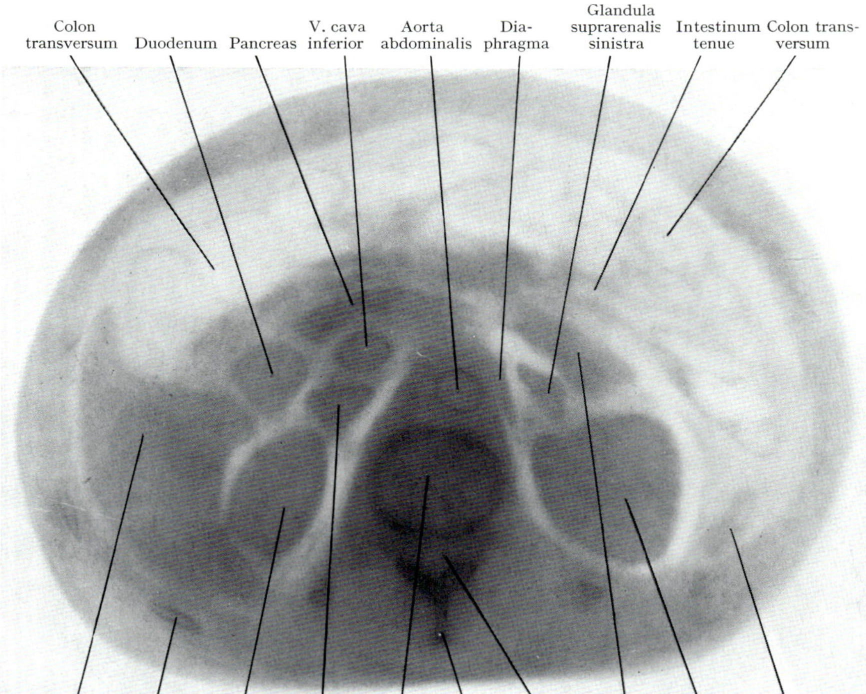

Fig. 312. Interpretation

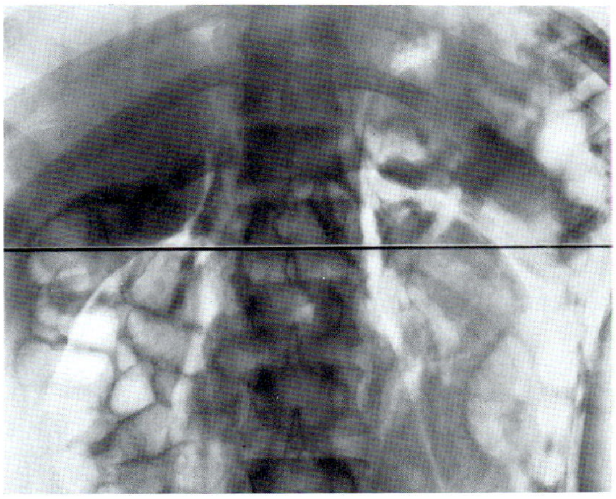

Fig. 313. Normal roentgenogram. Horizontal line showing the level tomographed

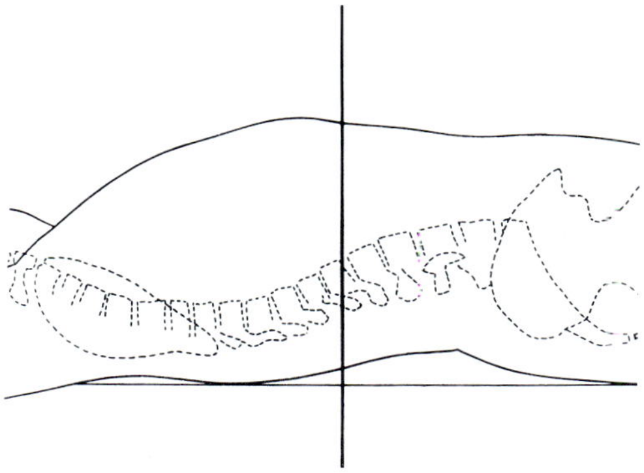

Fig. 314. Schematic drawing of the level tomographed

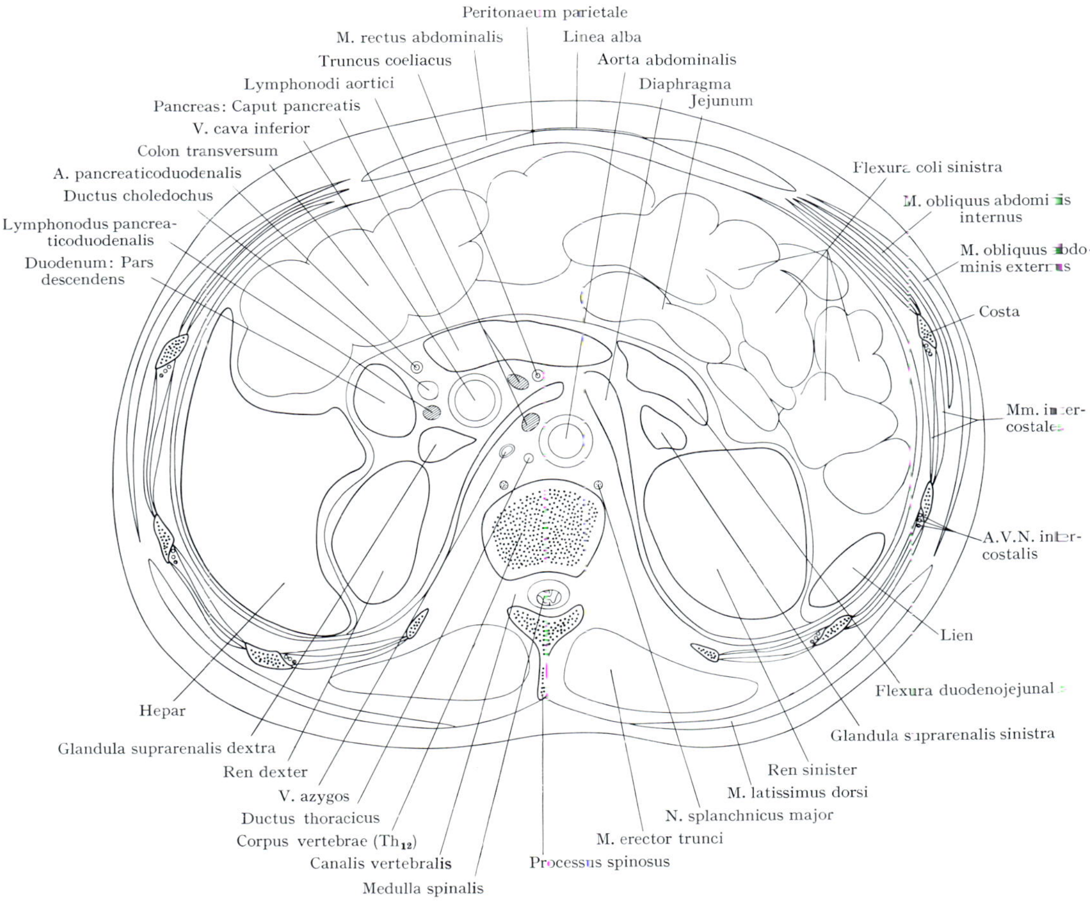

Fig. 315. Anatomical chart

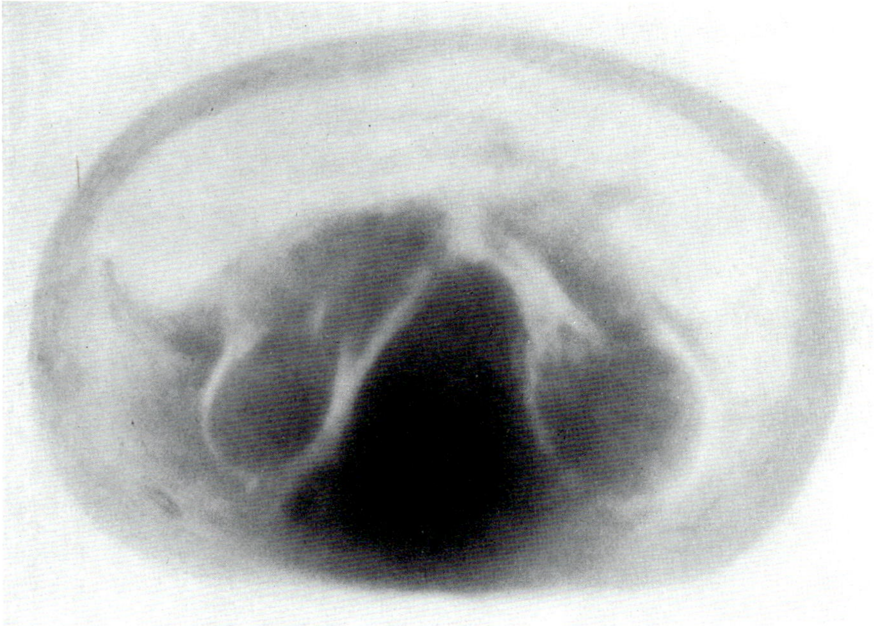

Fig. 316. Axial transverse tomogram

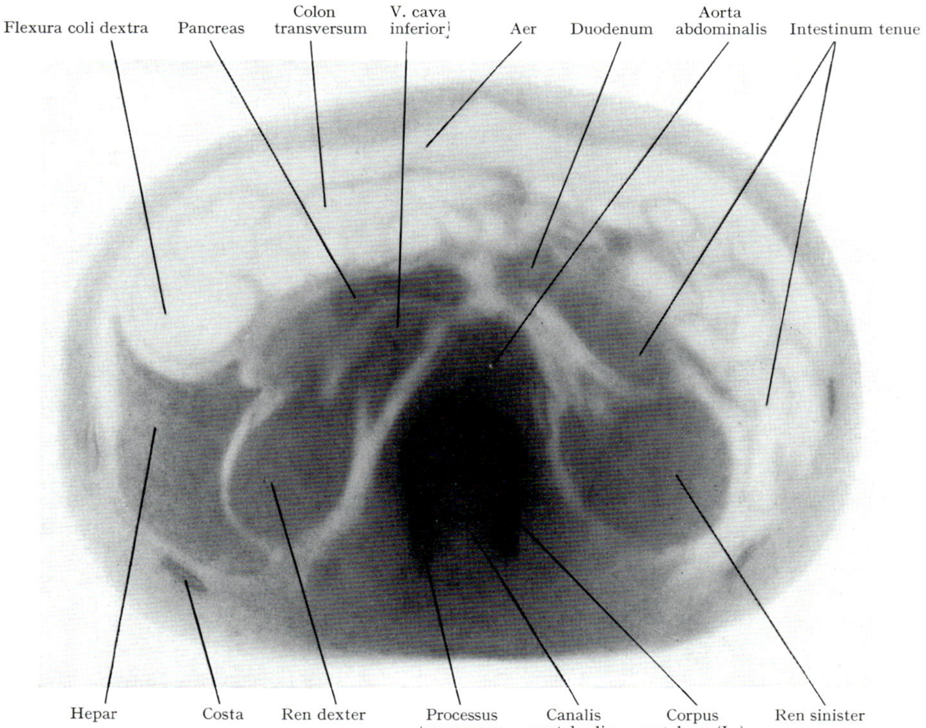

Fig. 317. Interpretation

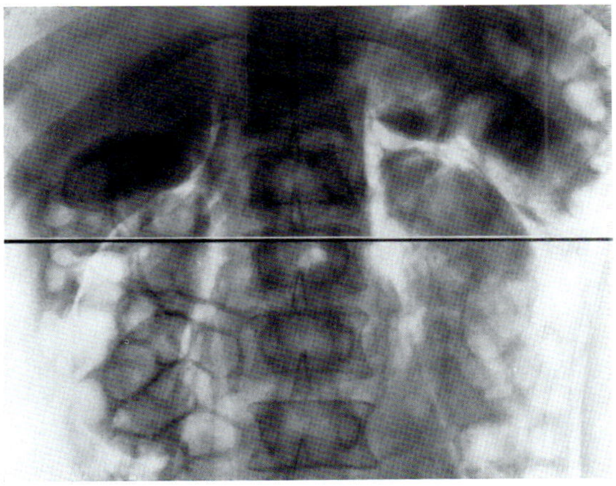

Fig. 318. Normal roentgenogram. Horizontal line showing the level tomographed

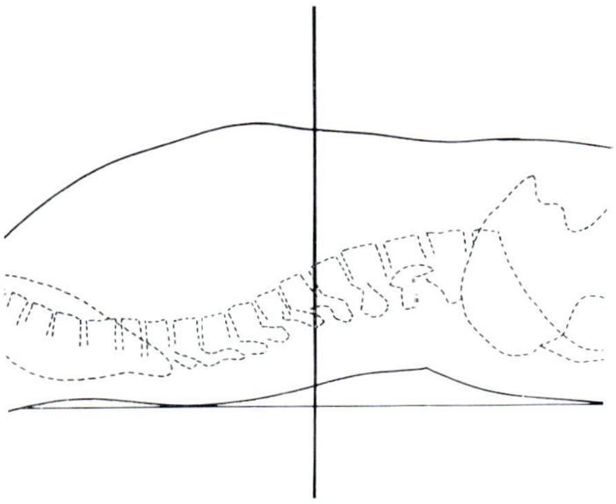

Fig. 319. Schematic drawing of the level tomographed

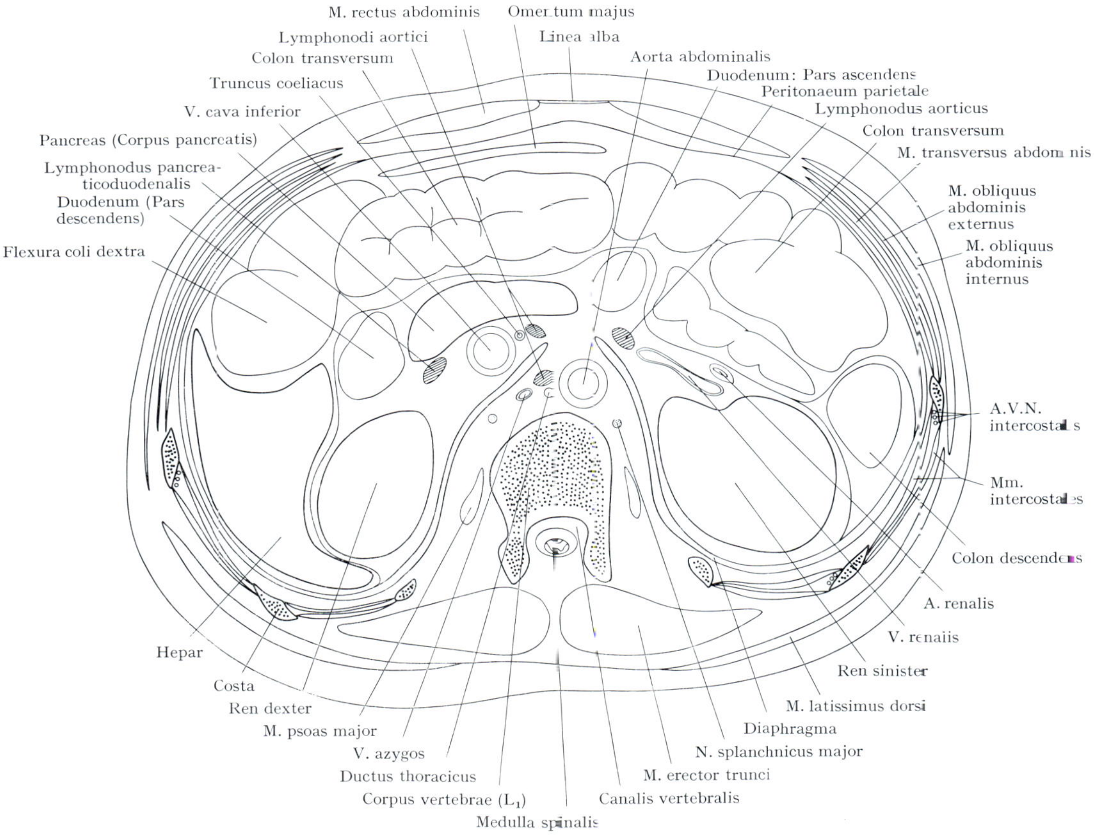

Fig. 320. Anatomical chart

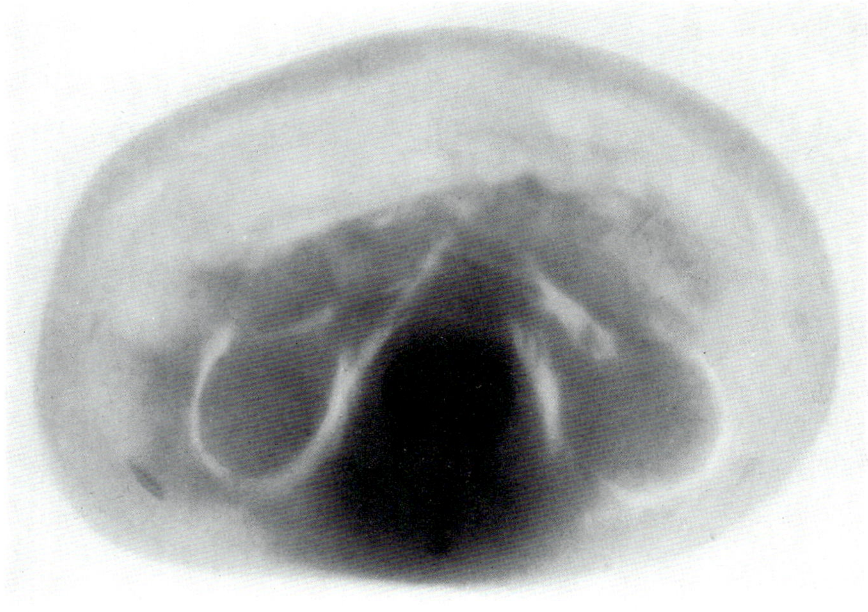

Fig. 321. Axial transverse tomogram

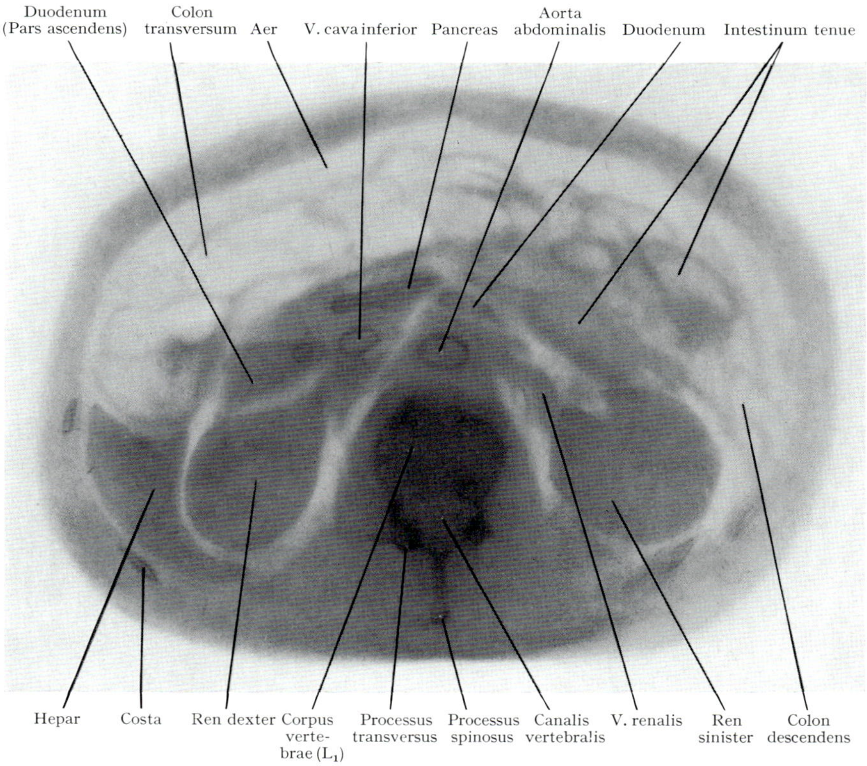

Fig. 322. Interpretation

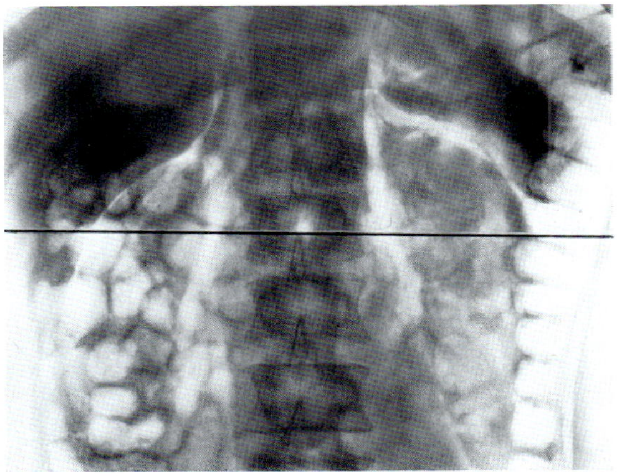

Fig. 323. Normal roentgenogram. Horizontal line showing the level tomographed

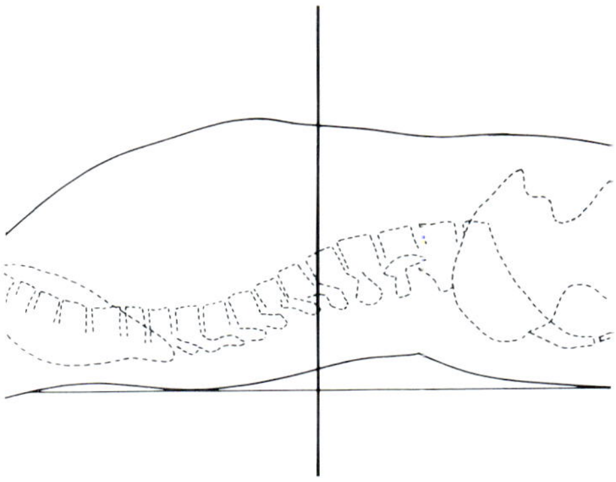

Fig. 324. Schematic drawing of the level tomographed

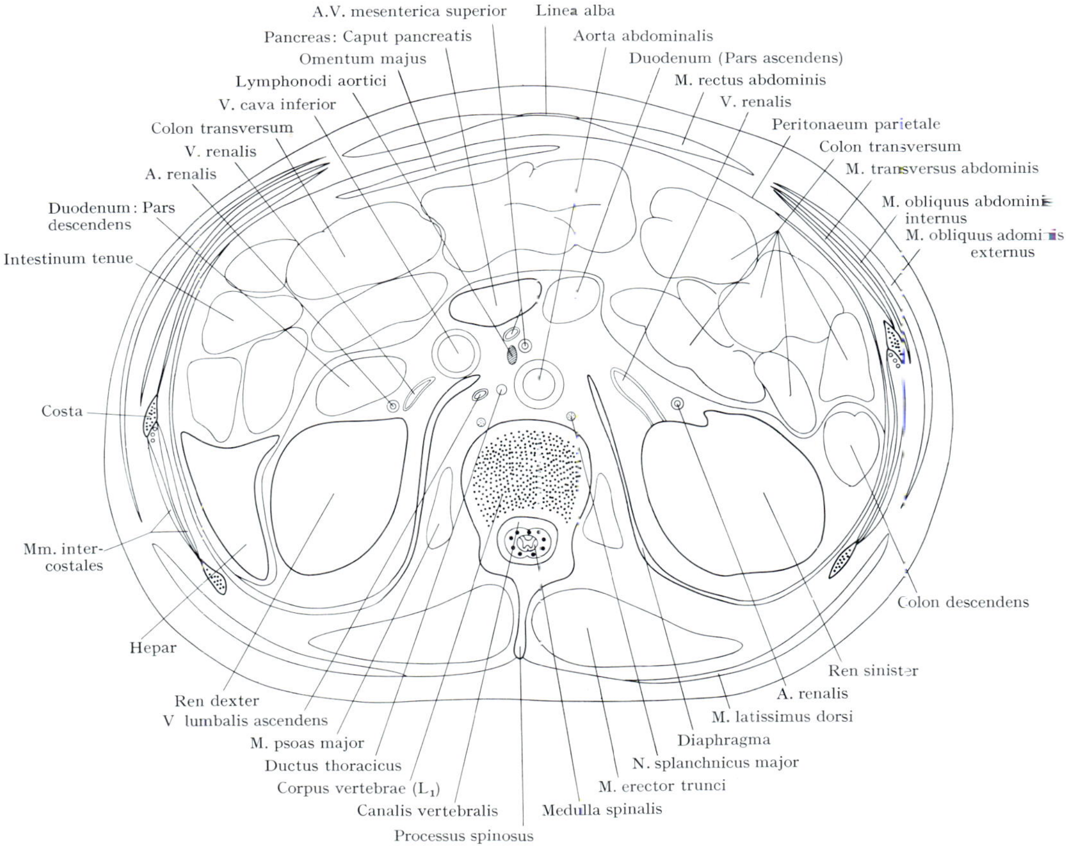

Fig. 325. Anatomical chart

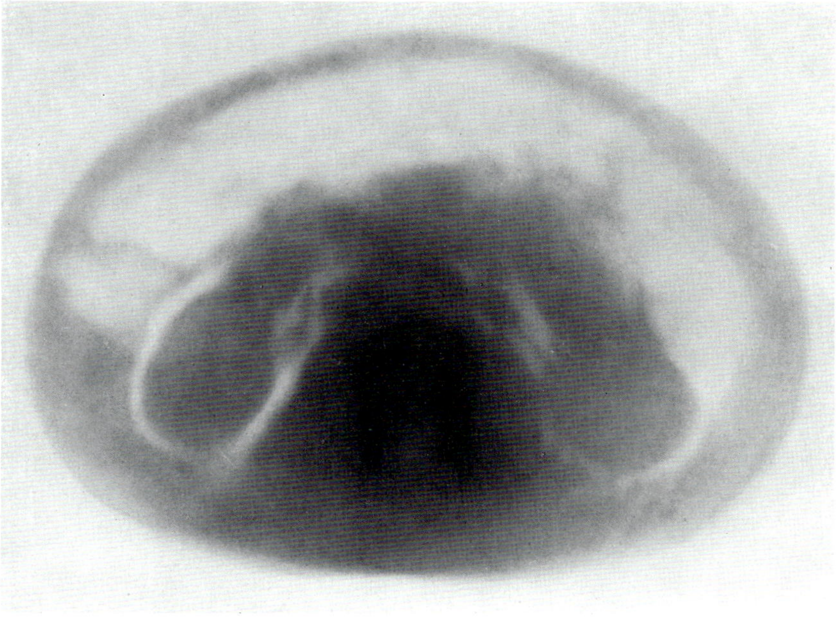

Fig. 326. Axial transverse tomogram

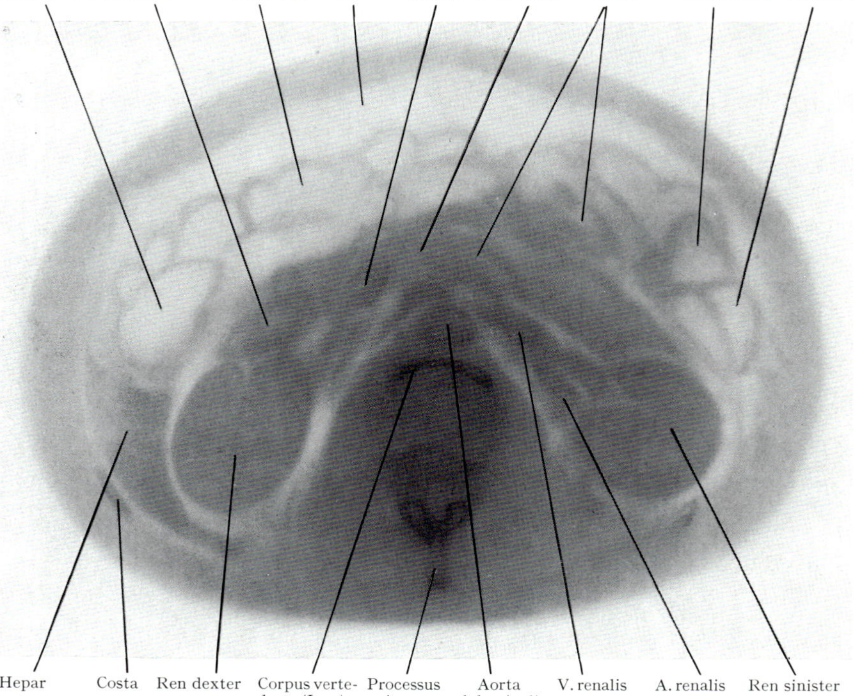

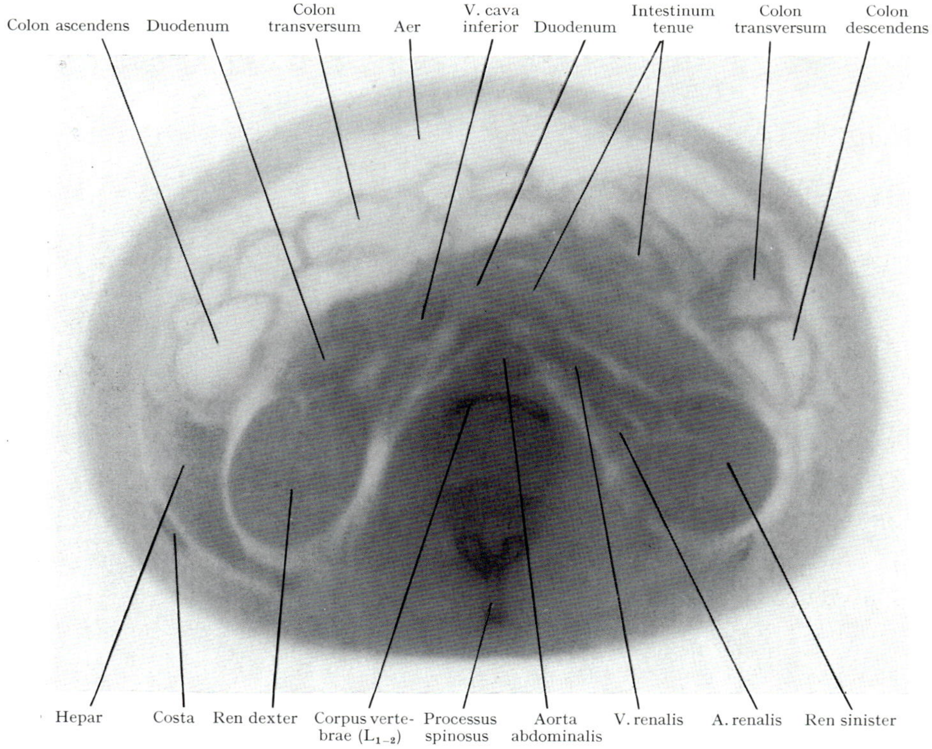

Fig. 327. Interpretation

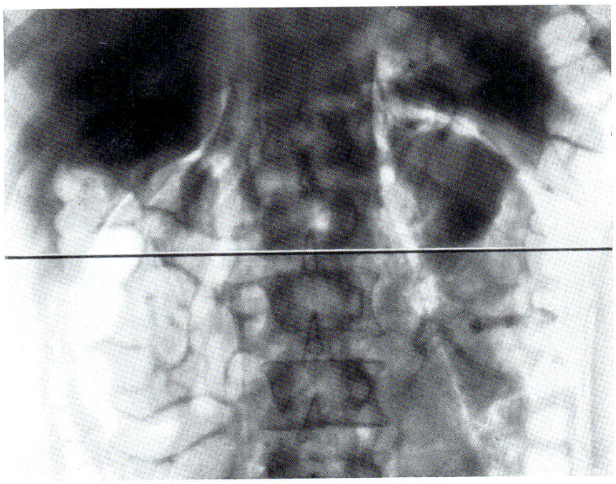

Fig. 328. Normal roentgenogram. Horizontal line showing the level tomographed

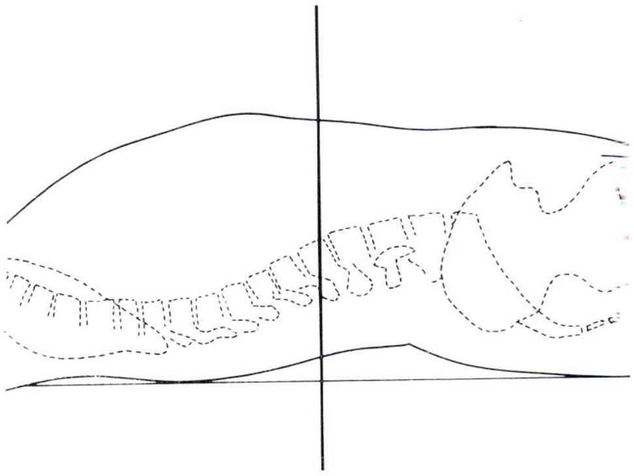

Fig. 329. Schematic drawing of the level tomographed

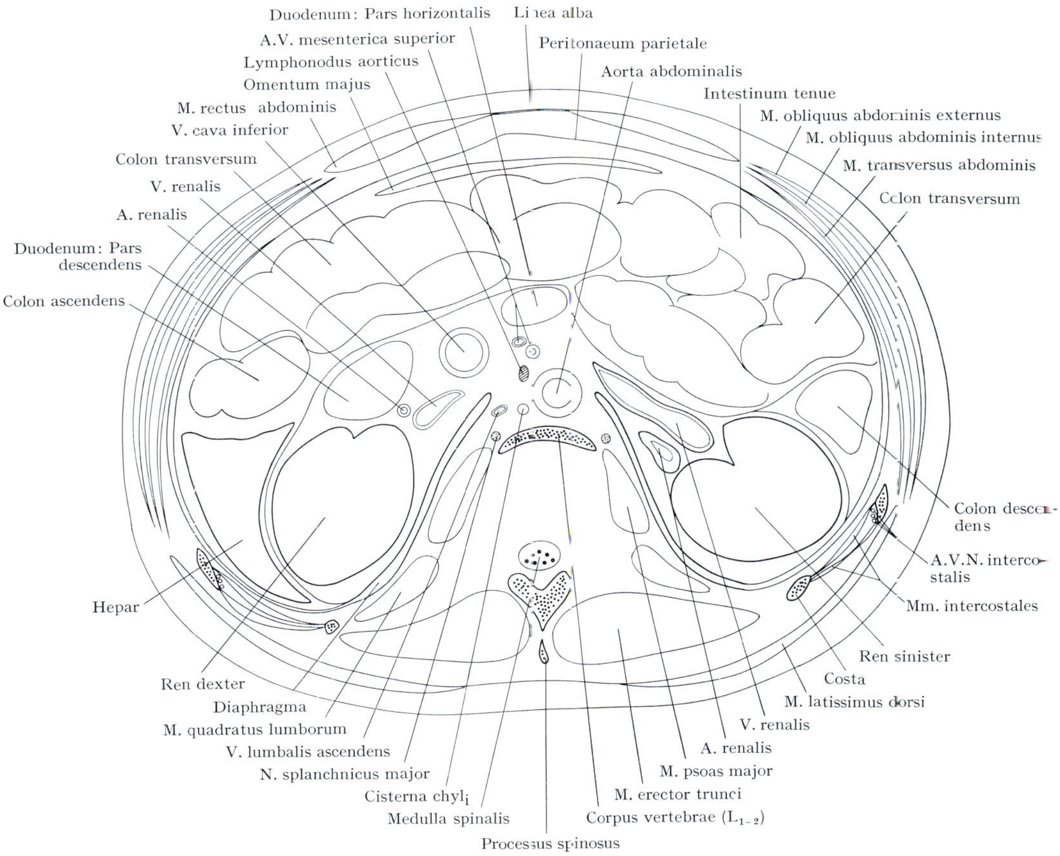

Fig. 330. Anatomical chart

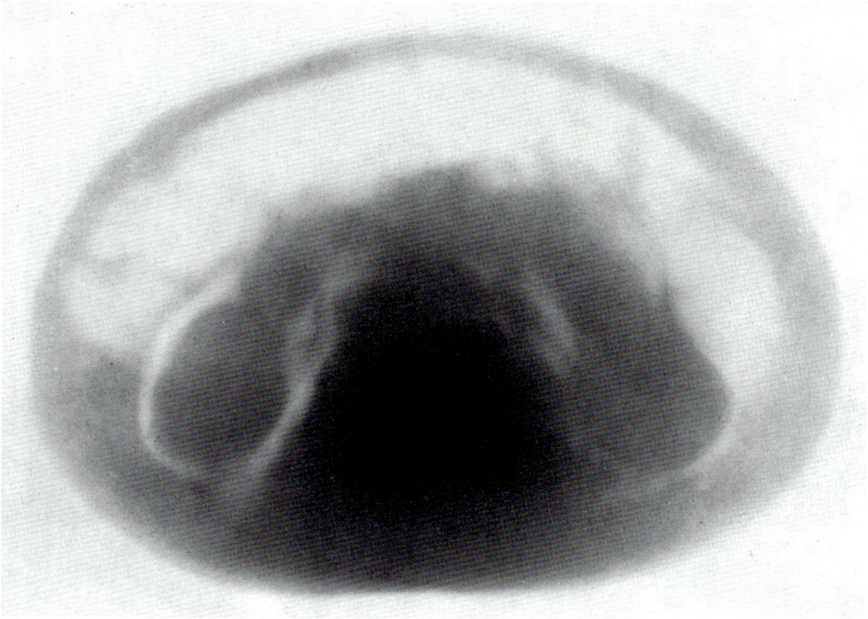

Fig. 331. Axial transverse tomogram

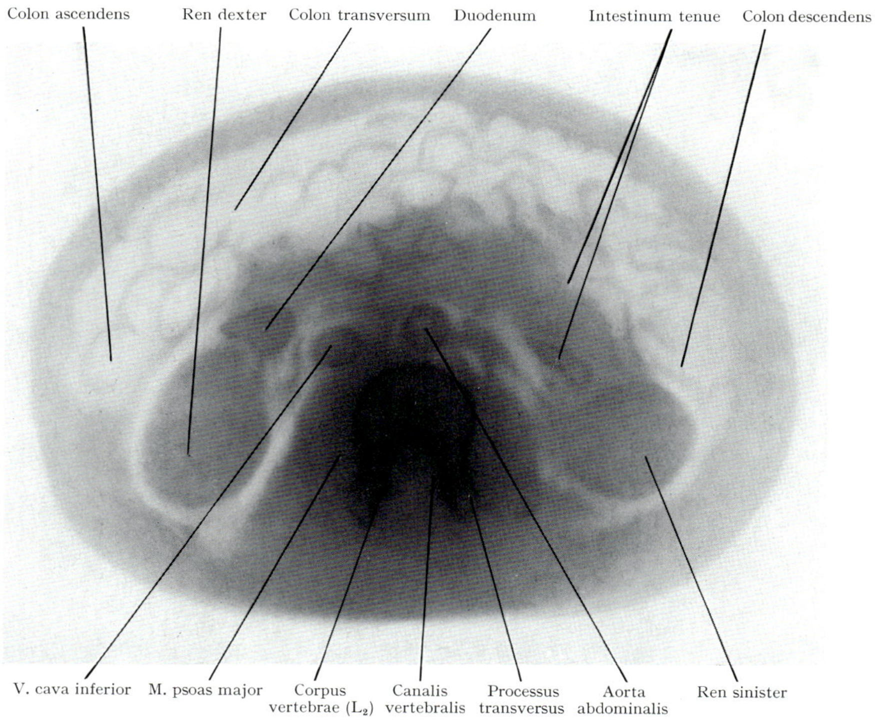

Fig. 332. Interpretation

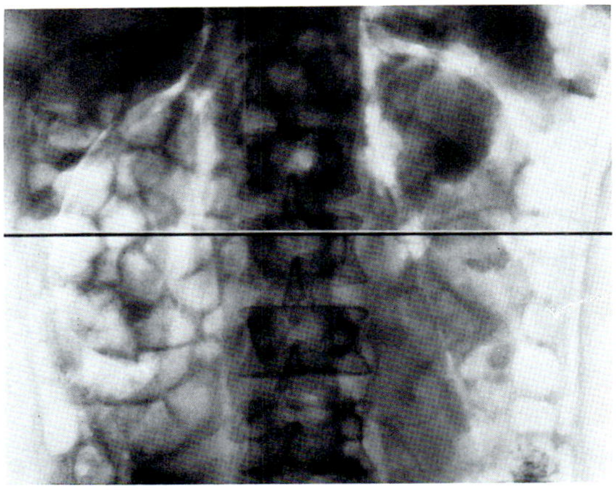

Fig. 333. Normal roentgenogram. Horizontal line showing the level tomographed

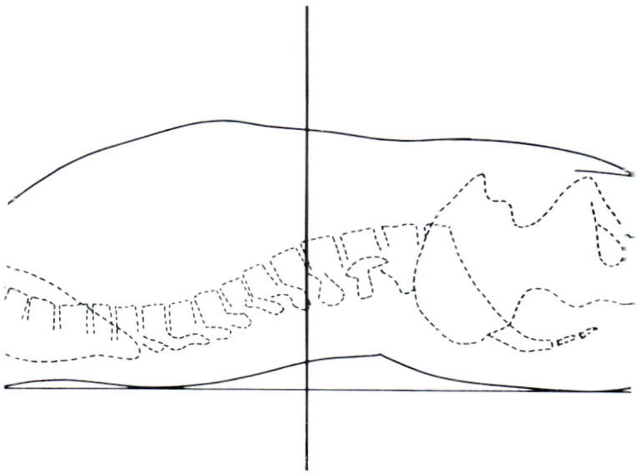

Fig. 334. Schematic drawing of the level tomographed

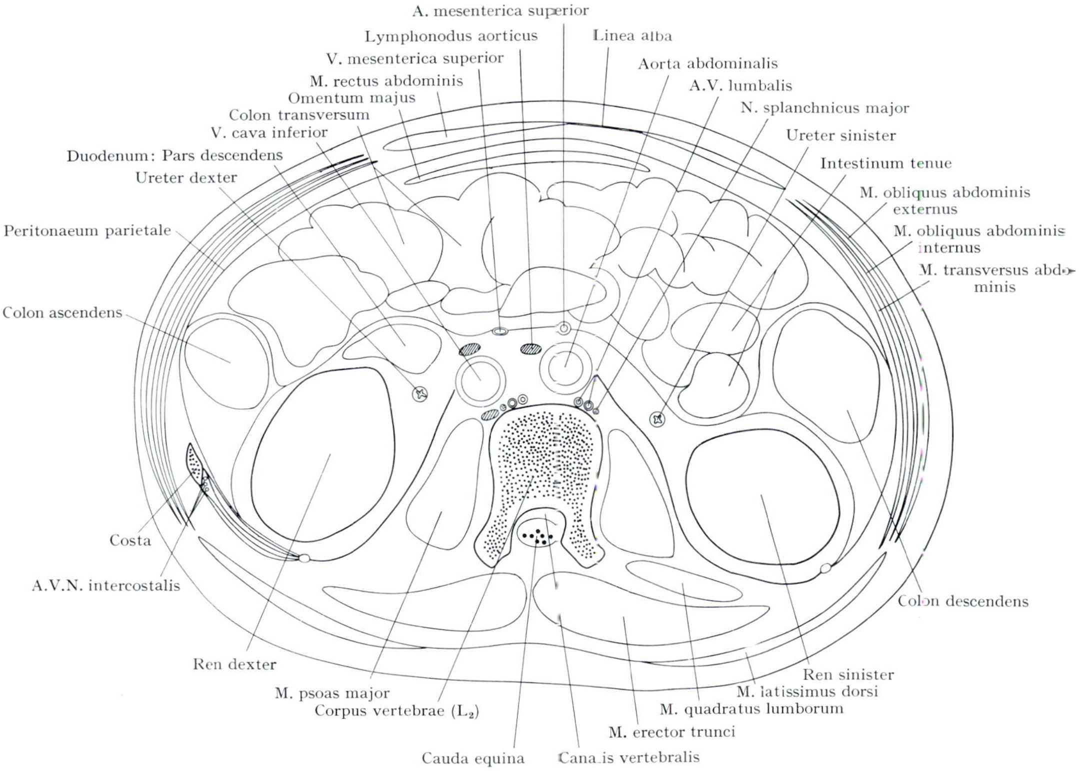

Fig. 335. Anatomical chart

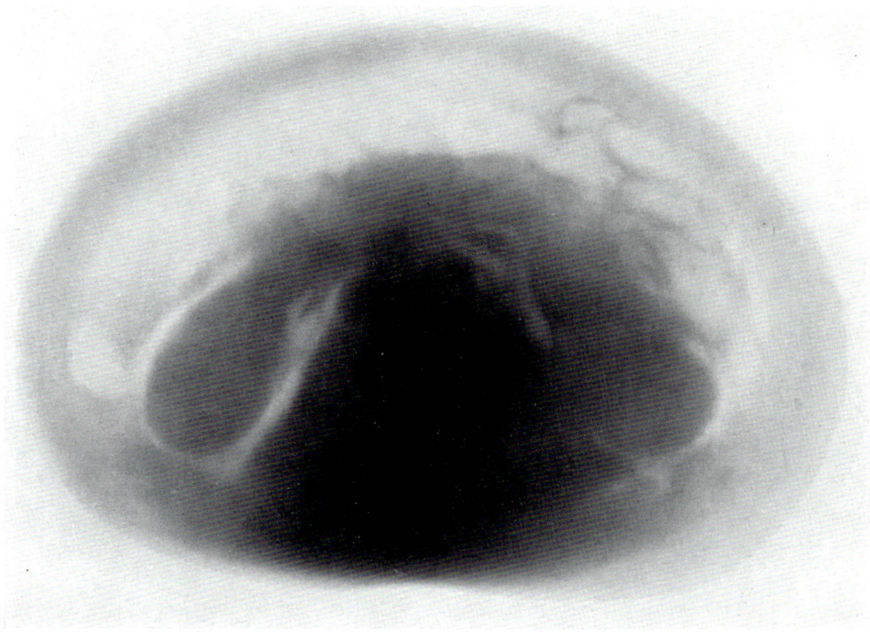

Fig. 336. Axial transverse tomogram

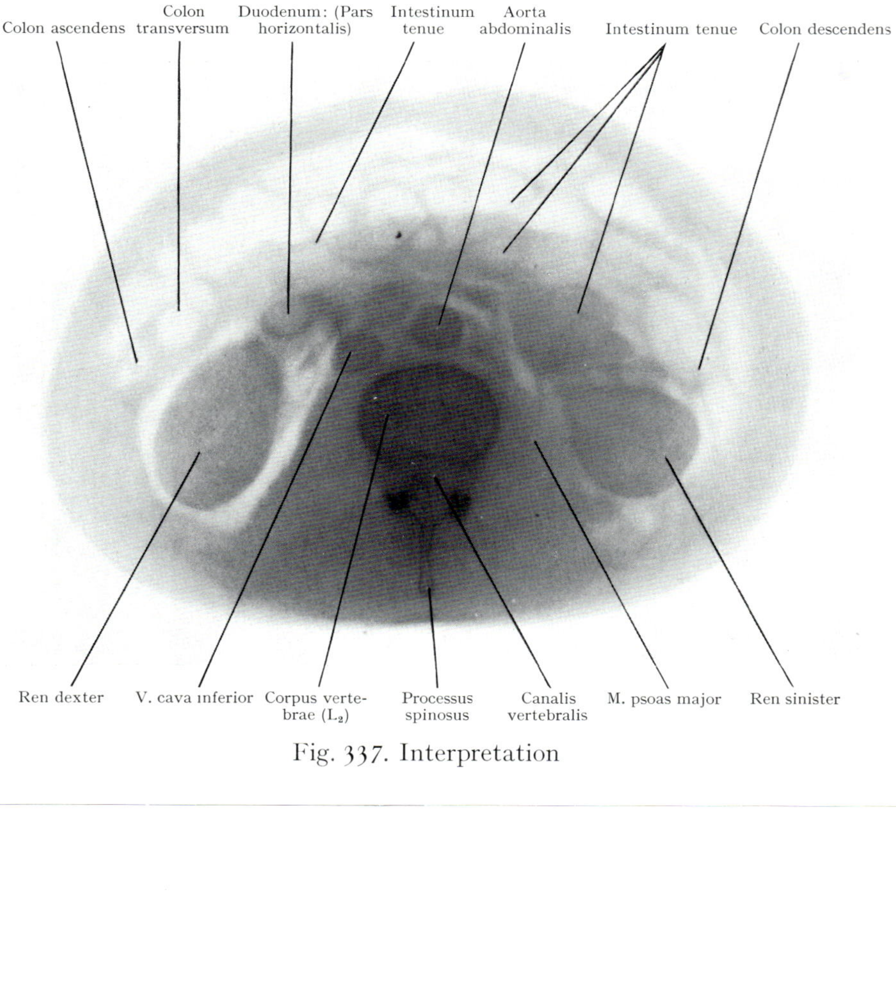

Fig. 337. Interpretation

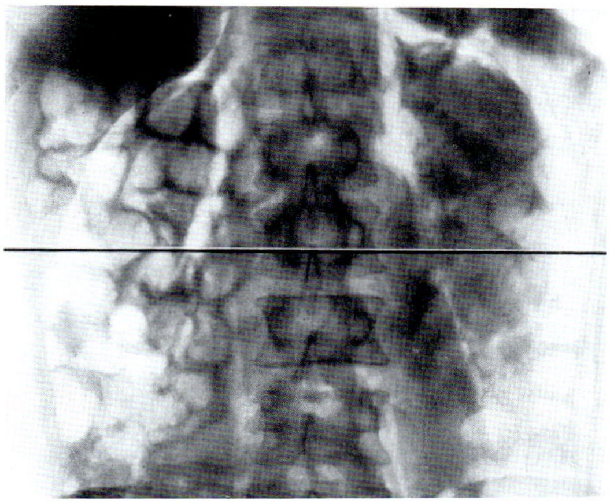

Fig. 338. Normal roentgenogram. Horizontal line showing the level tomographed

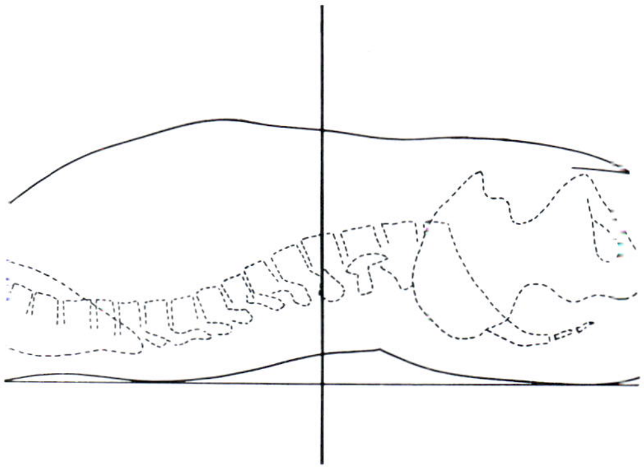

Fig. 339. Schematic drawing of the level tomographed

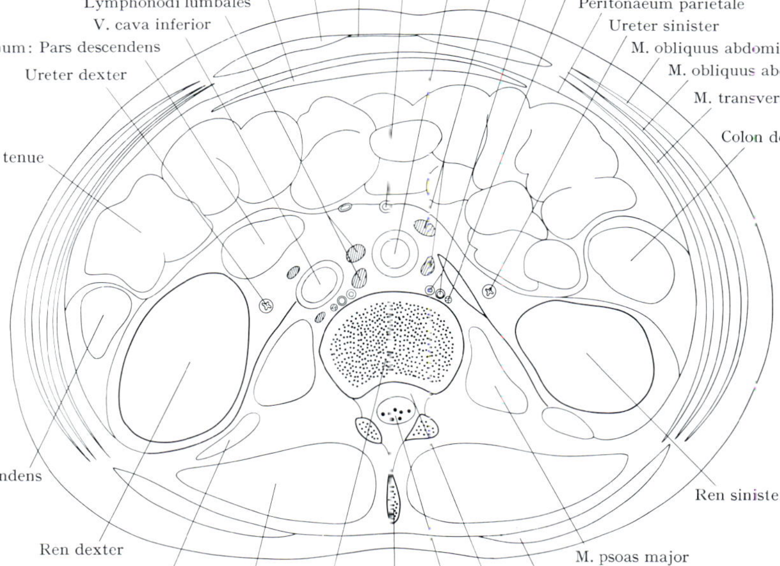

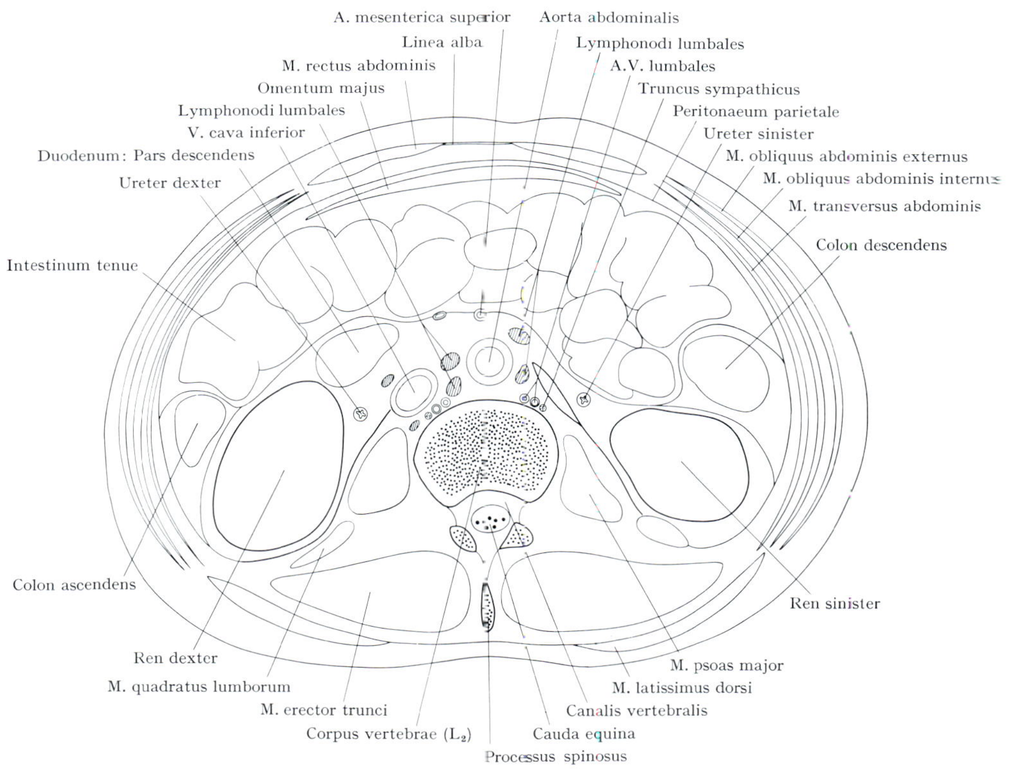

Fig. 340. Anatomical chart

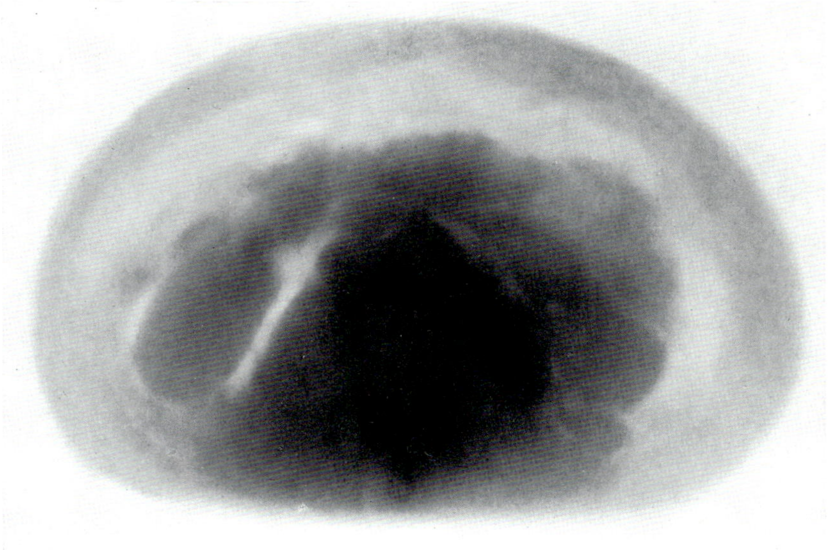

Fig. 341. Axial transverse tomogram

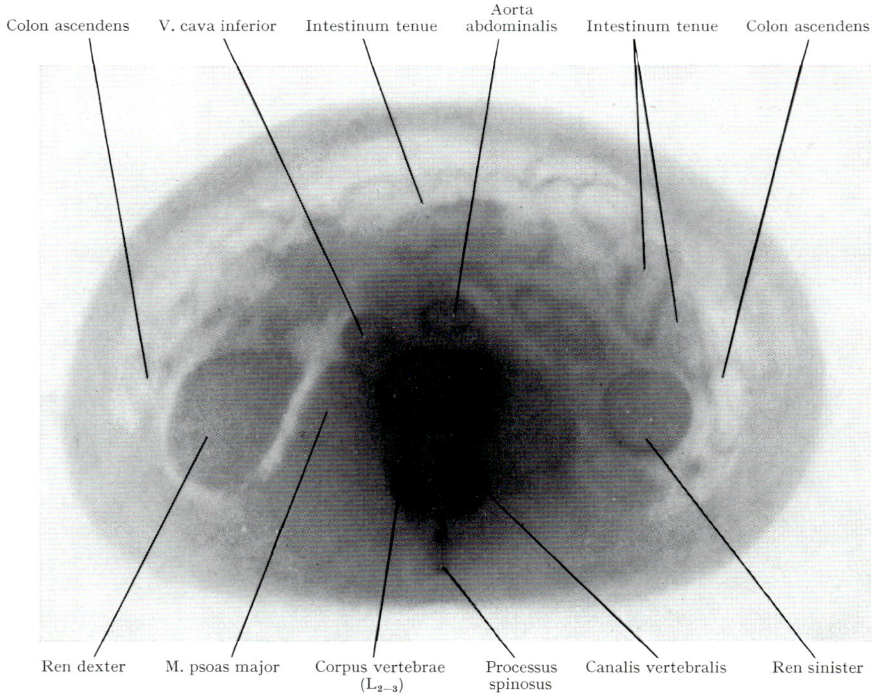

Fig. 342. Interpretation

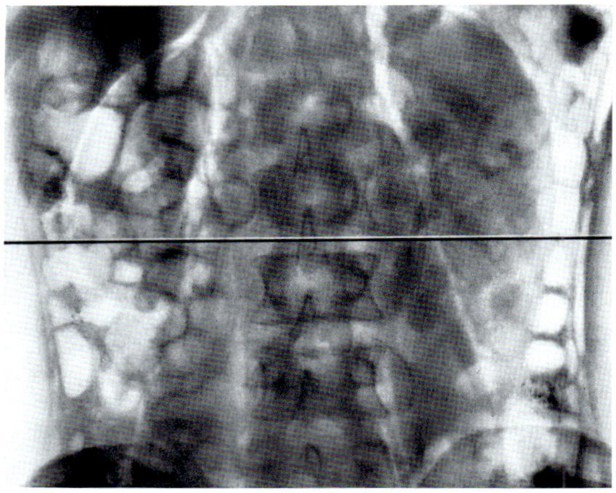

Fig. 343. Normal roentgenogram. Horizontal line showing the level tomographed

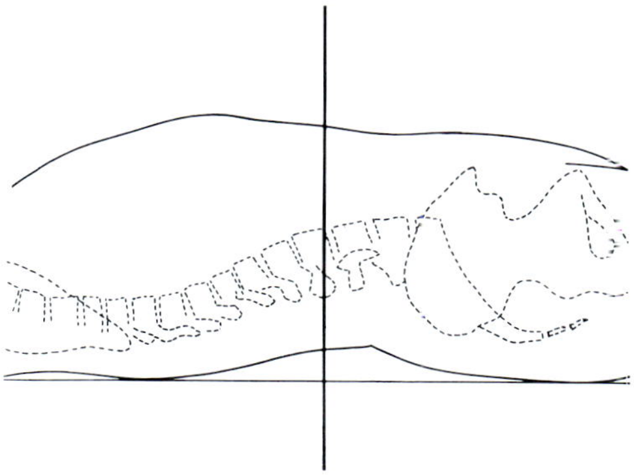

Fig. 344. Schematic drawing of the level tomographed

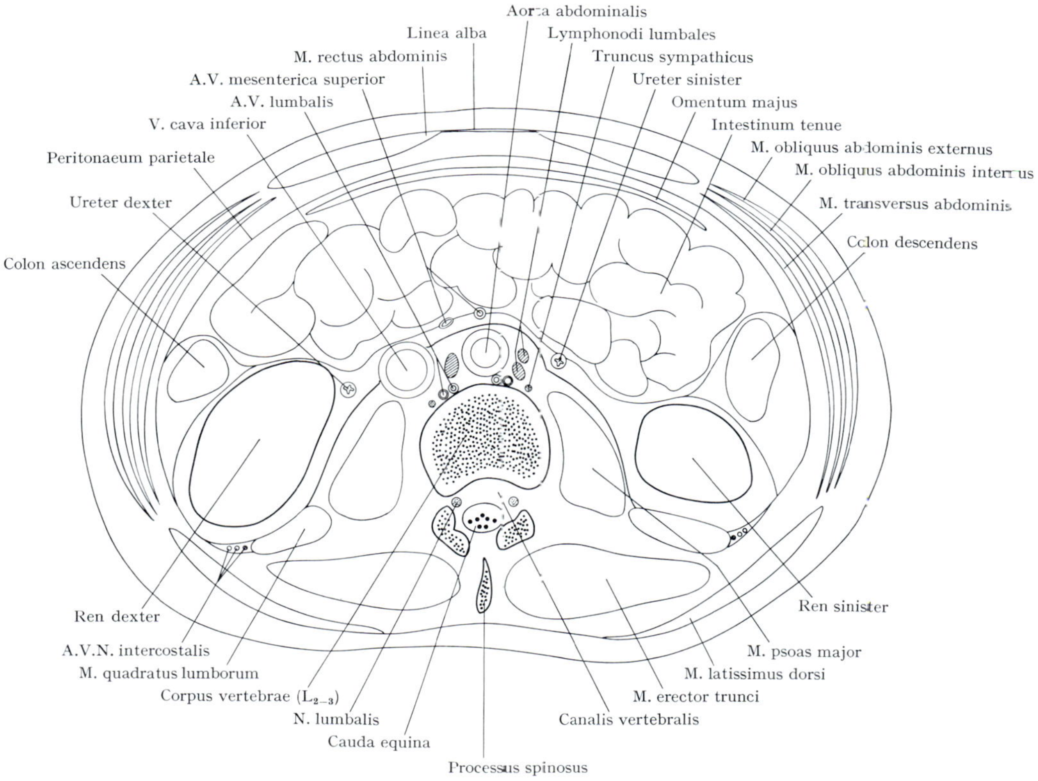

Fig. 345. Anatomical chart

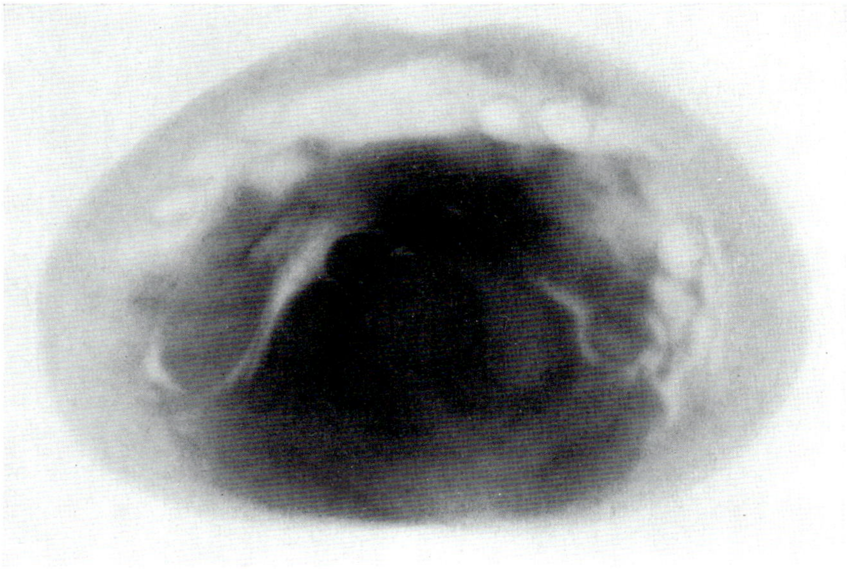

Fig. 346. Axial transverse tomogram

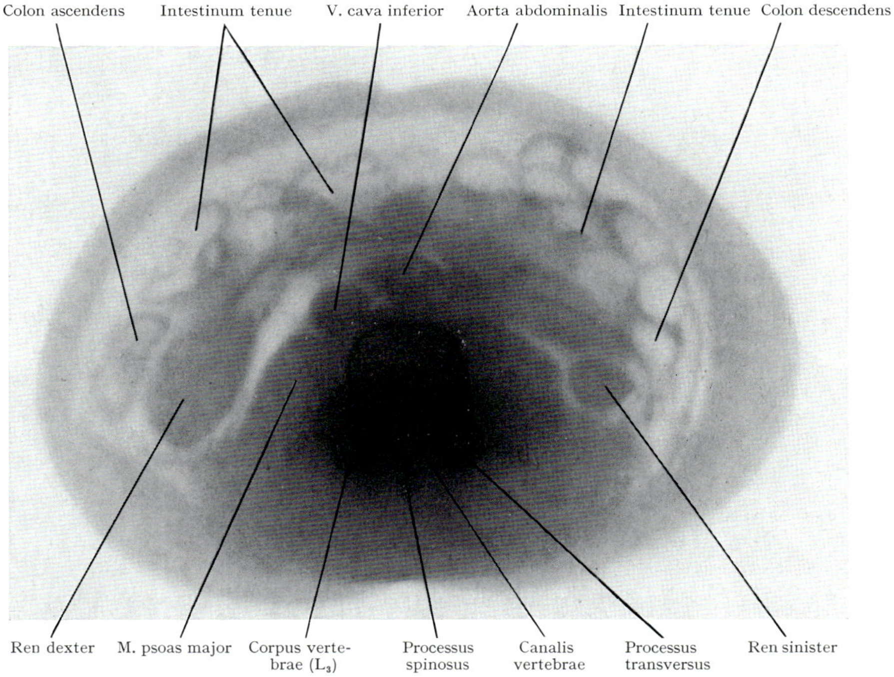

Fig. 347. Interpretation

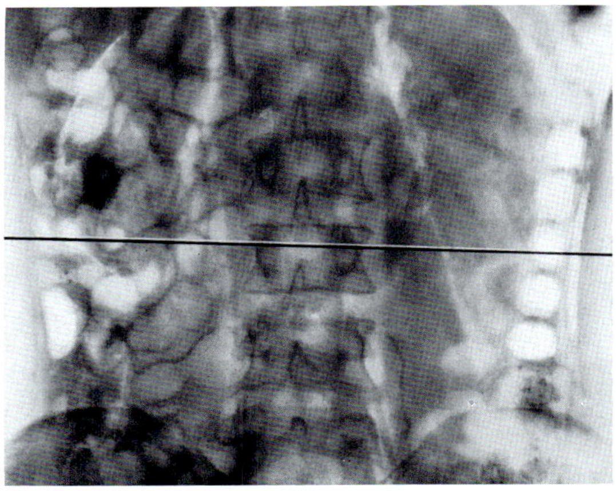

Fig. 348. Normal roentgenogram. Horizontal line showing the level tomographed

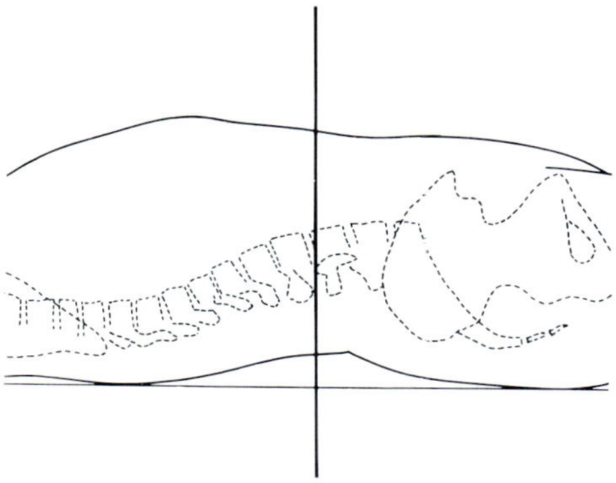

Fig. 349. Schematic drawing of the level tomographed

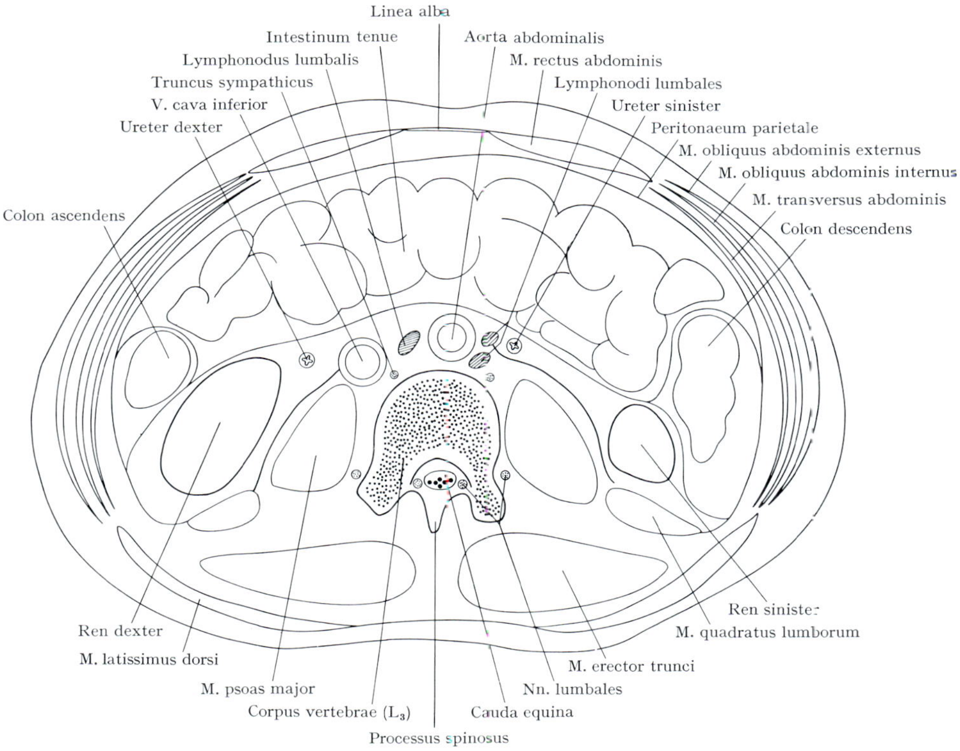

Fig. 350. Anatomical chart

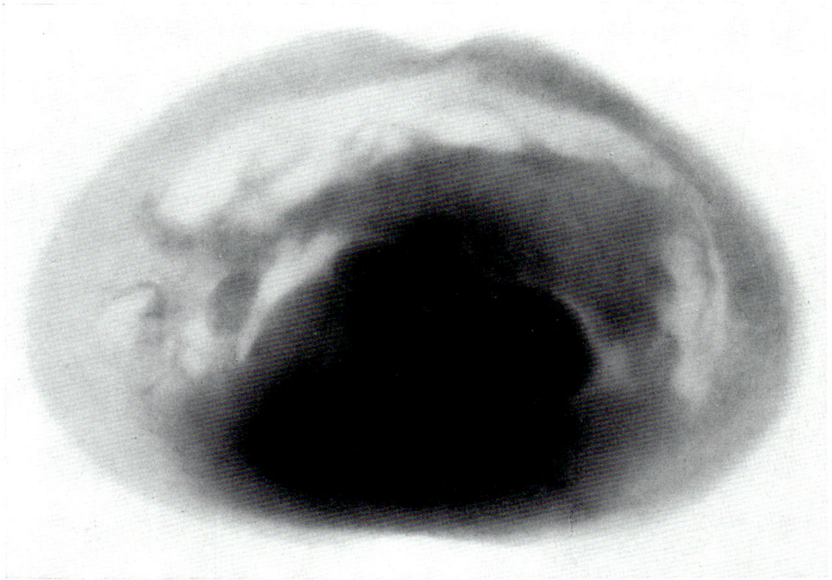

Fig. 351. Axial transverse tomogram

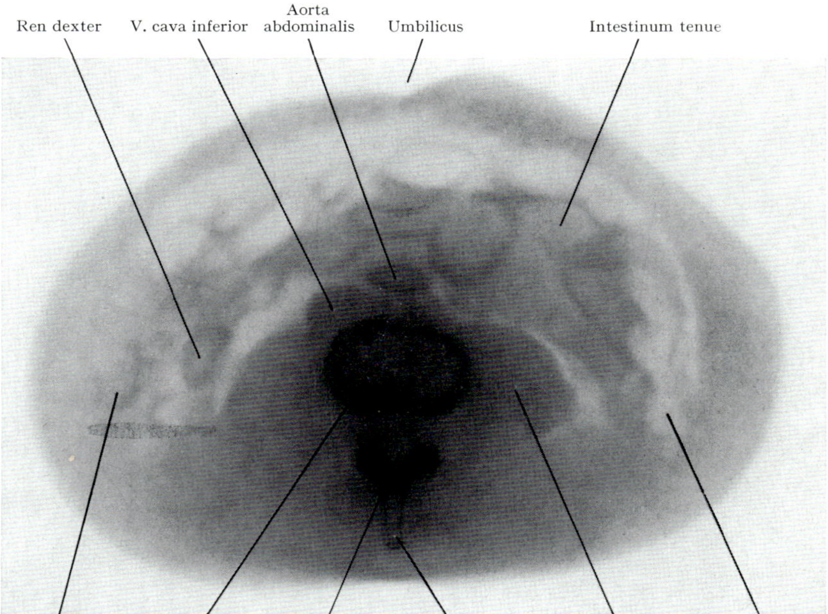

Fig. 352. Interpretation

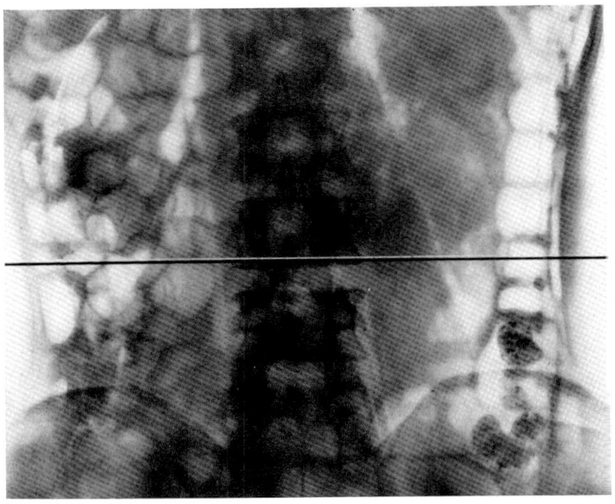

Fig. 353. Normal roentgenogram. Horizontal line showing the level tomographed

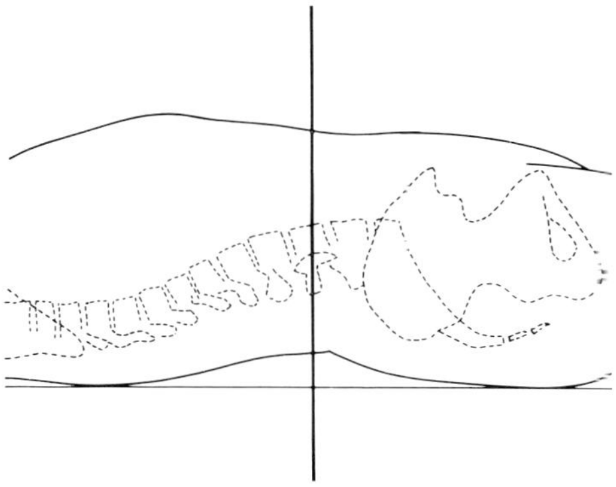

Fig. 354. Schematic drawing of the level tomographed

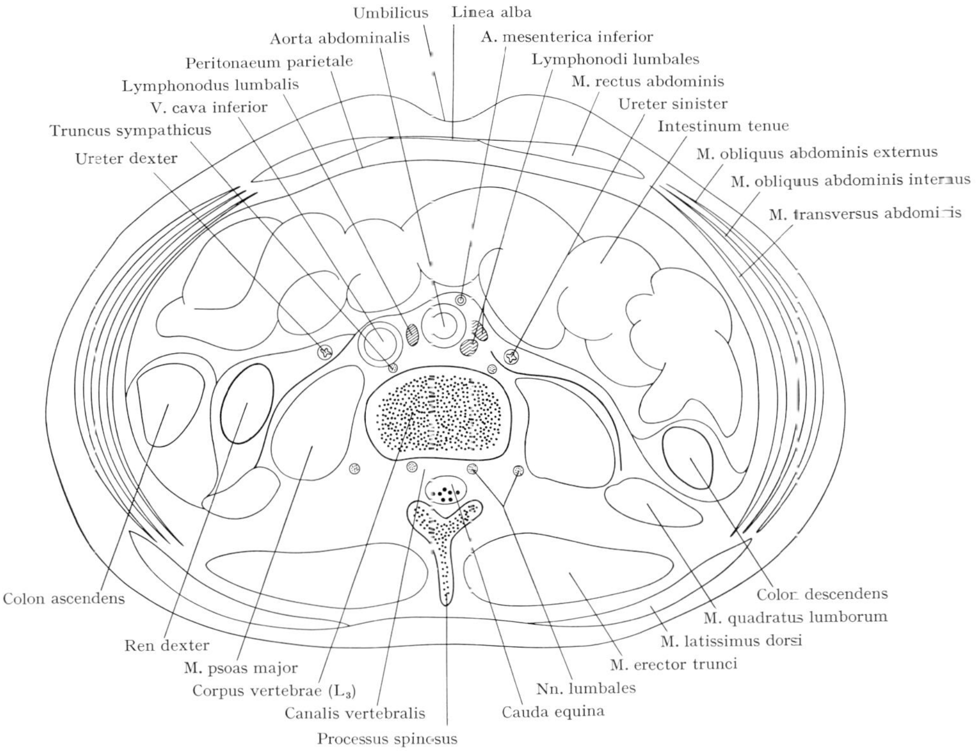

Fig. 355. Anatomical chart

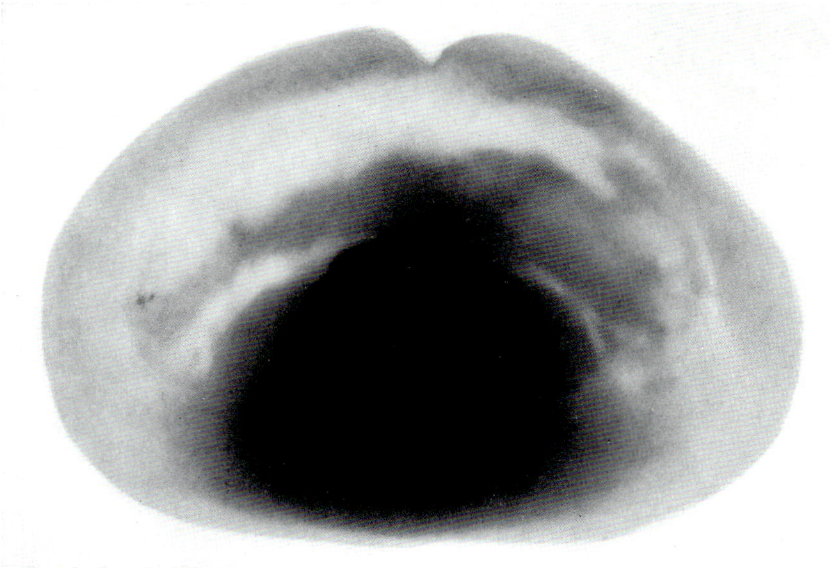

Fig. 356. Axial transverse tomogram

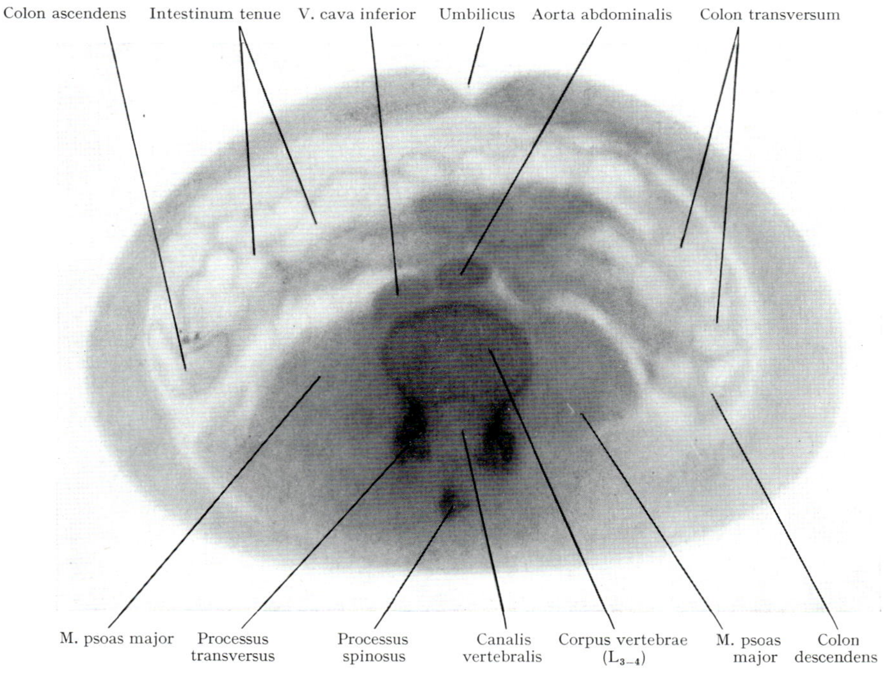

Fig. 357. Interpretation

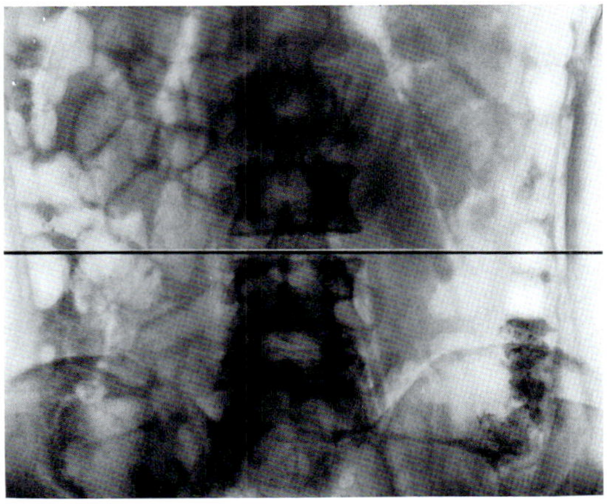

Fig. 358. Normal roentgenogram. Horizontal line showing the level tomographed

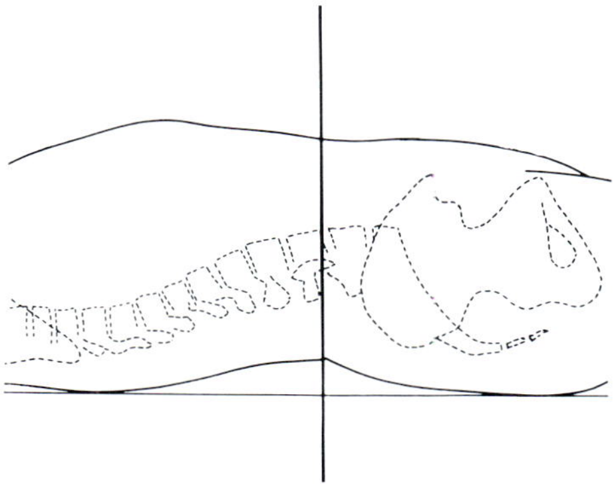

Fig. 359. Schematic drawing of the level tomographed

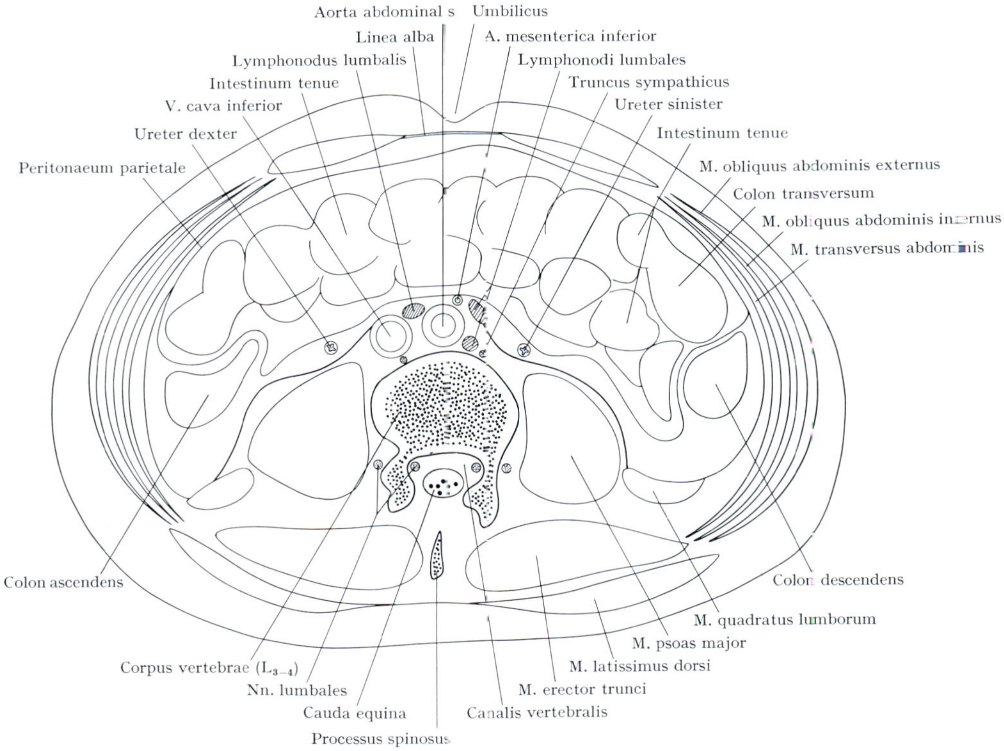

Fig. 360. Anatomical chart

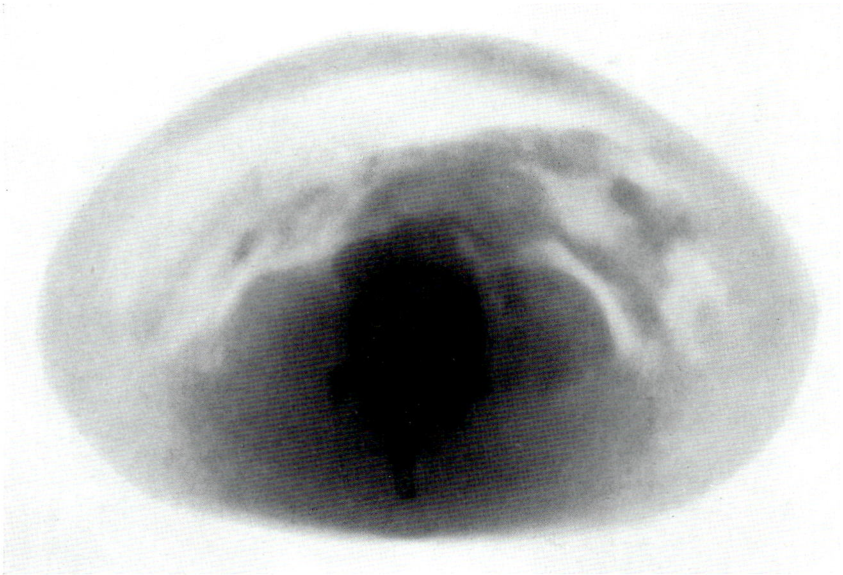

Fig. 361. Axial transverse tomogram

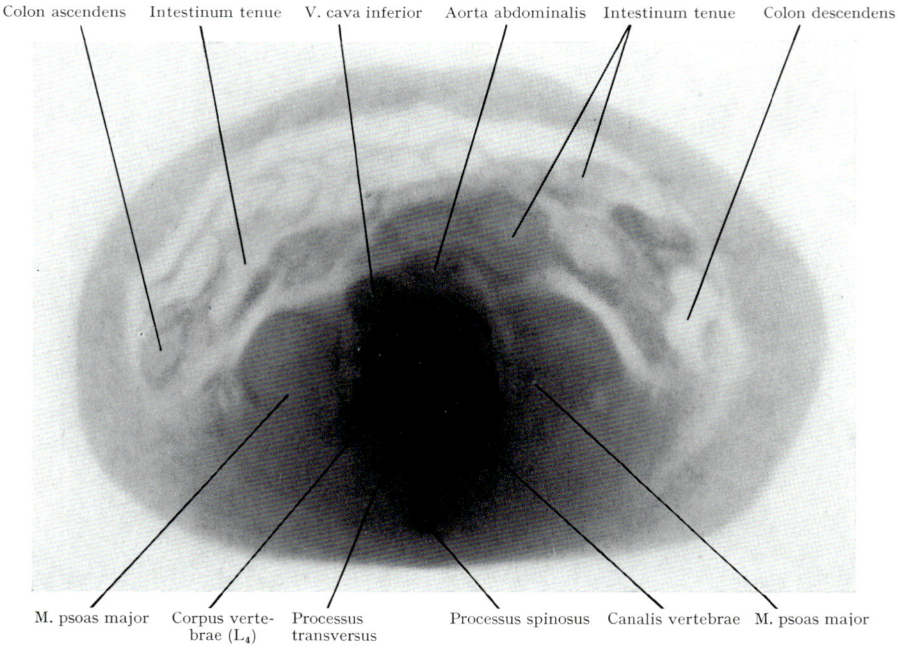

Fig. 362. Interpretation

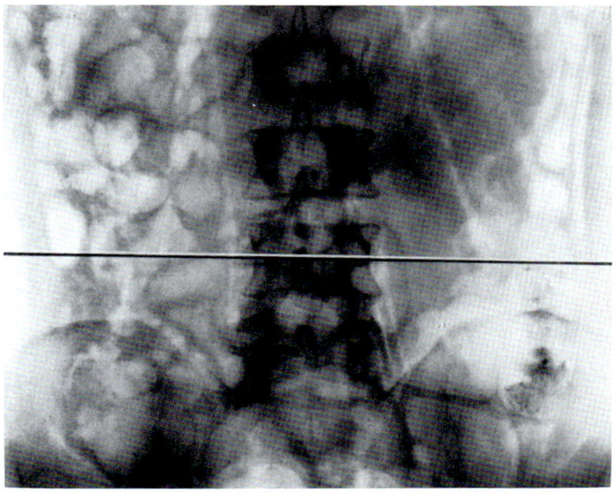

Fig. 363. Normal roentgenogram. Horizontal line showing the level tomographed

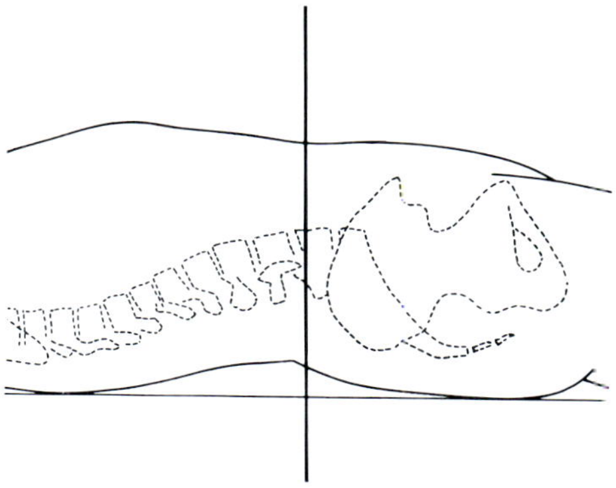

Fig. 364. Schematic drawing of the level tomographed

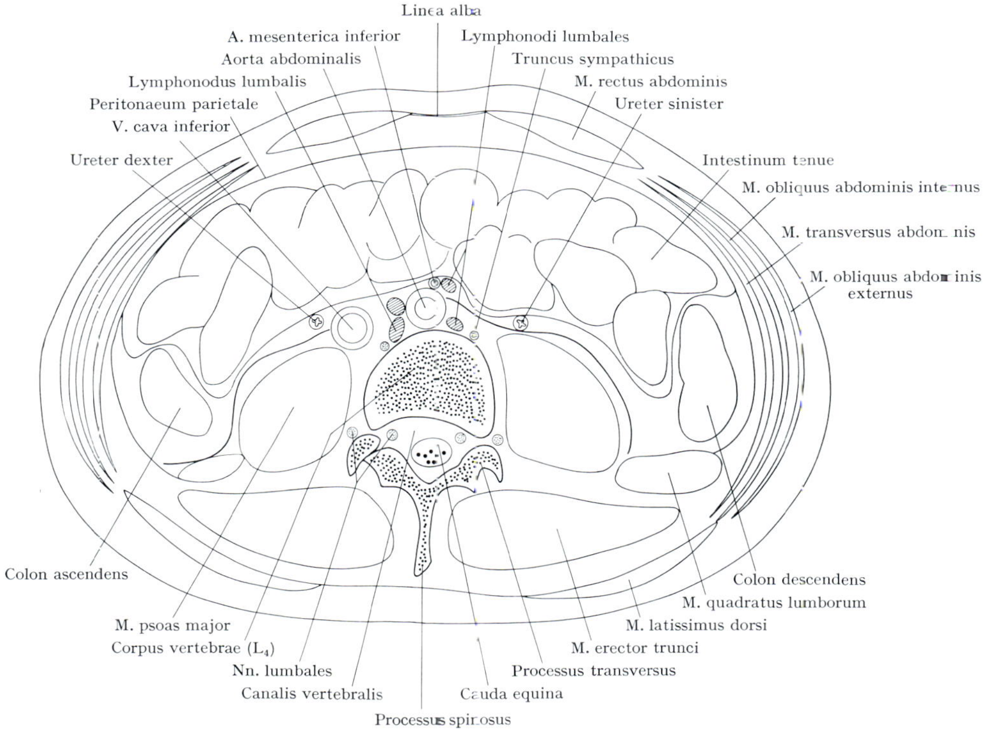

Fig. 365. Anatomical chart

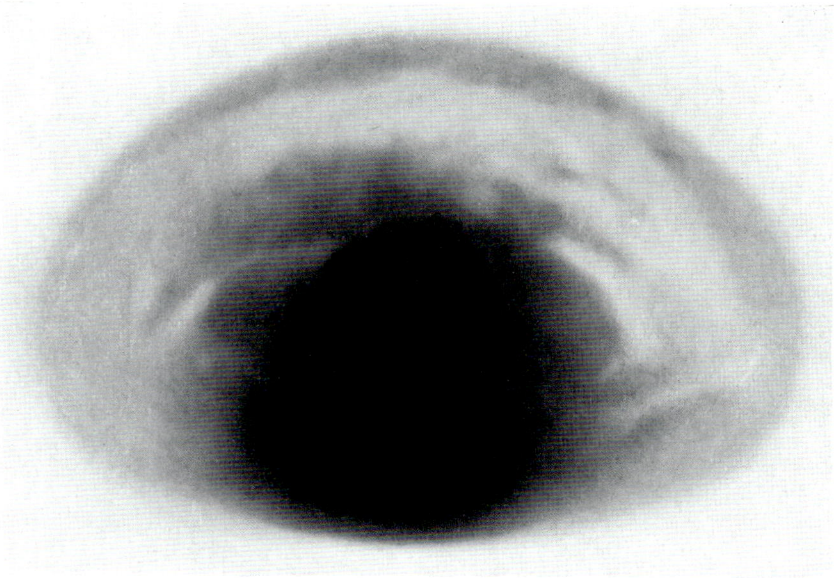

Fig. 366. Axial transverse tomogram

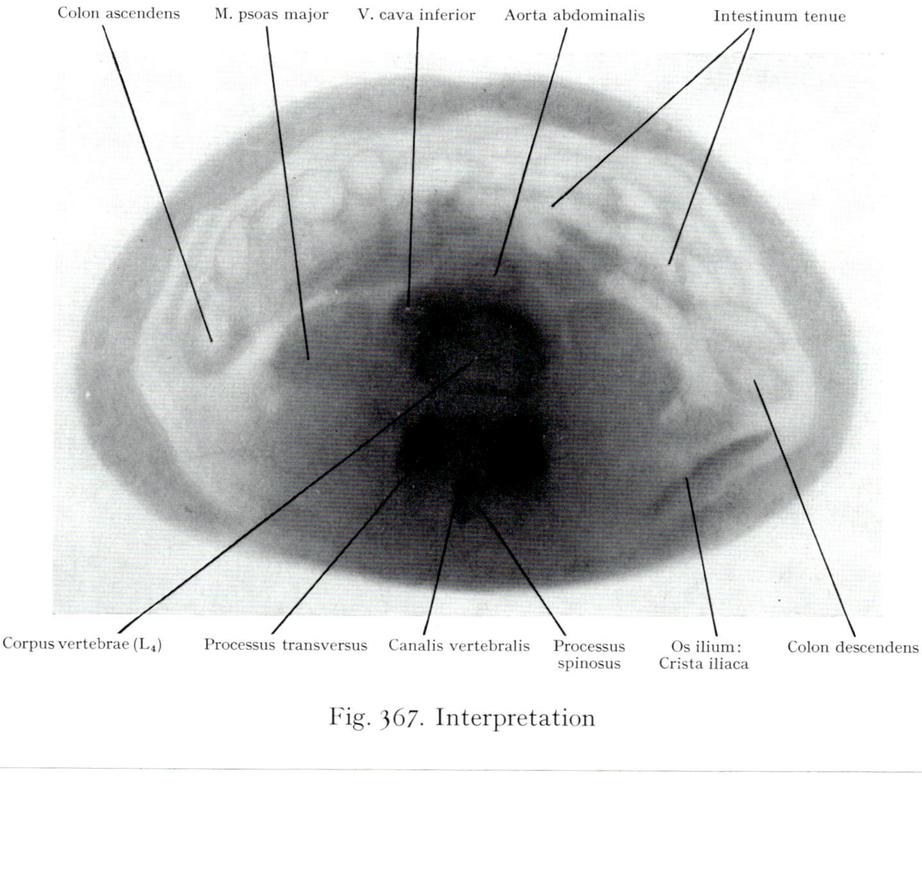

Fig. 367. Interpretation

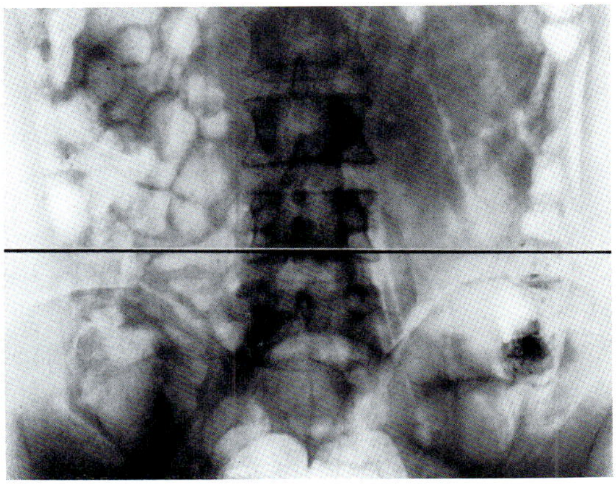

Fig. 368. Normal roentgenogram. Horizontal line showing the level tomographed

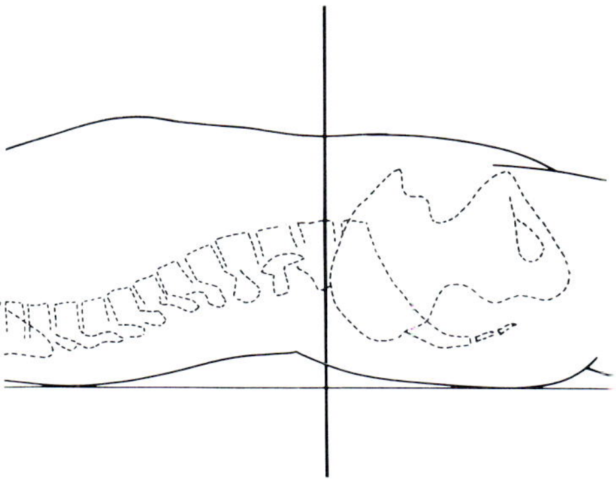

Fig. 369. Schematic drawing of the level tomographed

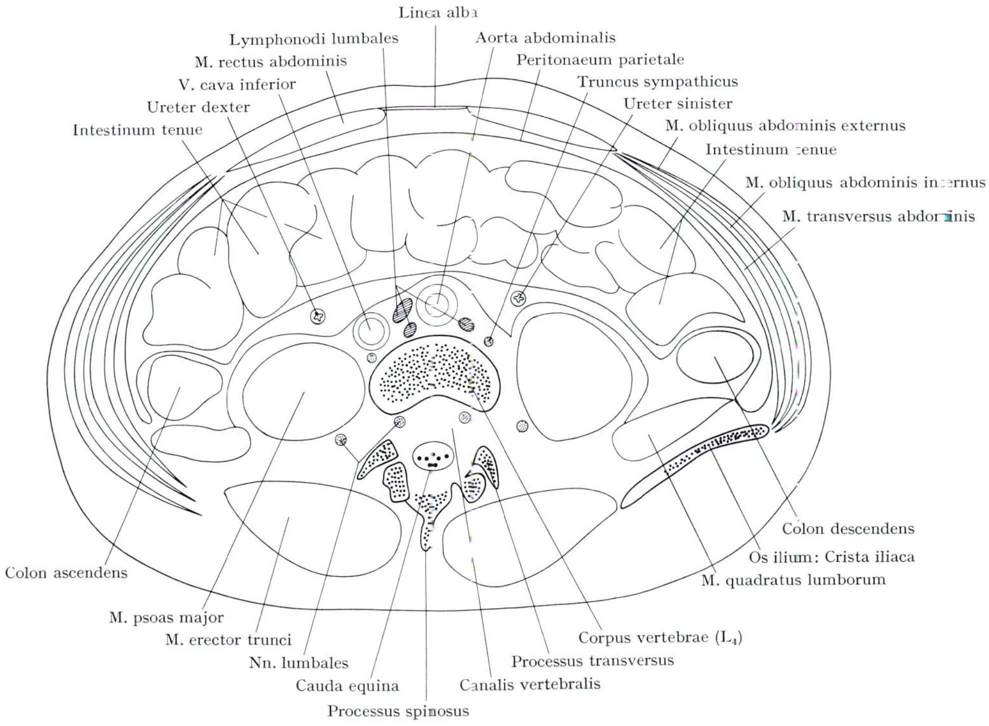

Fig. 370. Anatomical chart

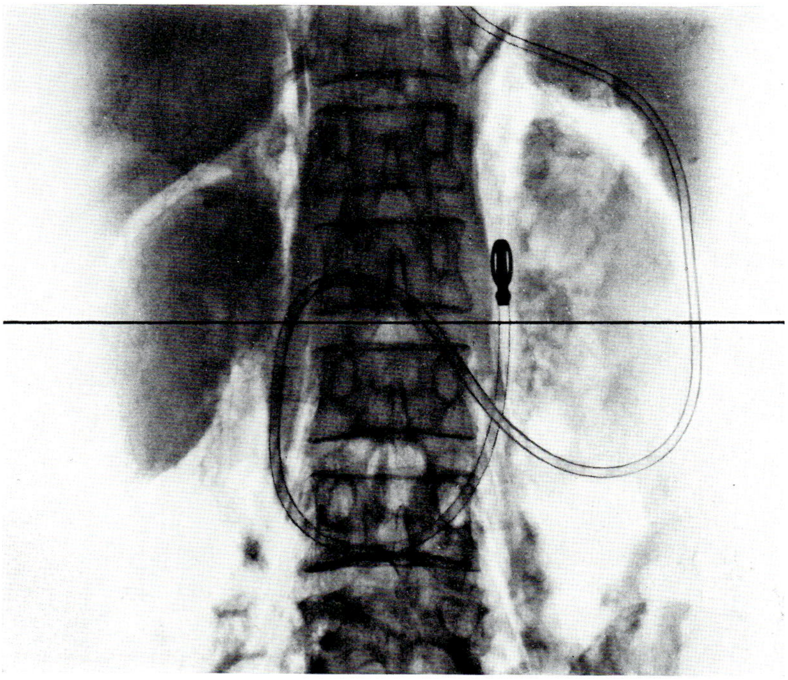

Fig. 371. Normal roentgenogram of the duodenum. The tip of the duodenal tube is located at the flexura duodenojejunalis. The retroperitoneal space is insufflated with air. The horizontal line shows the level tomographed

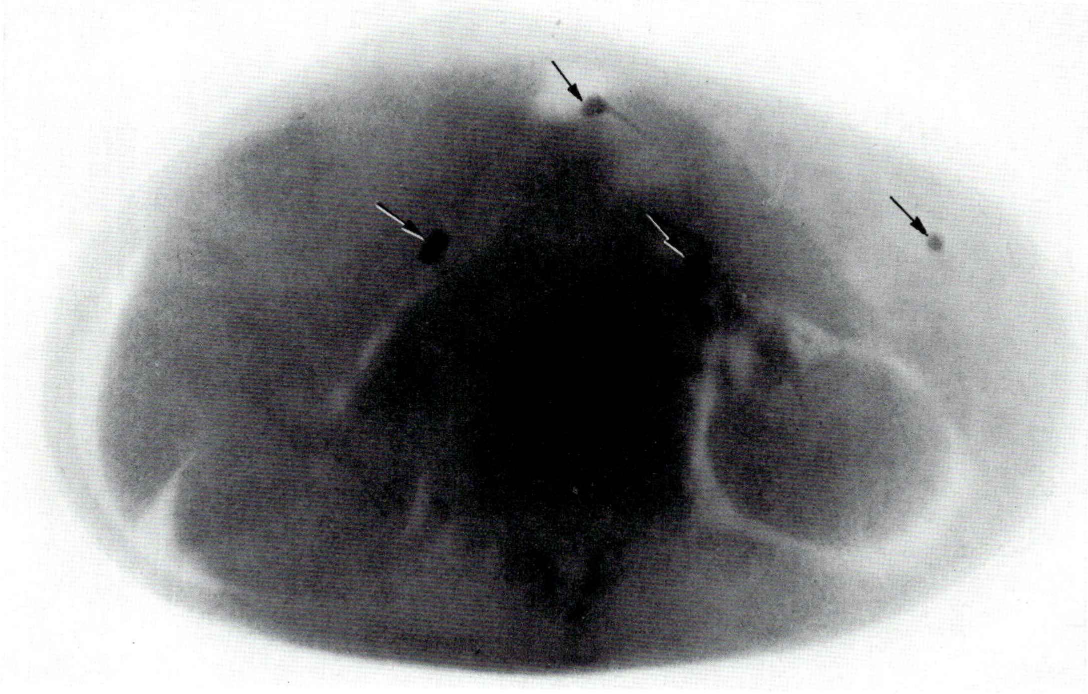

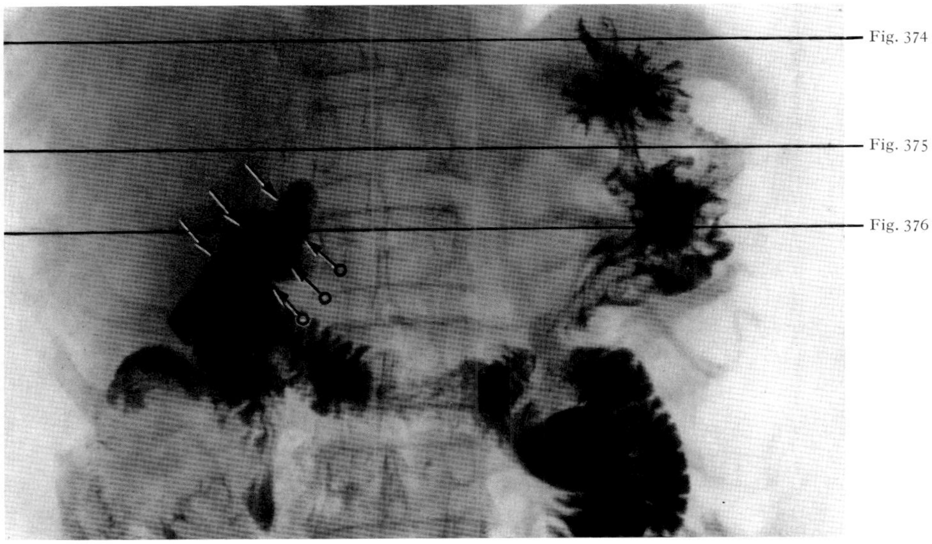

Fig. 373. Normal roentgenogram of the upper abdomen taken following the introduction of contrast media into the stomach, gallbladder and urinary pelvis, without air insufflation of the retroperitoneal space. Horizontal lines showing the levels tomographed

Fig. 372. Axial transverse tomogram shows the cross-section images of the duodenal tube seen (↗) in the body and pylorus of the stomach and in the descending and ascending duodenum (see Figs. 306—310, 311—315, 316—320, 321—325, 326—330)

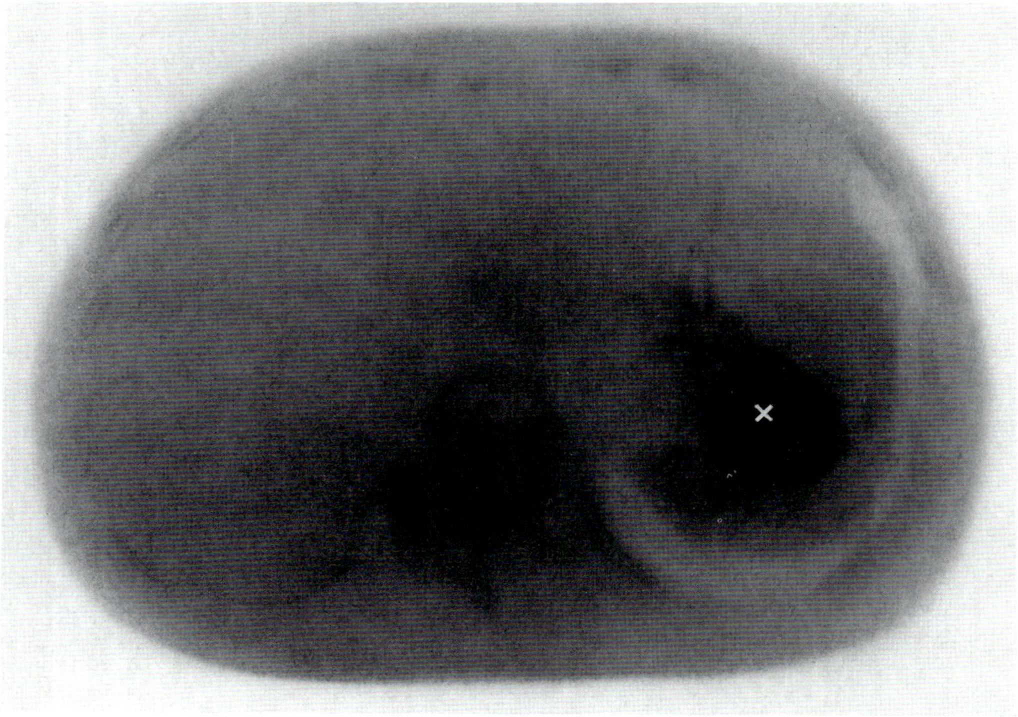

Fig. 374. Axial transverse tomogram shows the cardia (×) of the stomach (see Figs. 286—290)

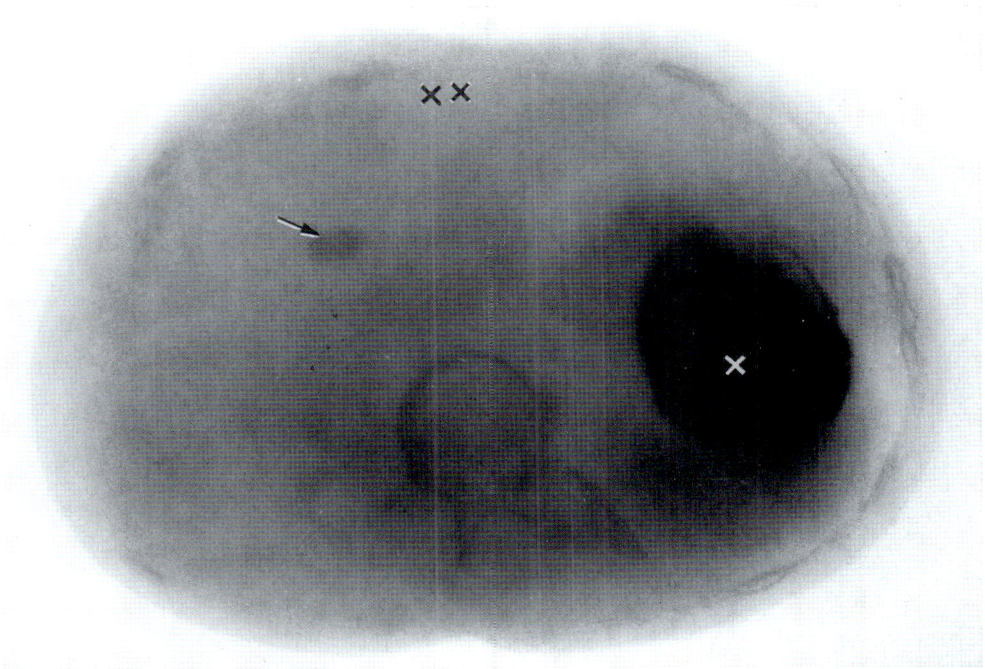

Fig. 375. Axial transverse tomogram shows the body (×) and pylorus (××) of the stomach and the upper part of the gallbladder (↗) (see Figs. 295, 300, 305, 310)

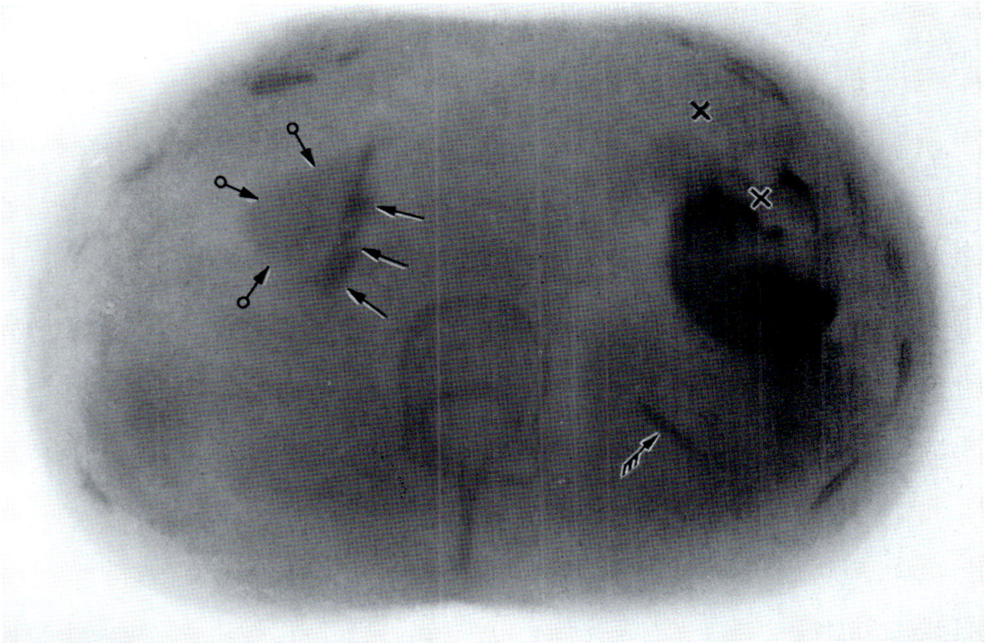

Fig. 376. Axial transverse tomogram shows the antrum (×) of the stomach, duodenum (↗), gallbladder (↗) and renal pelvis (↗) (see Figs. 310, 315)

Lower Abdomen

Six axial transverse tomograms of female subject with the rectum, the vagina and the bladder contrasted by air

and

Five axial transverse tomograms of male subject.

Appendices:

1. Axial transverse tomogram of urethra with catheter introduced
2. Axial transverse tomogram of iliac artery with catheter introduced.

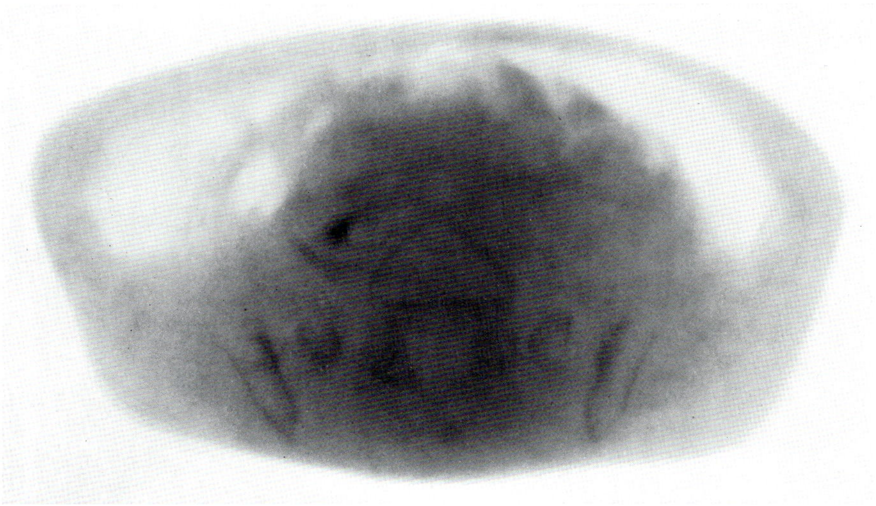

Fig. 377. Axial transverse tomogram

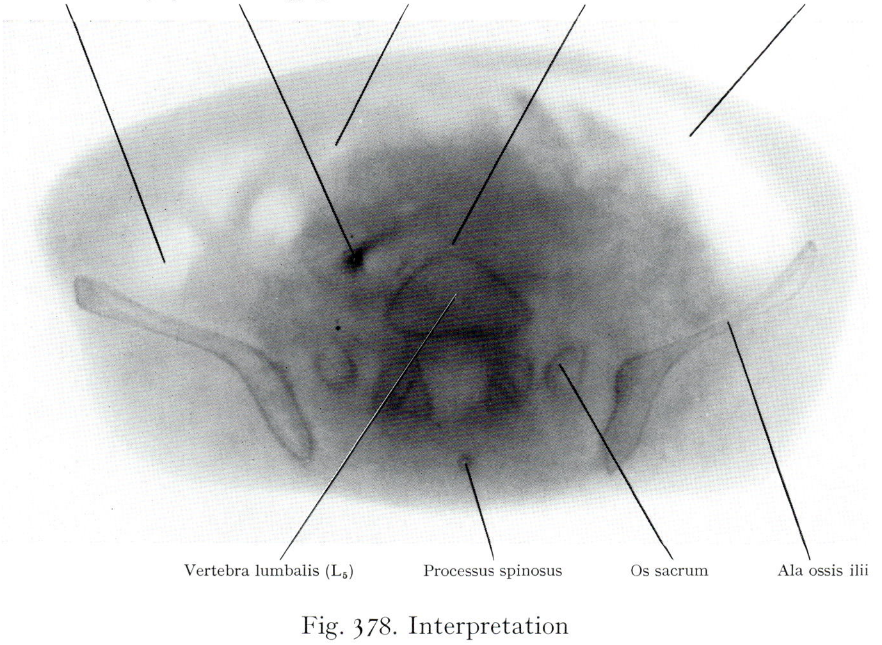

Fig. 378. Interpretation

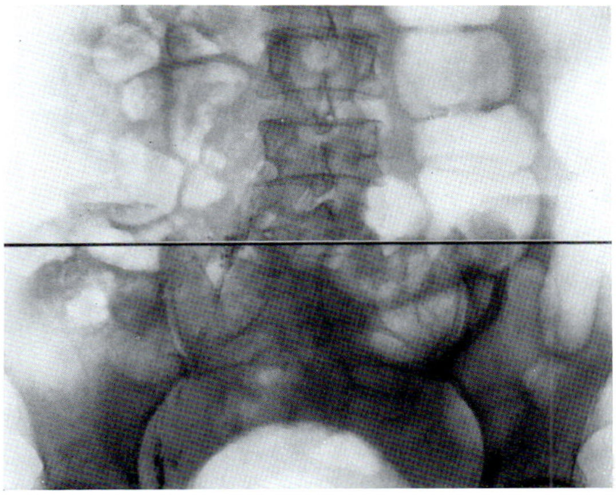

Fig. 379. Normal roentgenogram. Horizontal line showing the level tomographed

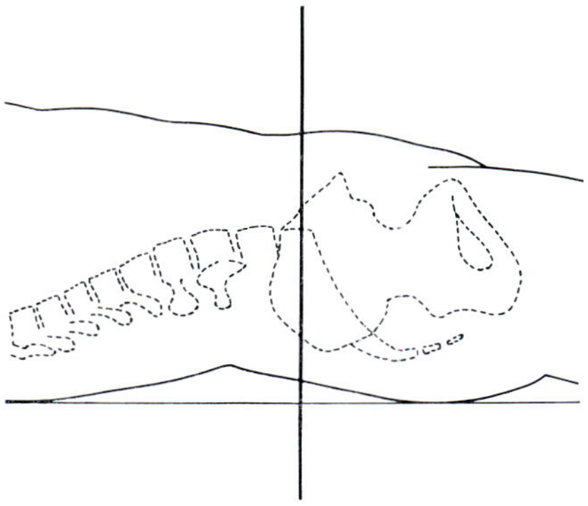

Fig. 380. Schematic drawing of the level tomographed

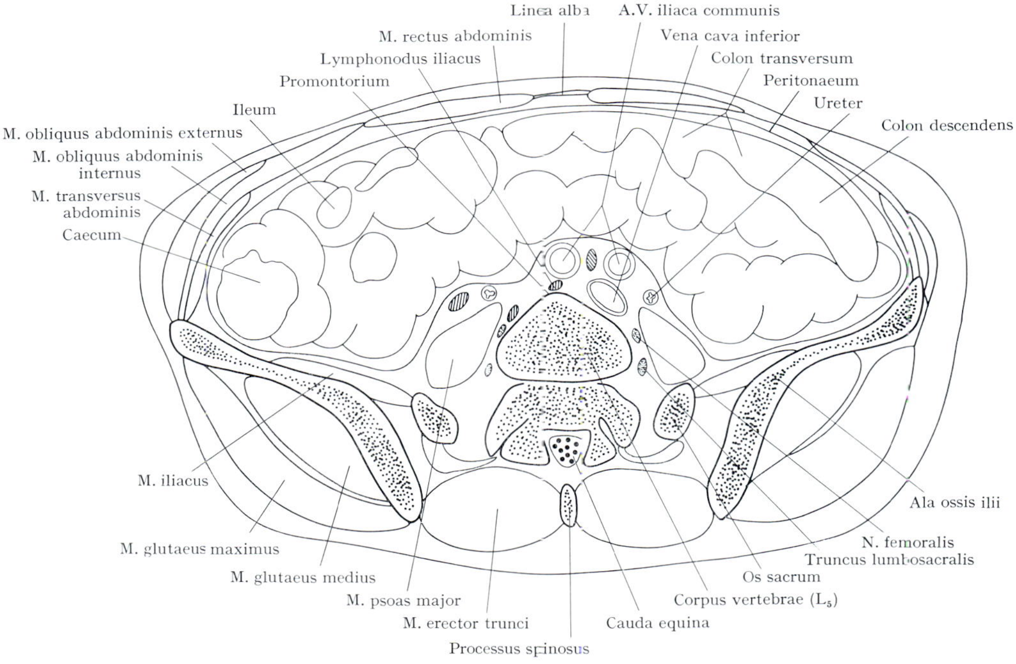

Fig. 381. Anatomical chart

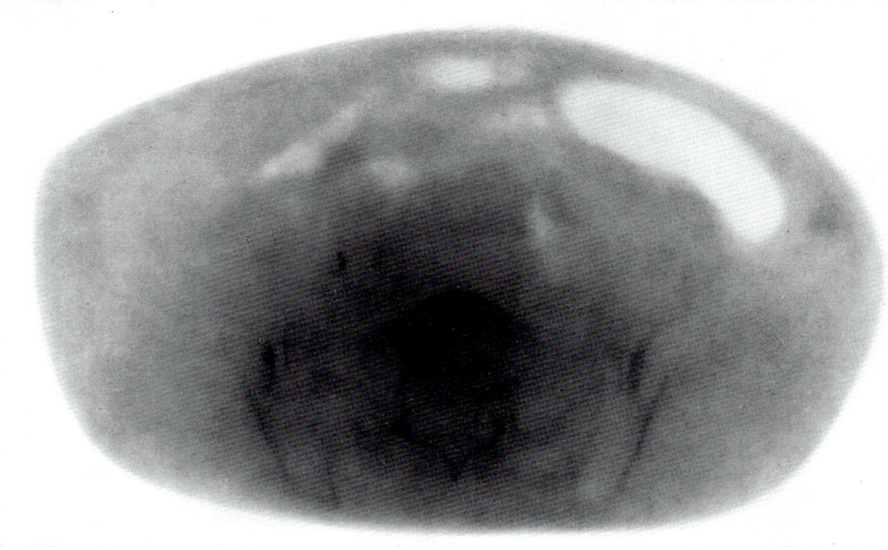

Fig. 382. Axial transverse tomogram

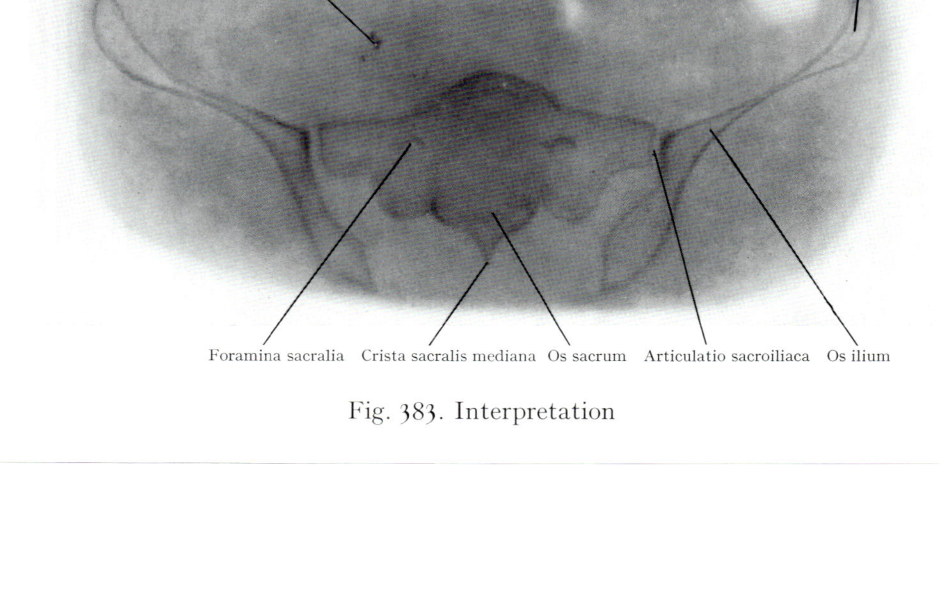

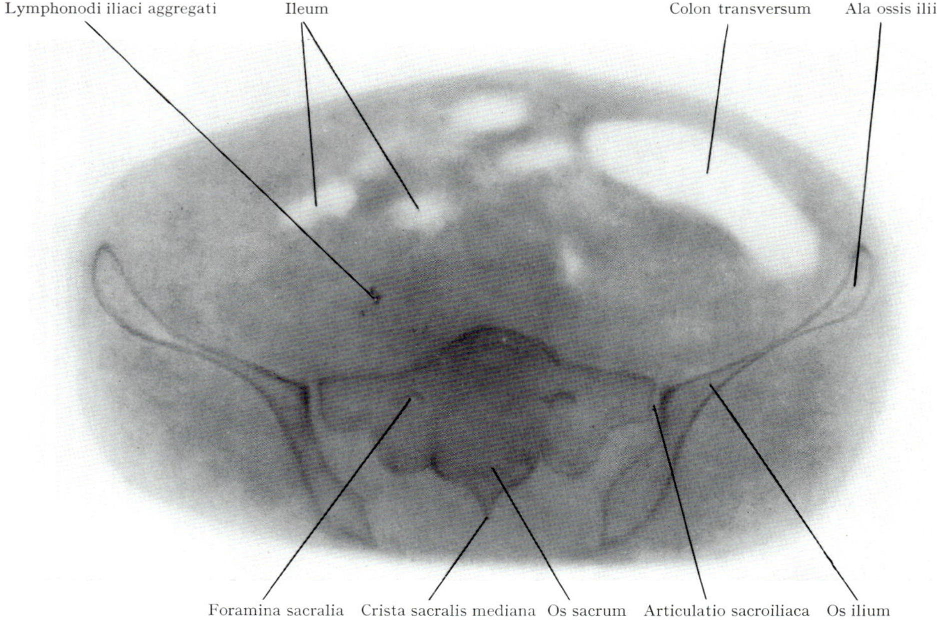

Fig. 383. Interpretation

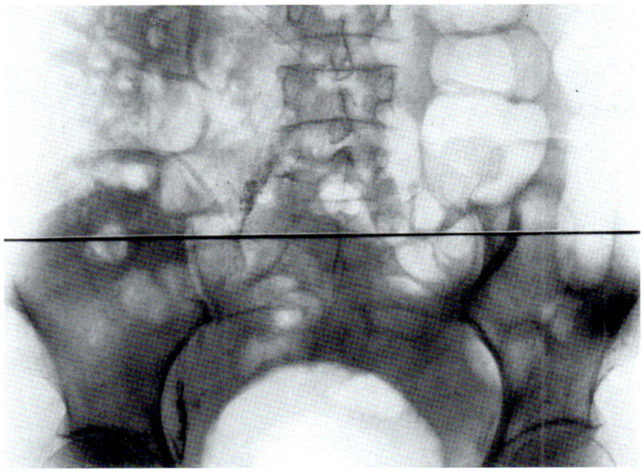

Fig. 384. Normal roentgenogram. Horizontal line showing the level tomographed

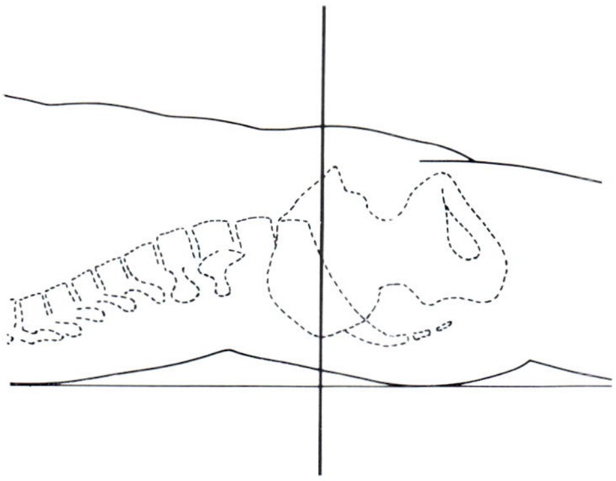

Fig. 385. Schematic drawing of the level tomographed

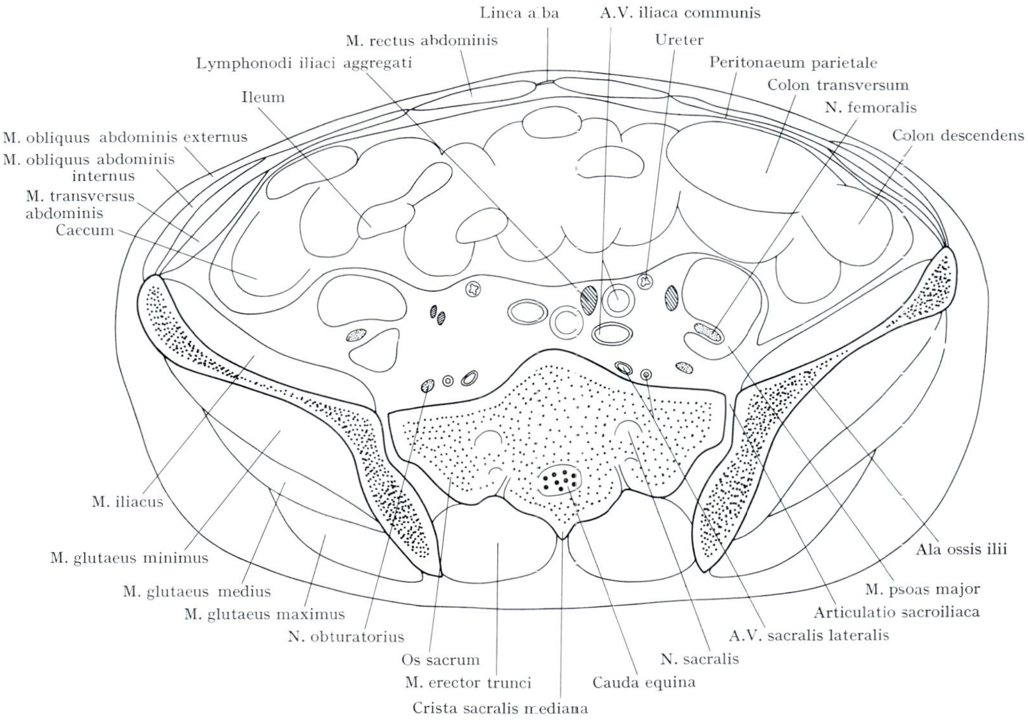

Fig. 386. Anatomical chart

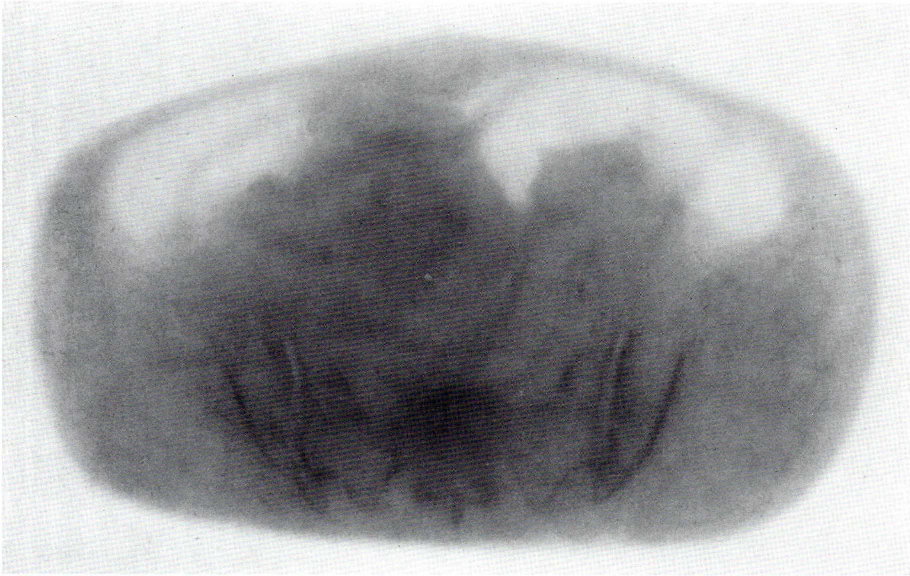

Fig. 387. Axial transverse tomogram

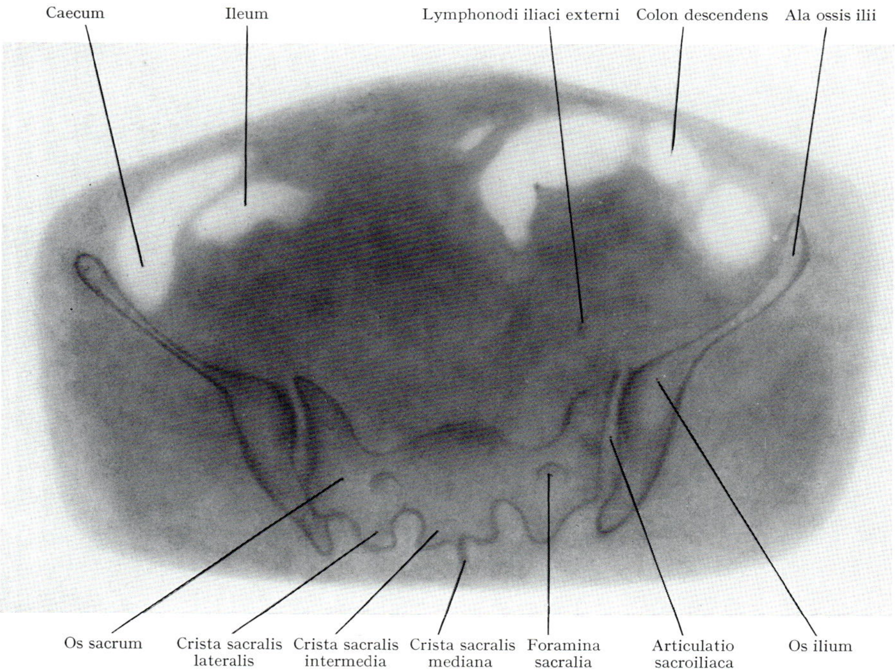

Fig. 388. Interpretation

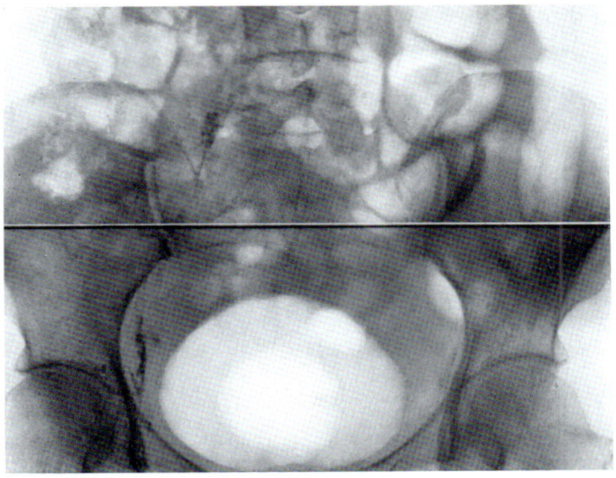

Fig. 389. Normal roentgenogram. Horizontal line showing the level tomographed

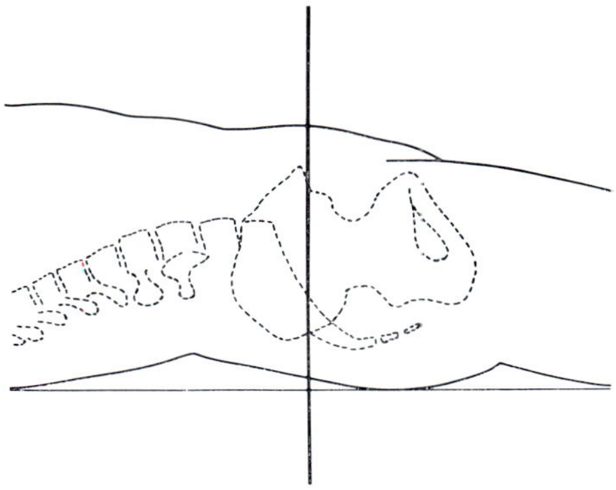

Fig. 390. Schematic drawing of the level tomographed

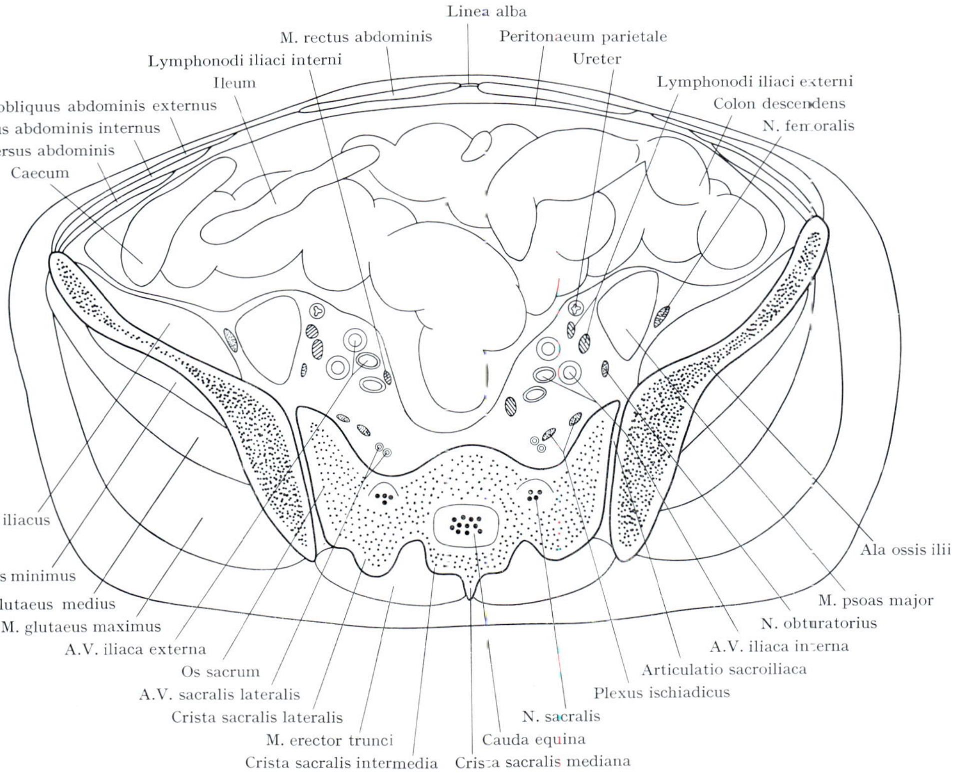

Fig. 391. Anatomical chart

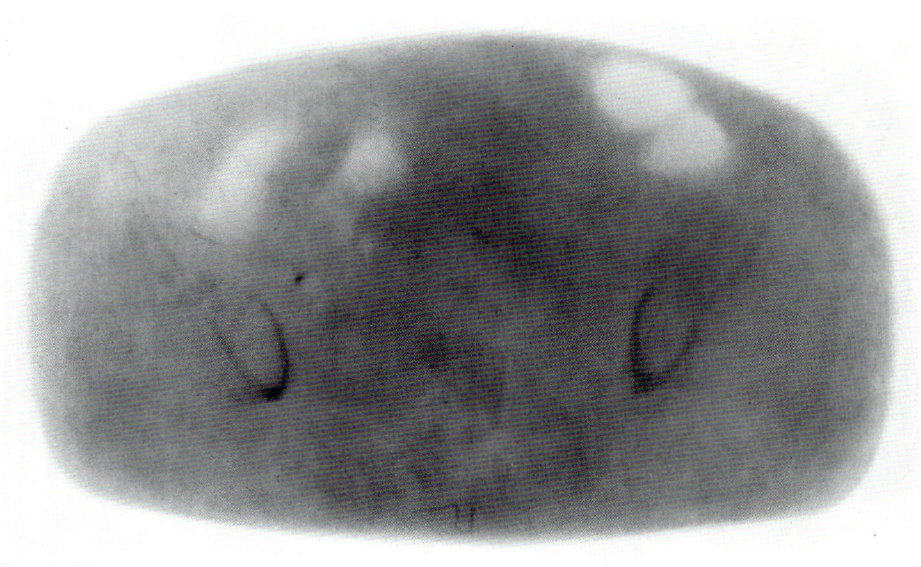

Fig. 392. Axial transverse tomogram

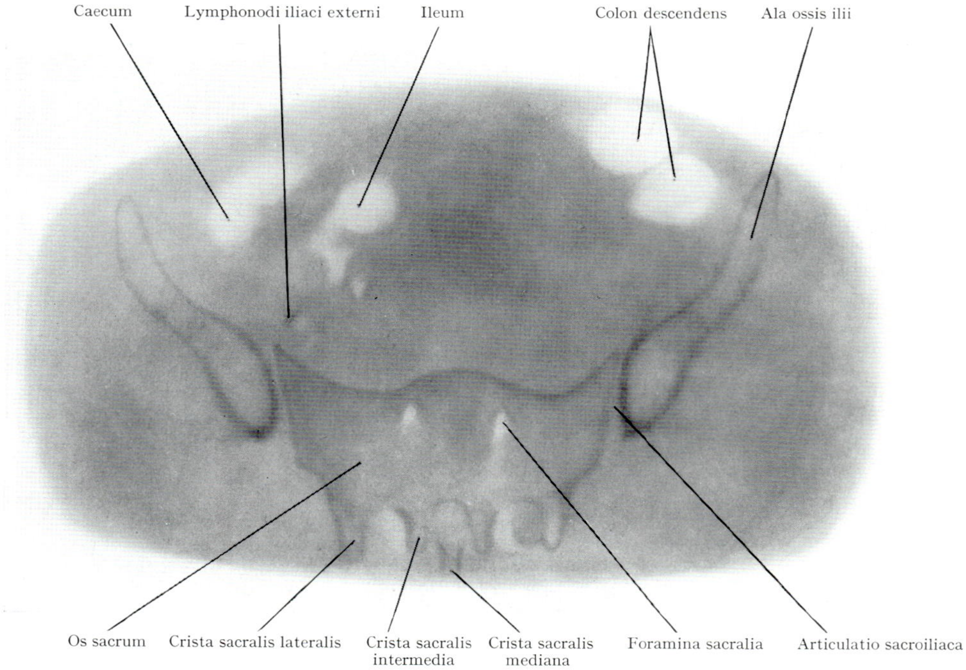

Fig. 393. Interpretation

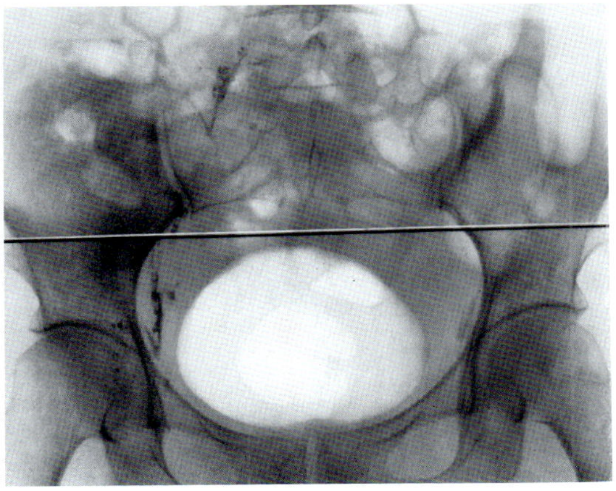

Fig. 394. Normal roentgenogram. Horizontal line showing the level tomographed

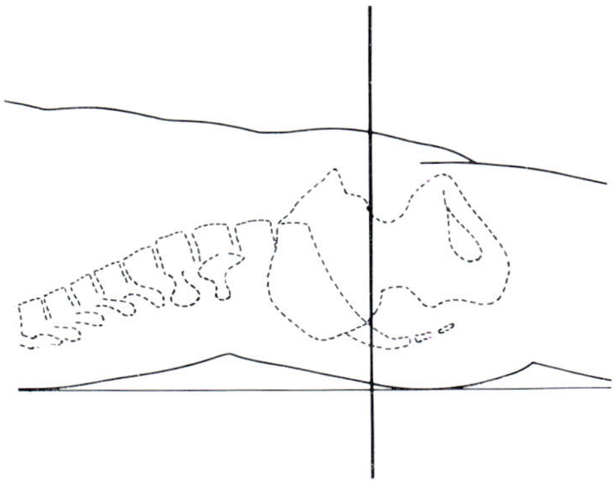

Fig. 395. Schematic drawing of the level tomographed

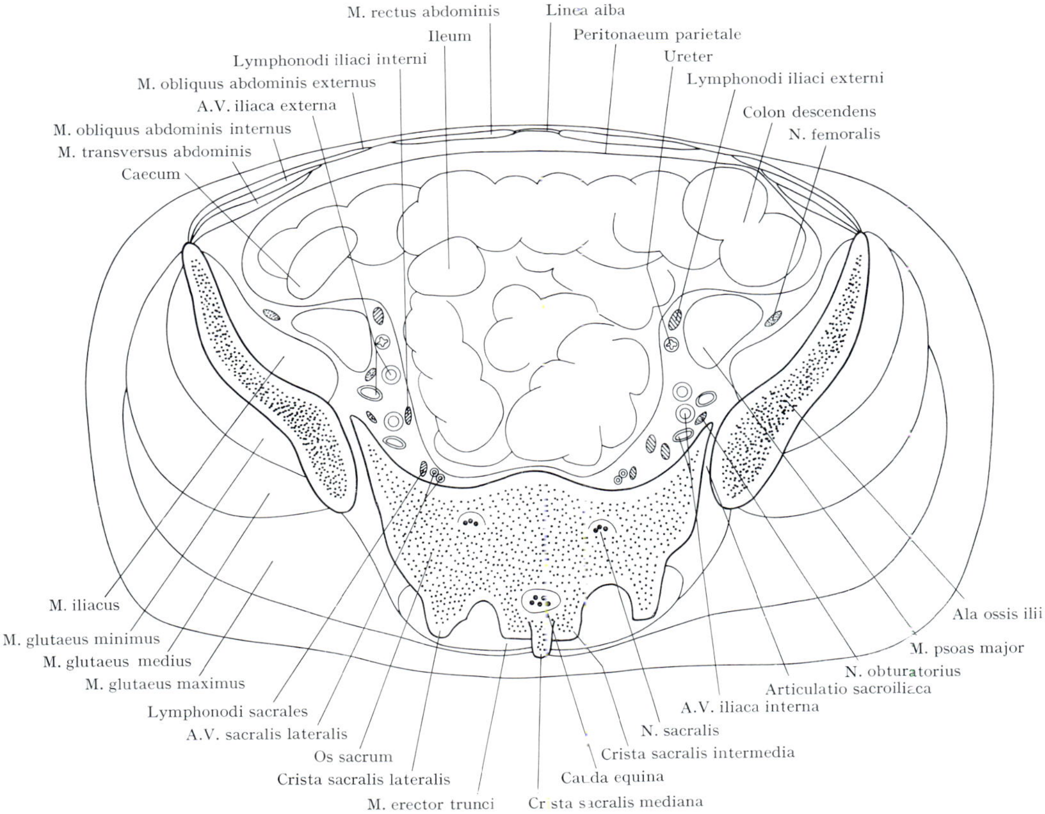

Fig. 396. Anatomical chart

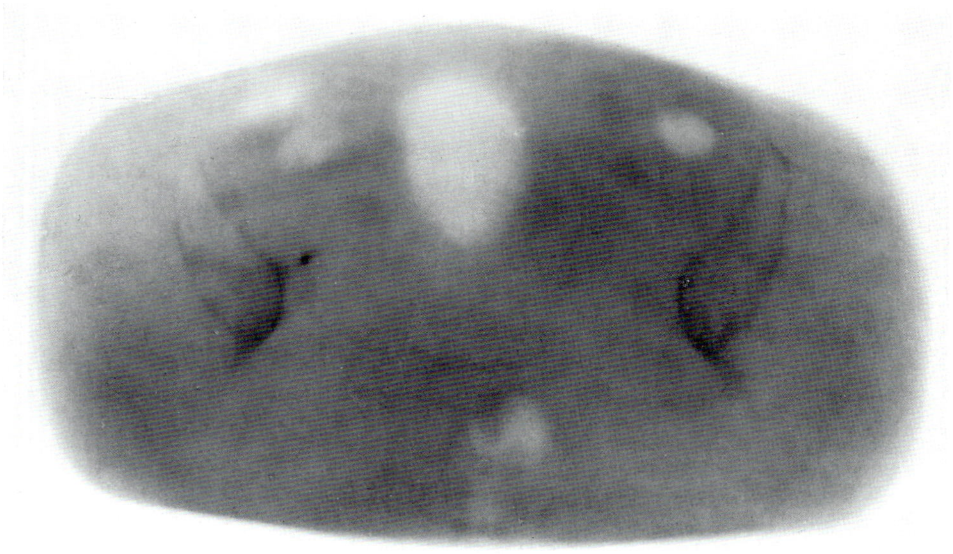

Fig. 397. Axial transverse tomogram

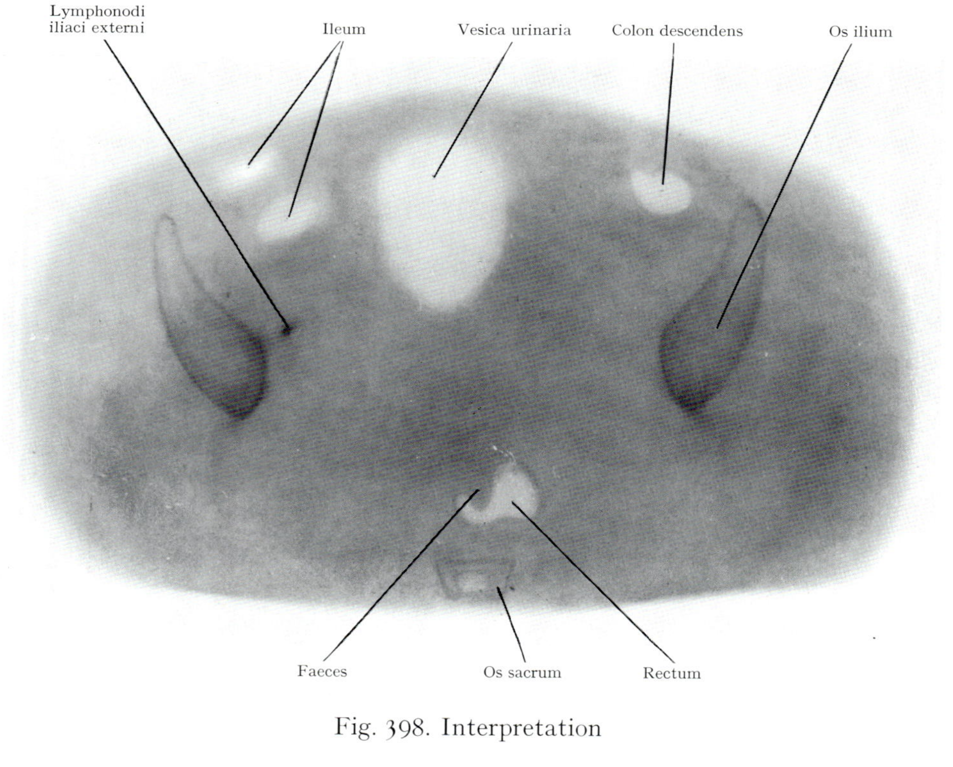

Fig. 398. Interpretation

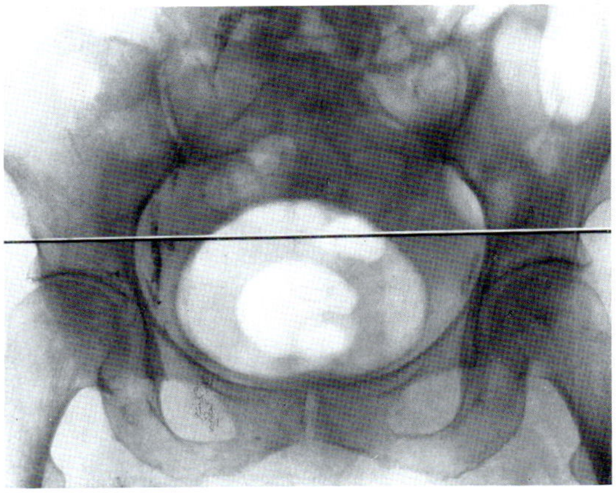

Fig. 399. Normal roentgenogram. Horizontal line showing the level tomographed

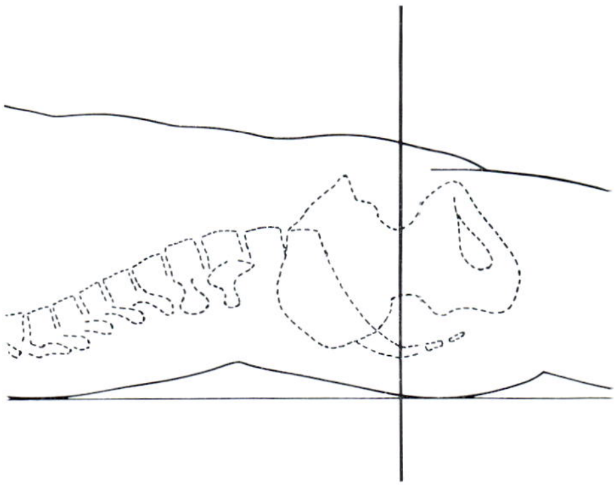

Fig. 400. Schematic drawing of the level tomographed

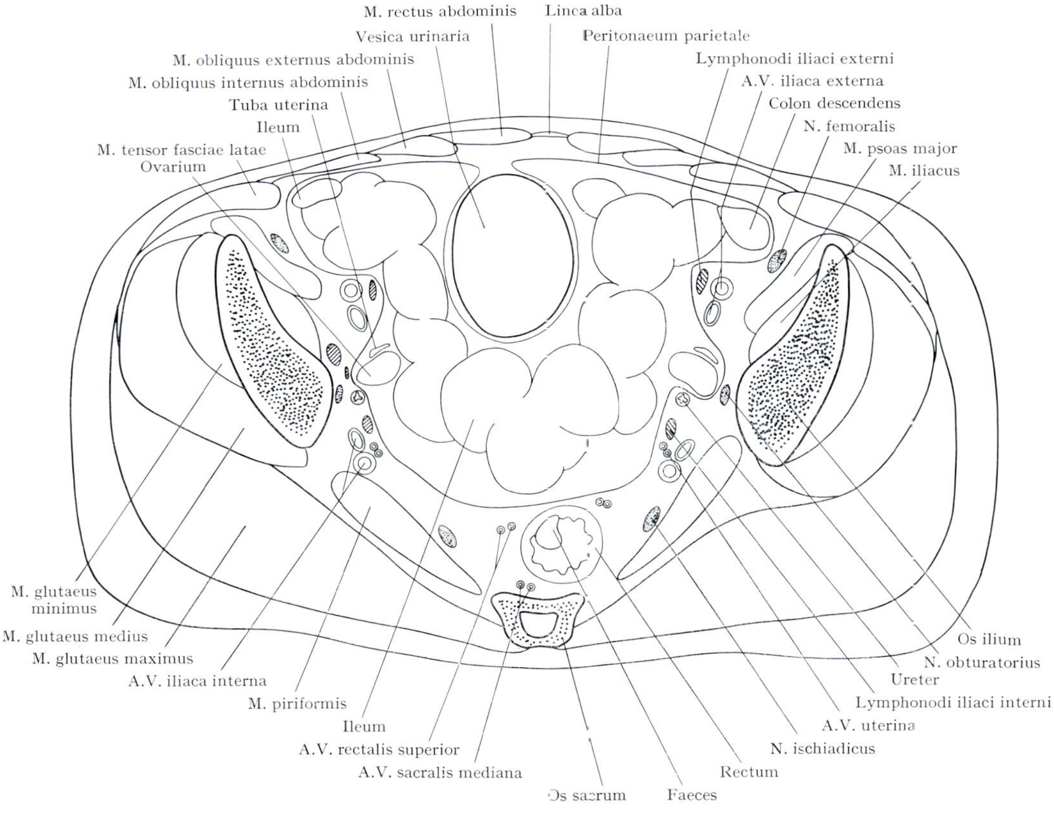

Fig. 401. Anatomical chart

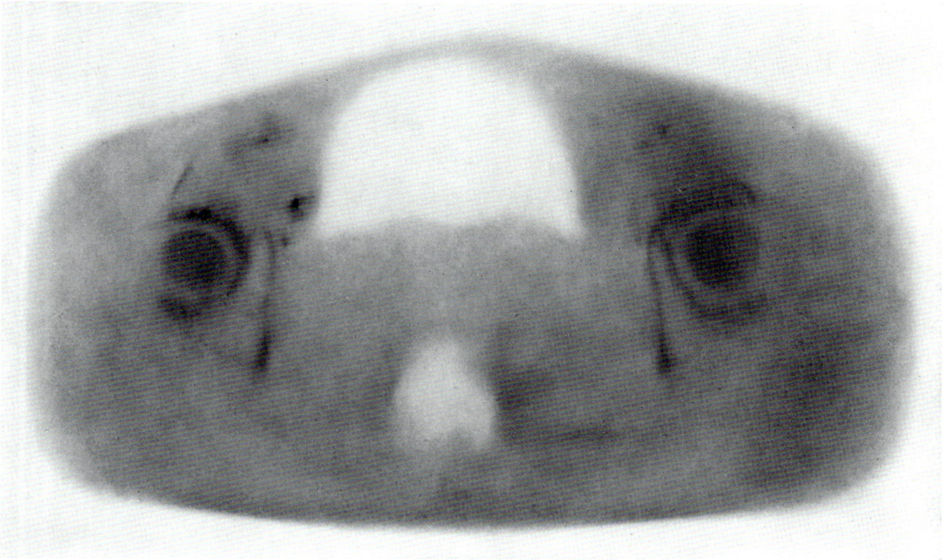

Fig. 402. Axial transverse tomogram

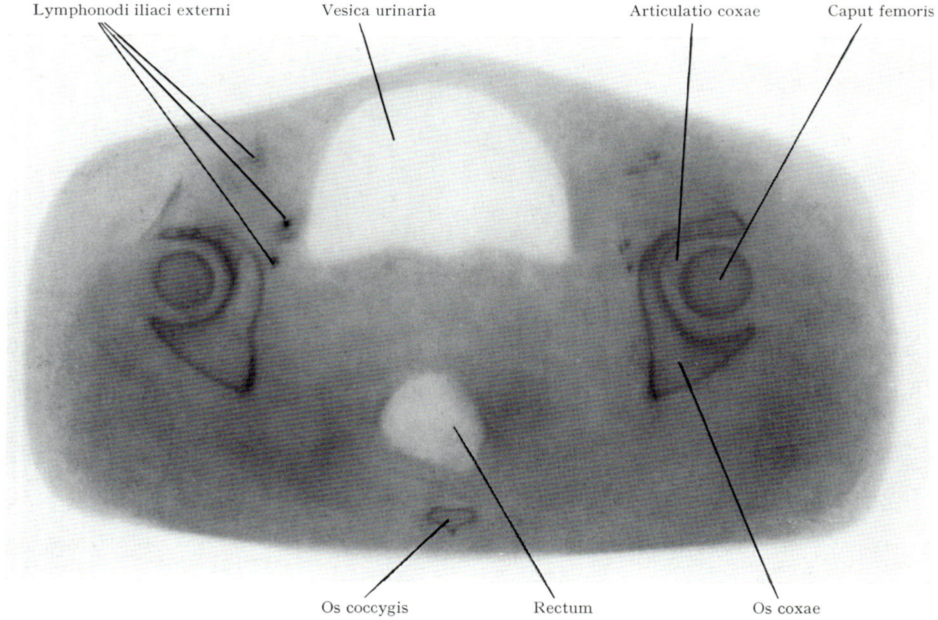

Fig. 403. Interpretation

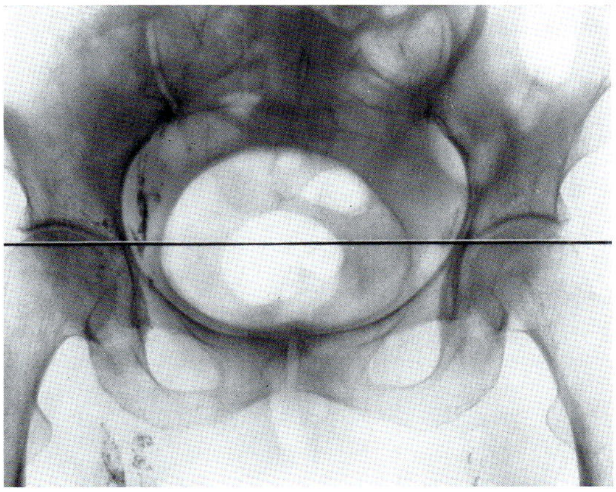

Fig. 404. Normal roentgenogram. Horizontal line showing the level tomographed

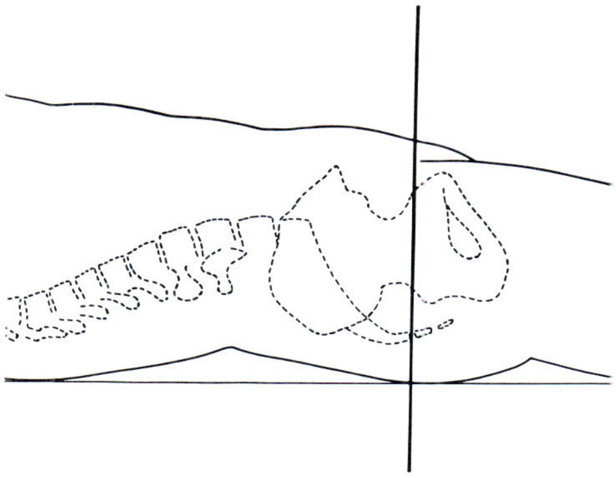

Fig. 405. Schematic drawing of the level tomographed

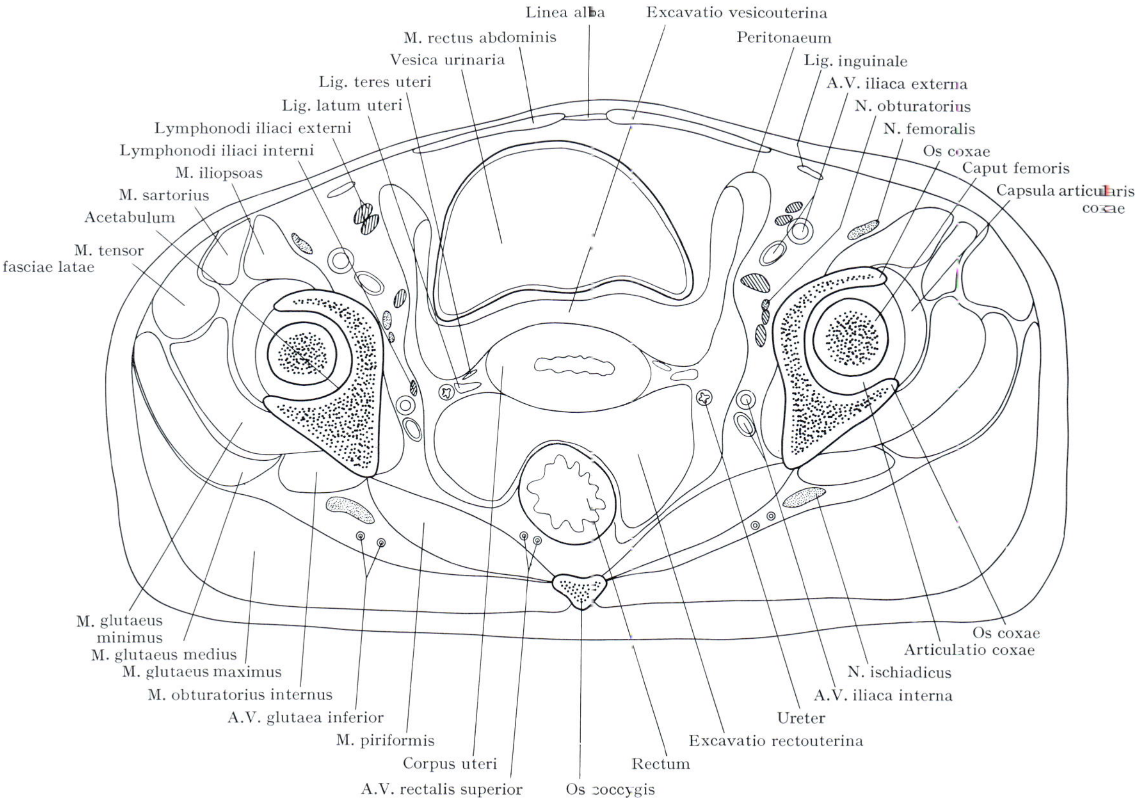

Fig. 406. Anatomical chart

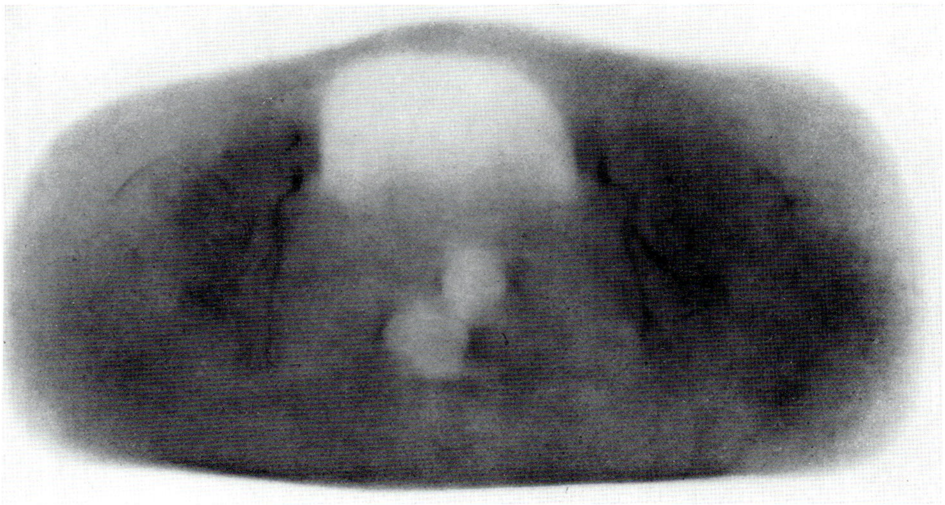

Fig. 407. Axial transverse tomogram

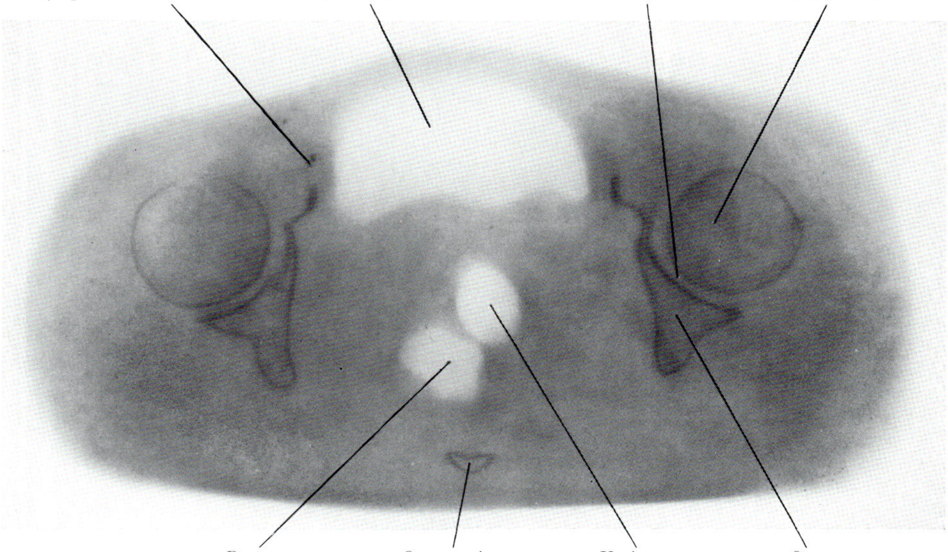

Fig. 408. Interpretation

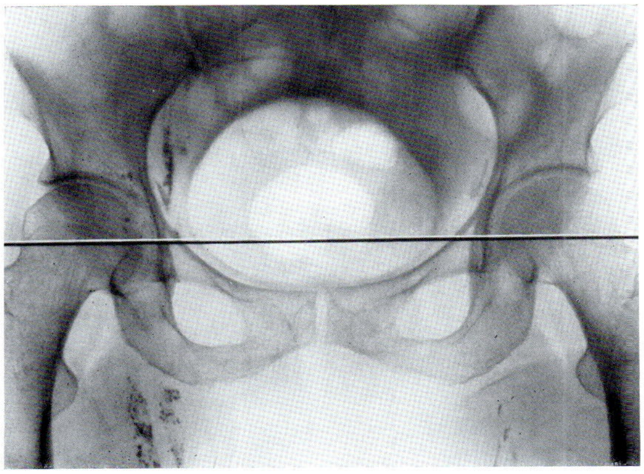

Fig. 409. Normal roentgenogram. Horizontal line showing the level tomographed

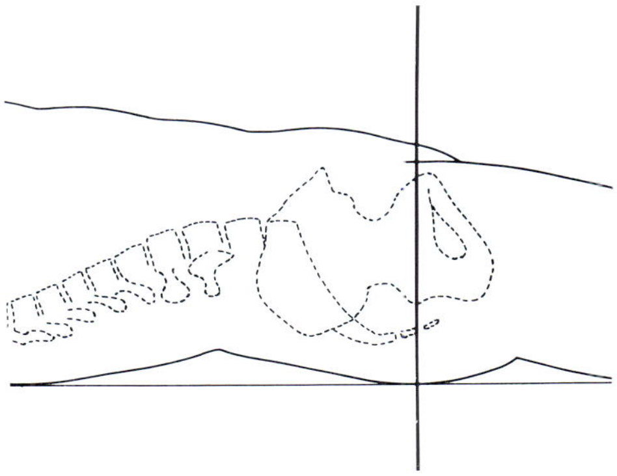

Fig. 410. Schematic drawing of the level tomographed

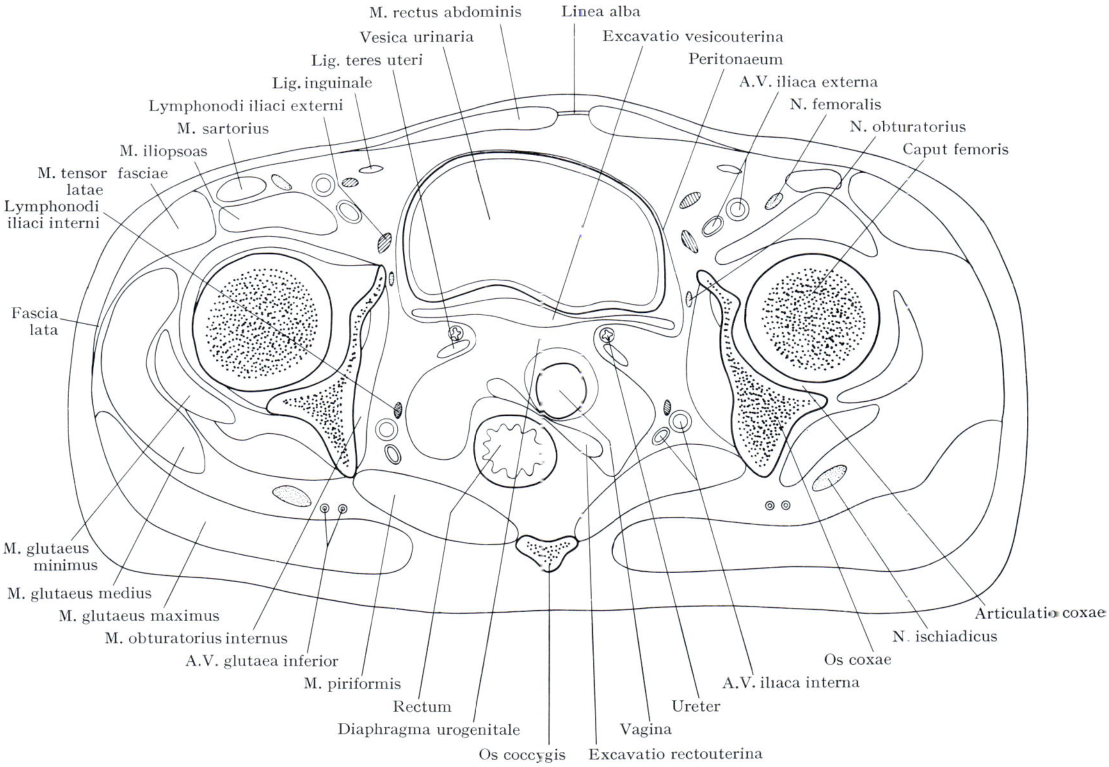

Fig. 411. Anatomical chart

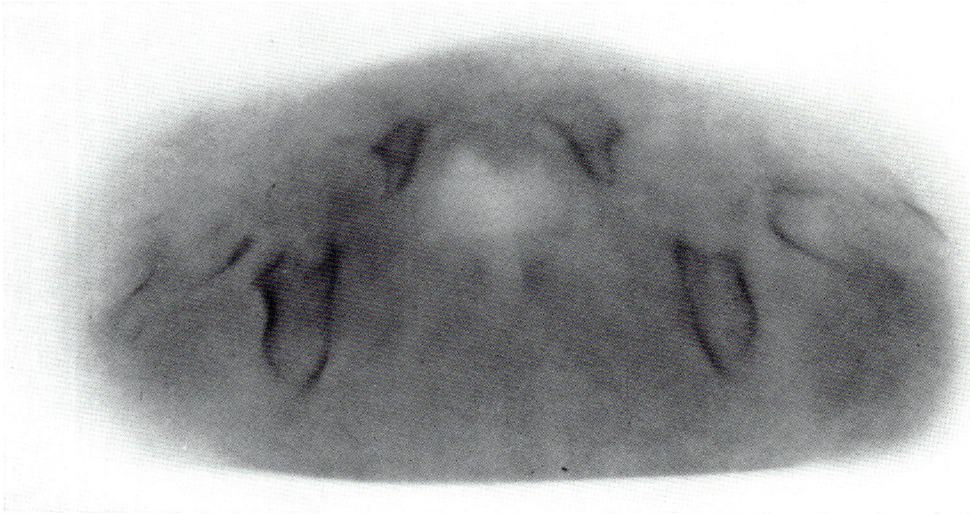

Fig. 412. Axial transverse tomogram

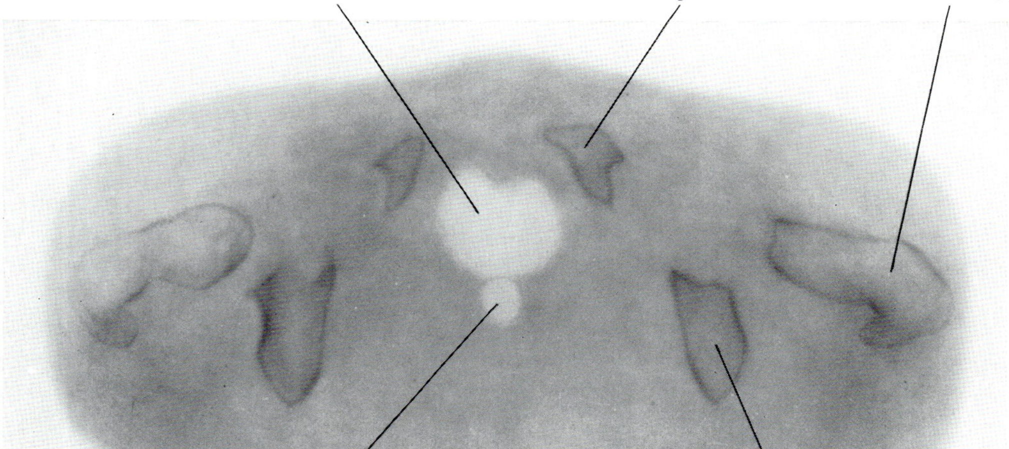

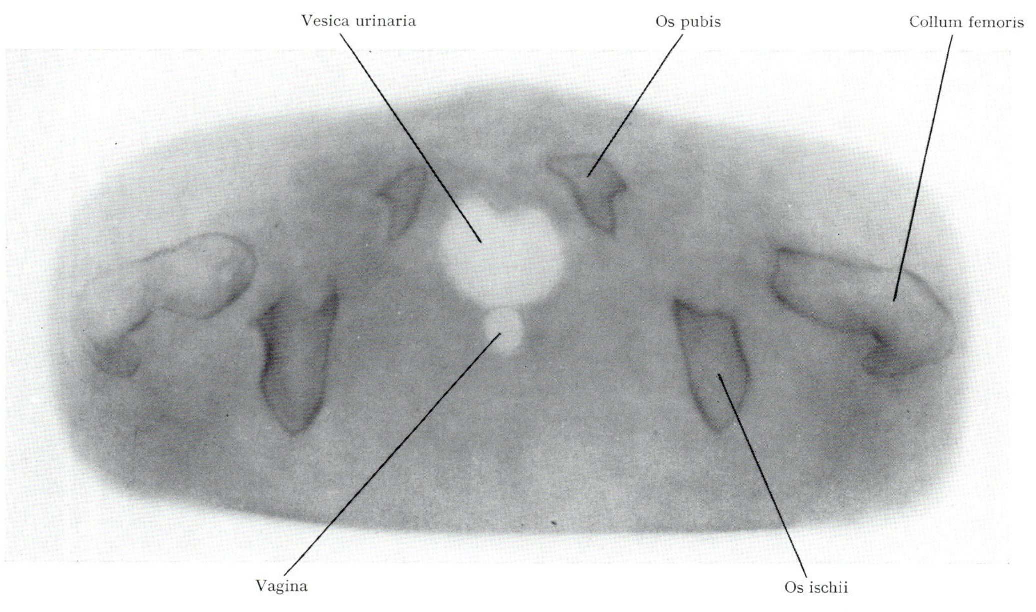

Fig. 413. Interpretation

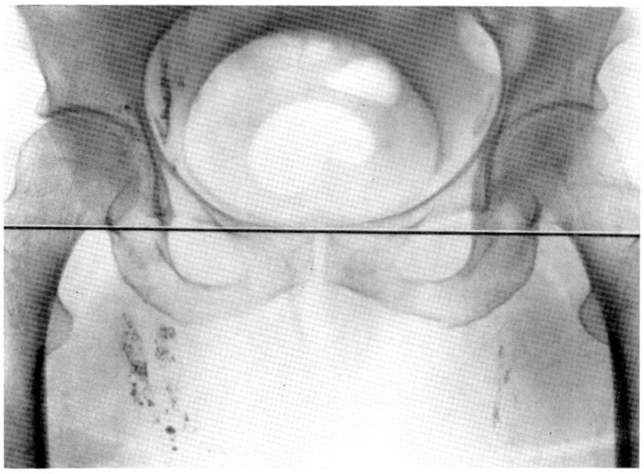

Fig. 414. Normal roentgenogram. Horizontal line showing the level tomographed

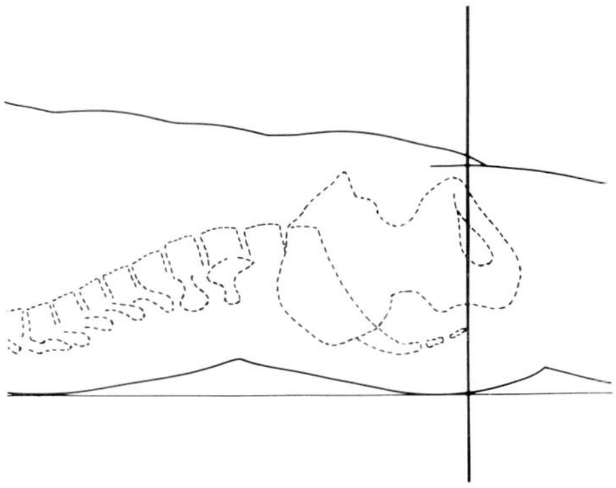

Fig. 415. Schematic drawing of the level tomographed

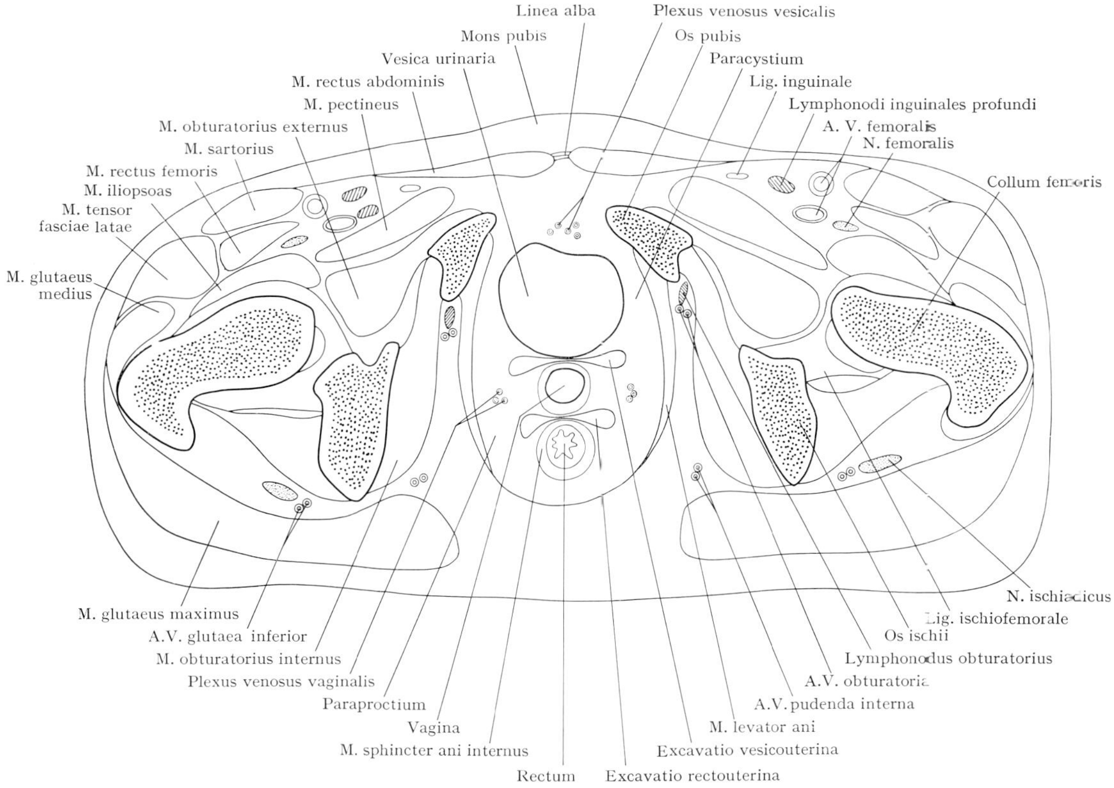

Fig. 416. Anatomical chart

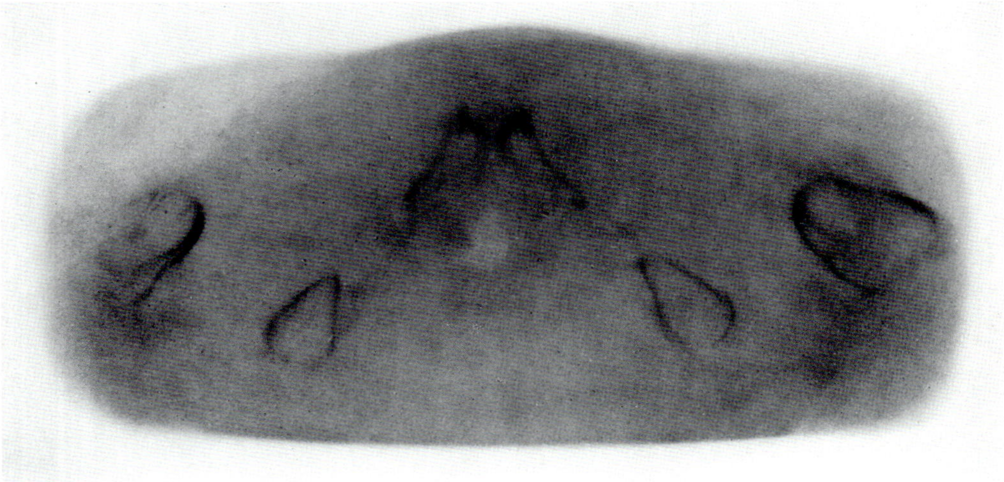

Fig. 417. Axial transverse tomogram

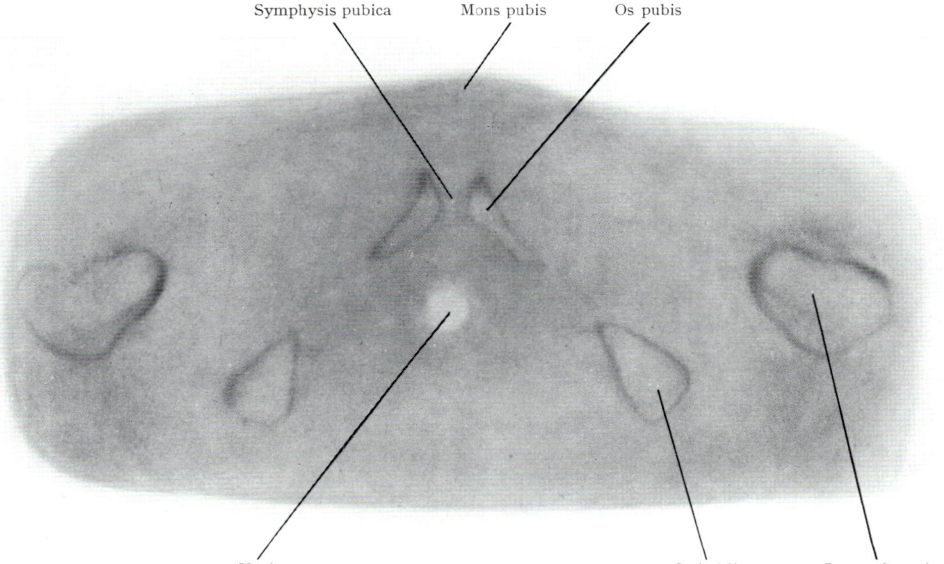

Fig. 418. Interpretation

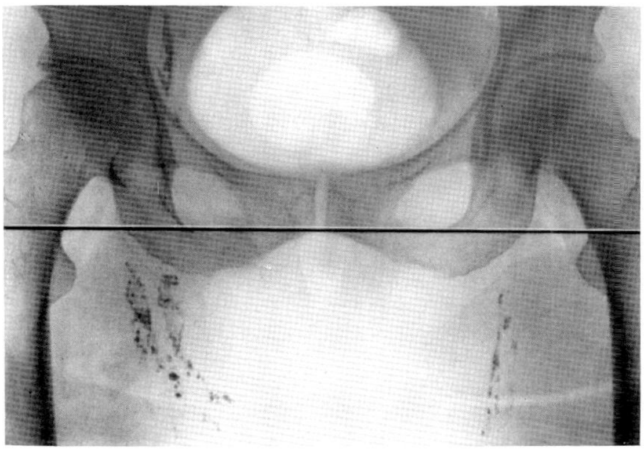

Fig. 419. Normal roentgenogram. Horizontal line showing the level tomographed

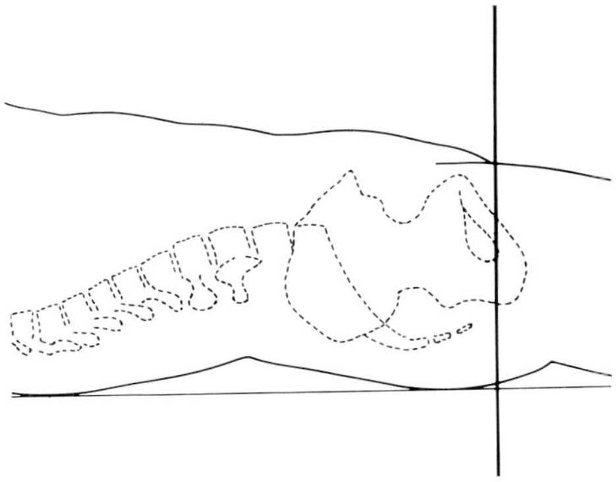

Fig. 420. Schematic drawing of the level tomographed

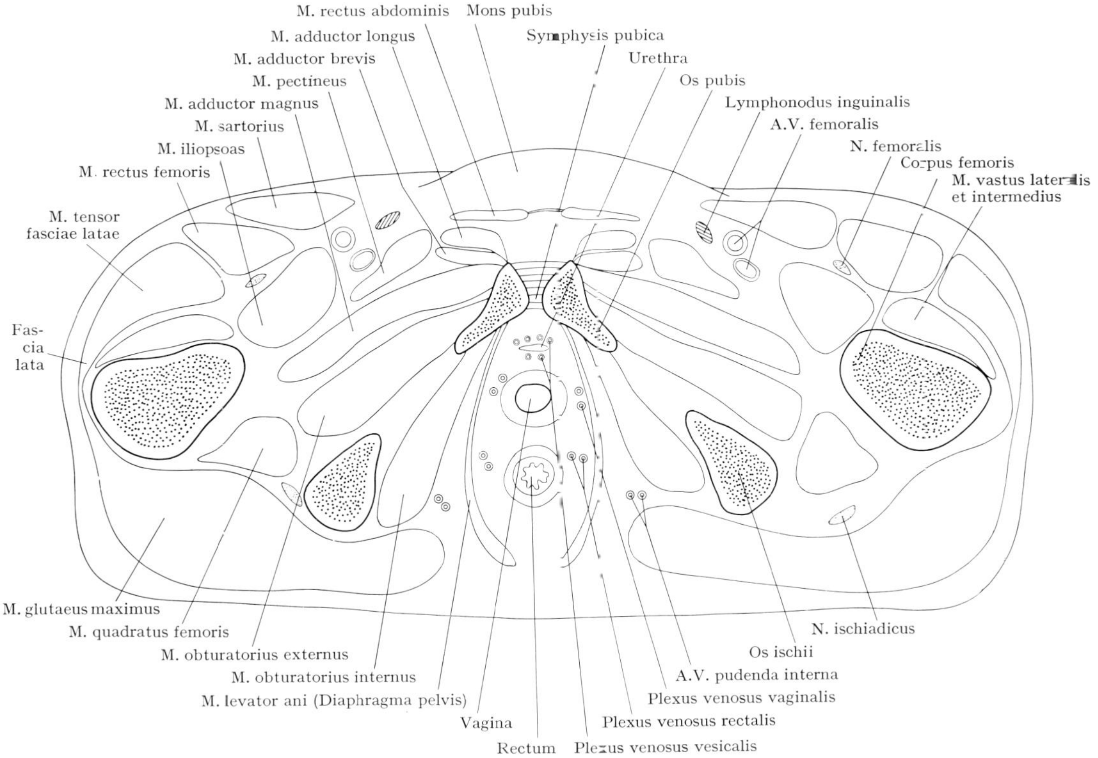

Fig. 421. Anatomical chart

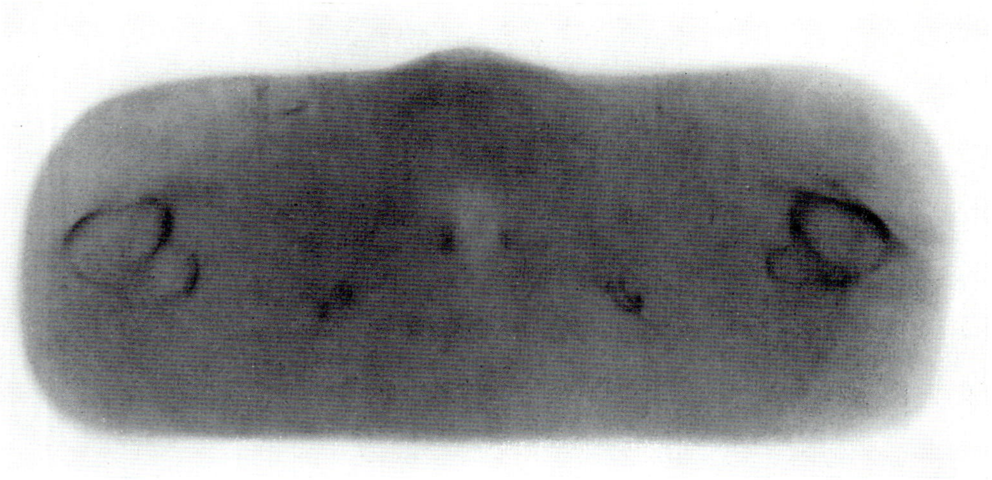

Fig. 422. Axial transverse tomogram

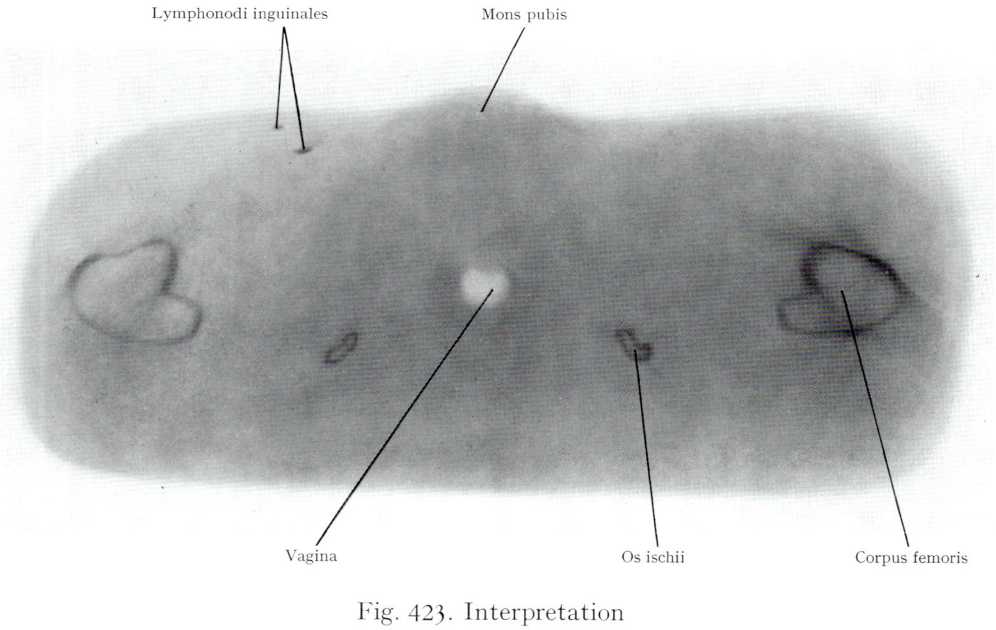

Fig. 423. Interpretation

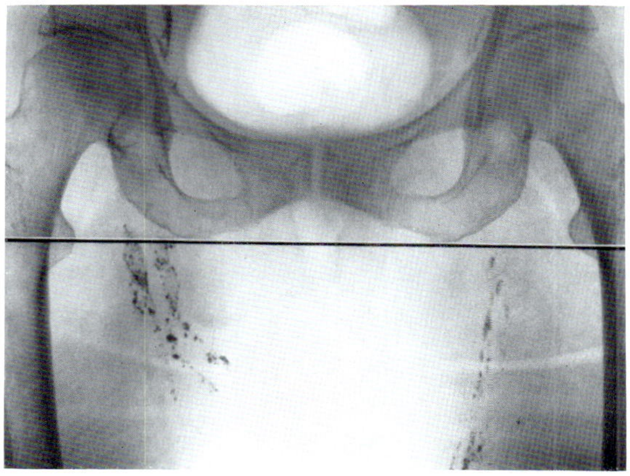

Fig. 424. Normal roentgenogram. Horizontal line showing the level tomographed

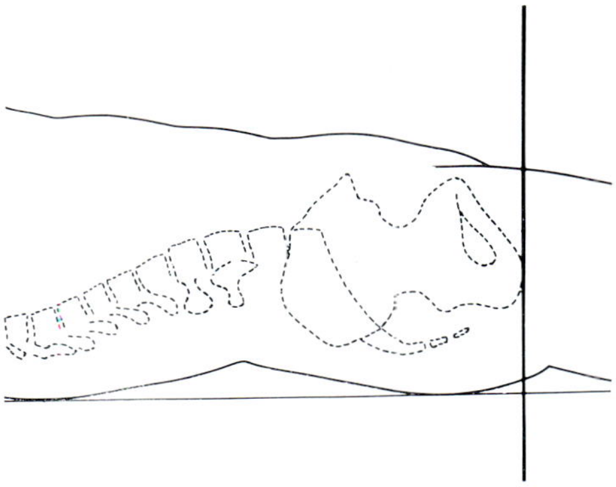

Fig. 425. Schematic drawing of the level tomographed

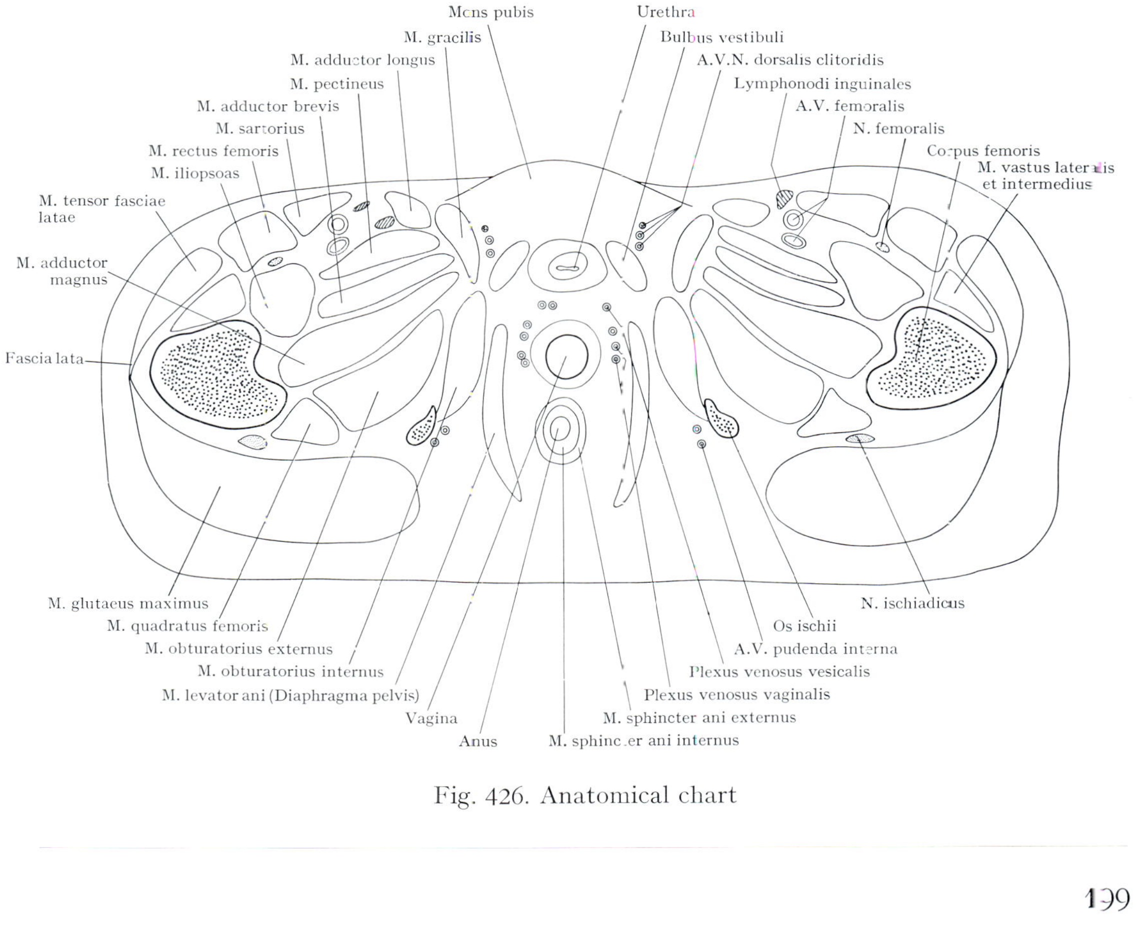

Fig. 426. Anatomical chart

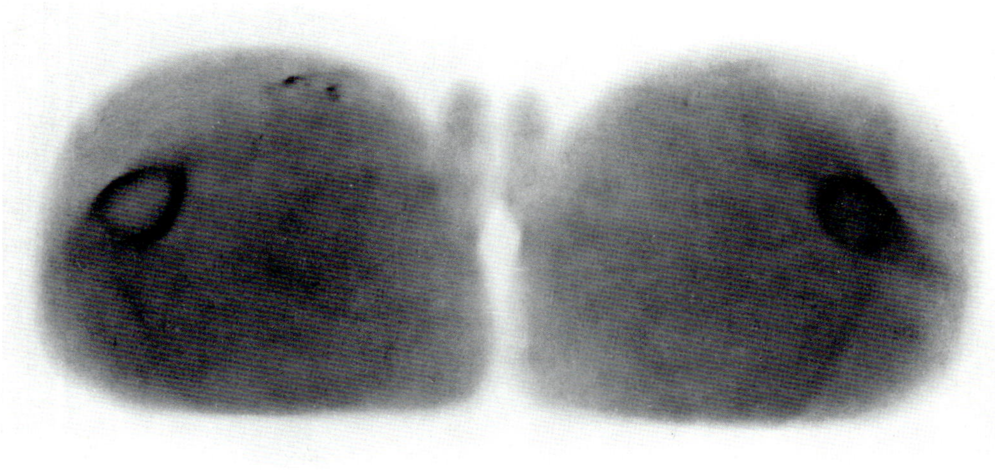

Fig. 427. Axial transverse tomogram

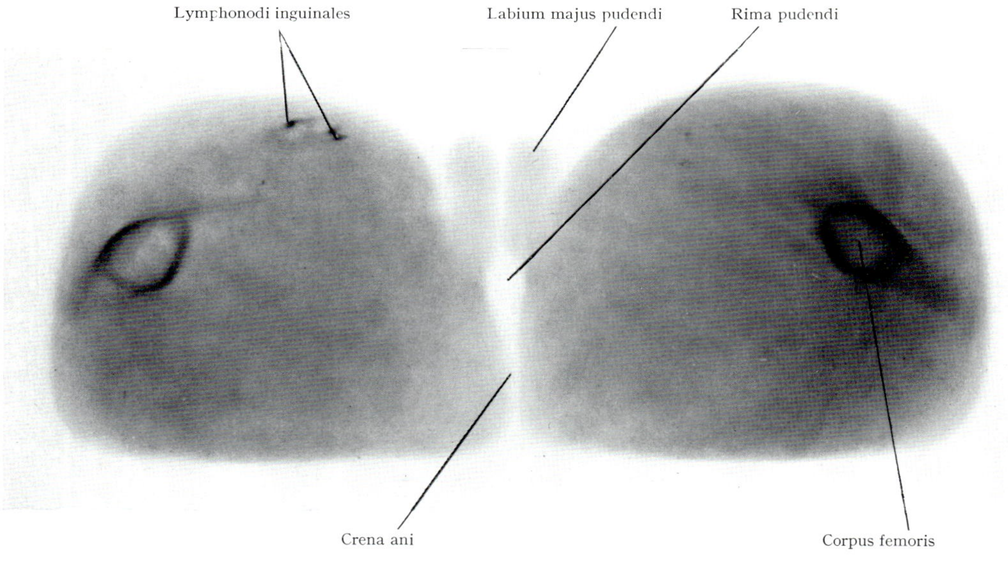

Fig. 428. Interpretation

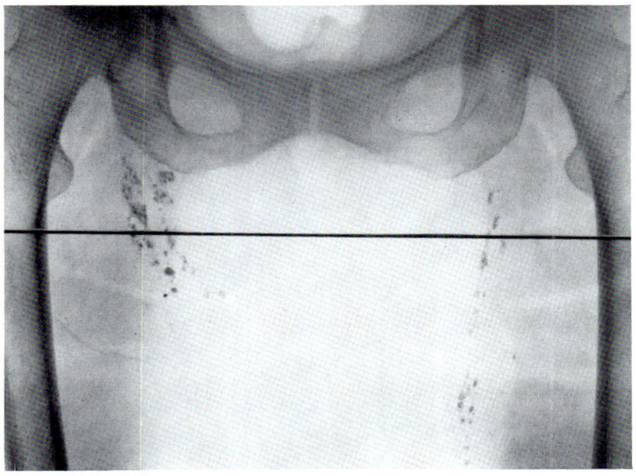

Fig. 429. Normal roentgenogram. Horizontal line showing the level tomographed

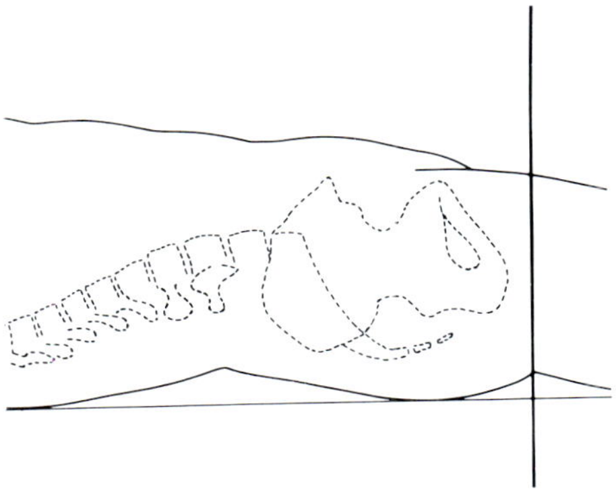

Fig. 430. Schematic drawing of the level tomographed

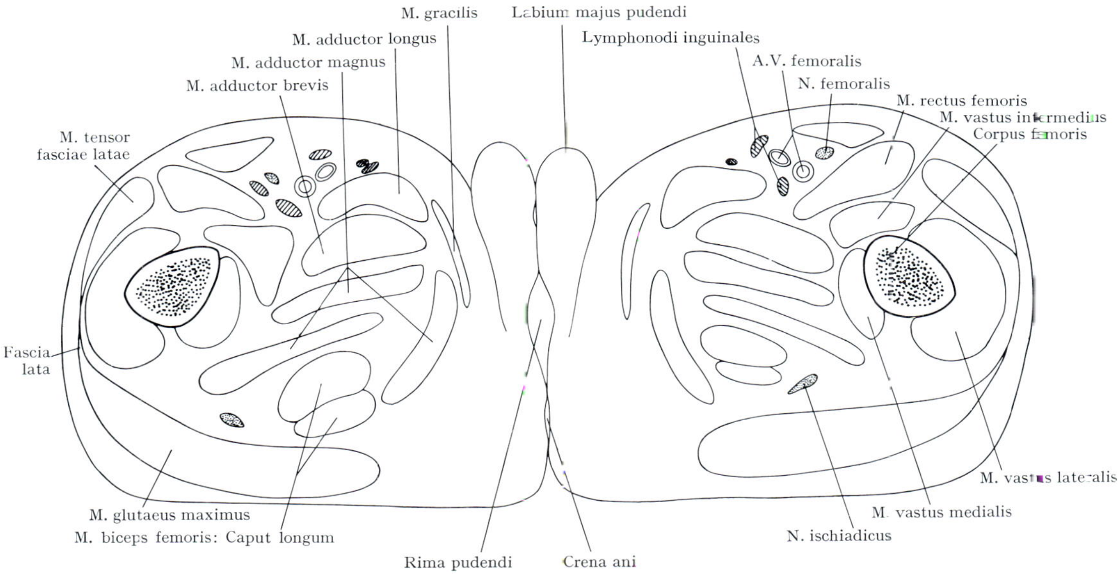

Fig. 431. Anatomical chart

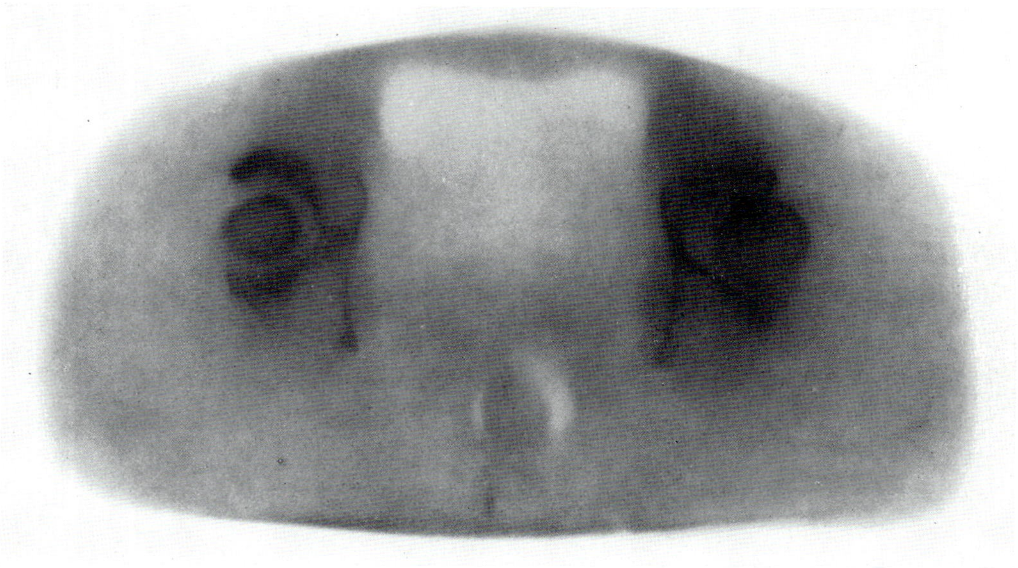

Fig. 432. Axial transverse tomogram

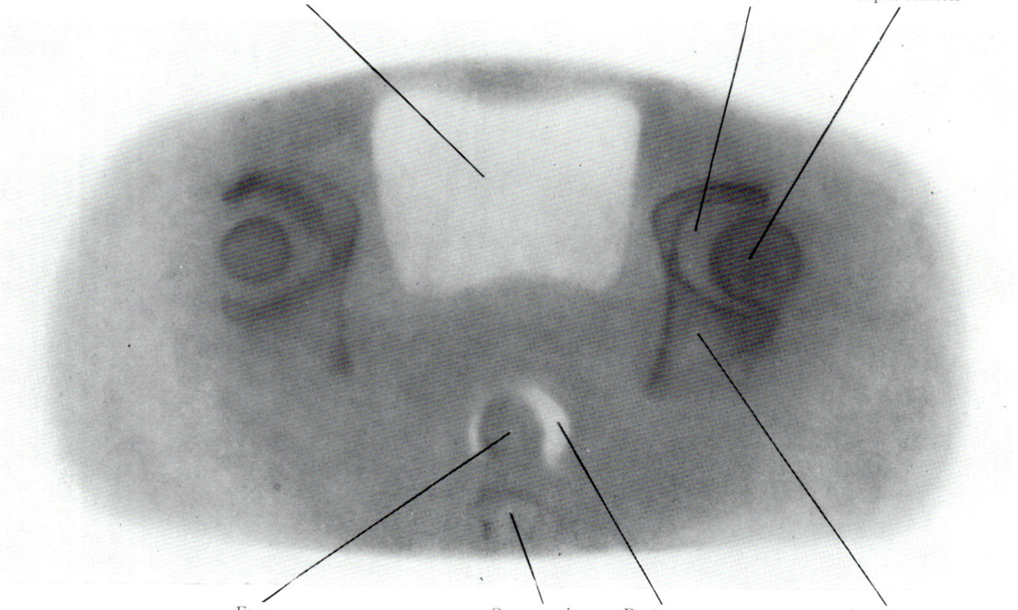

Fig. 433. Interpretation

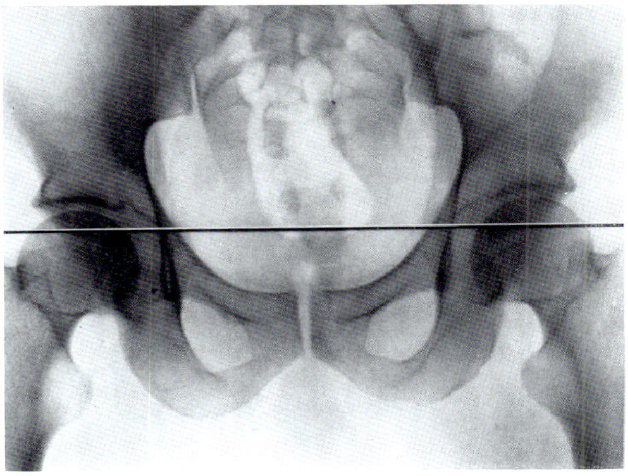

Fig. 434. Normal roentgenogram. Horizontal line showing the level tomographed

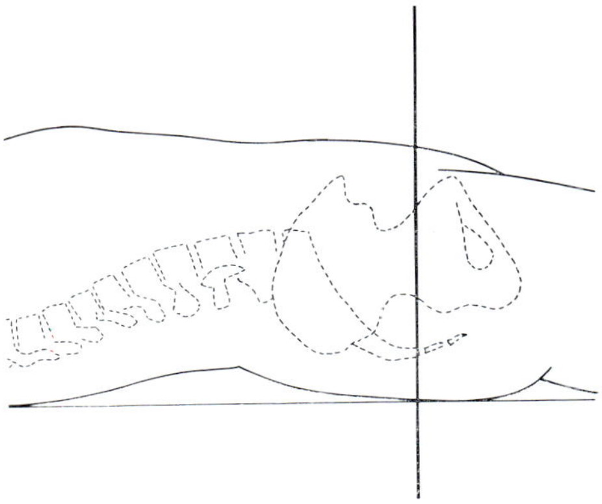

Fig. 435. Schematic drawing of the level tomographed

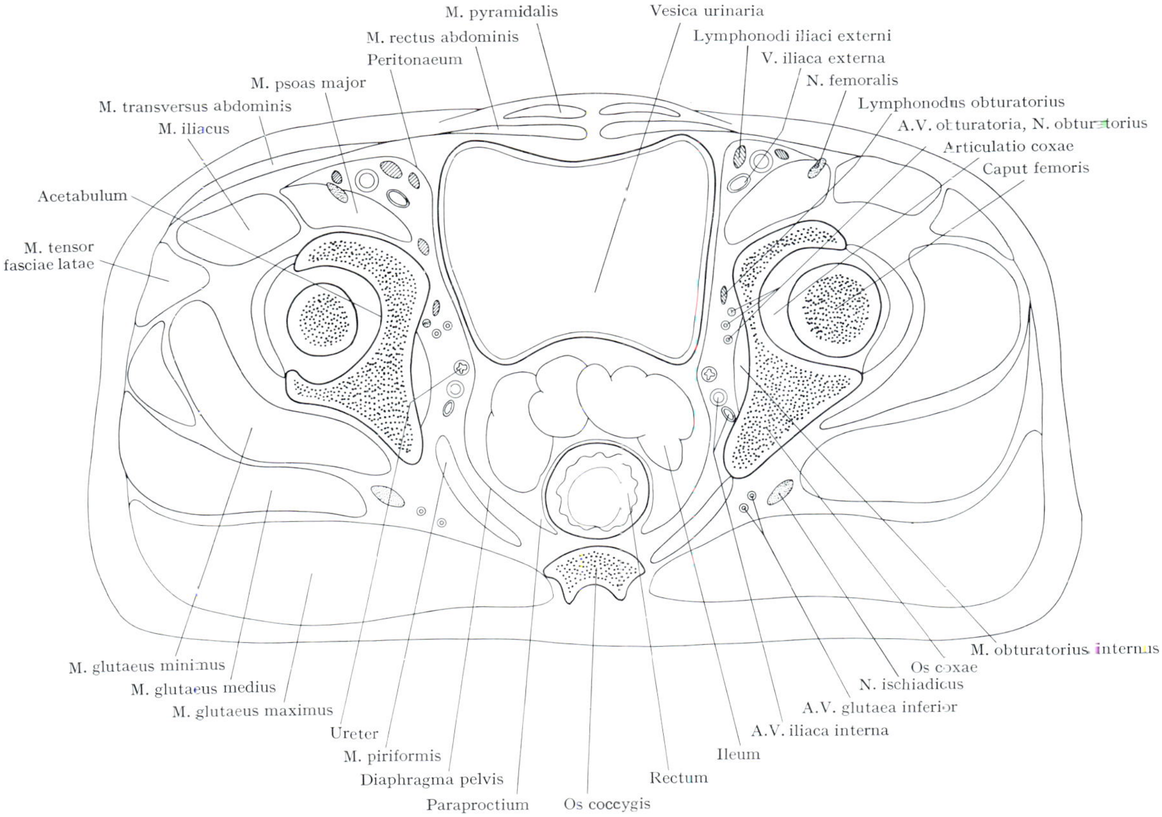

Fig. 436. Anatomical chart

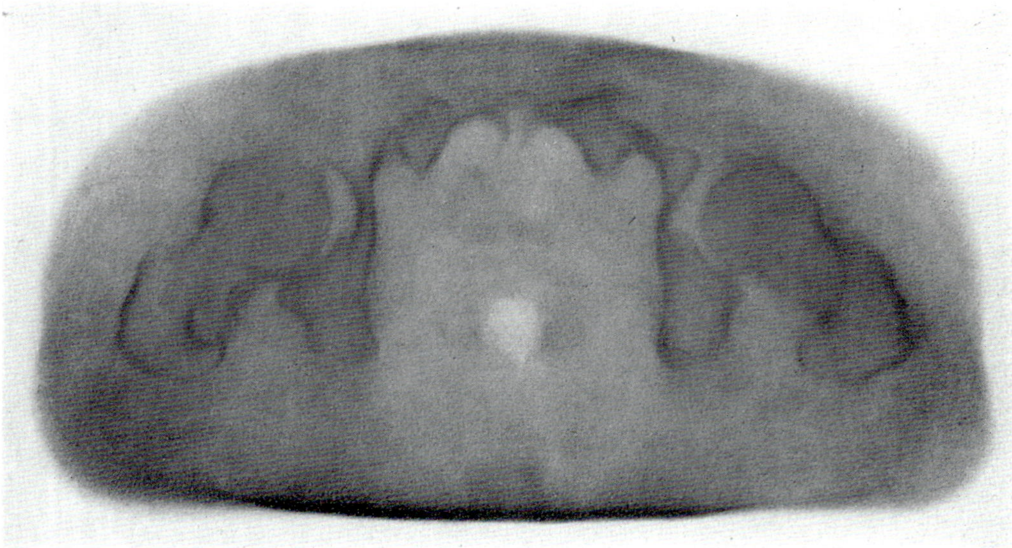

Fig. 437. Axial transverse tomogram

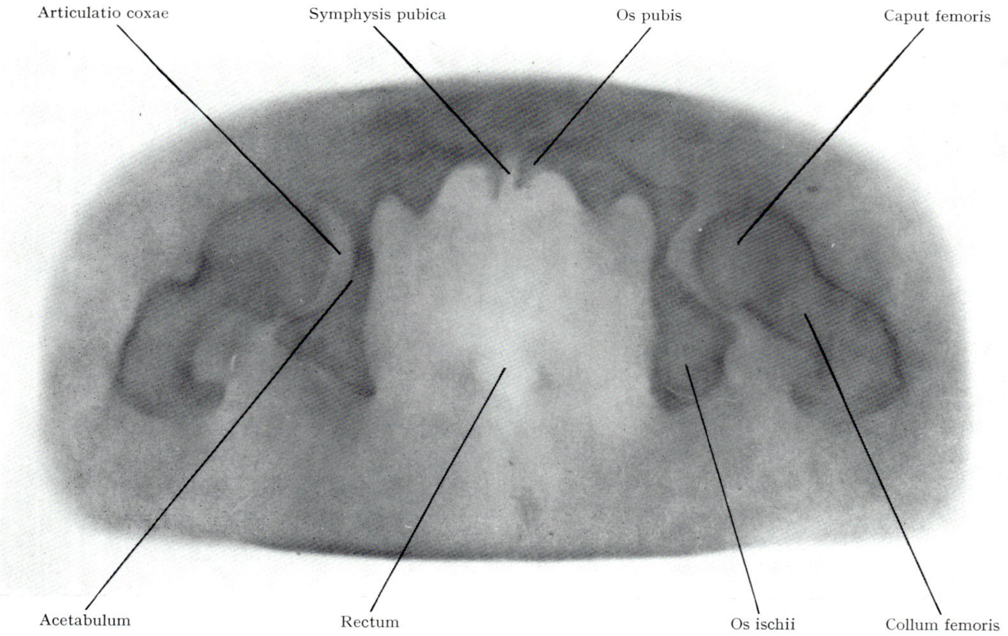

Fig. 438. Interpretation

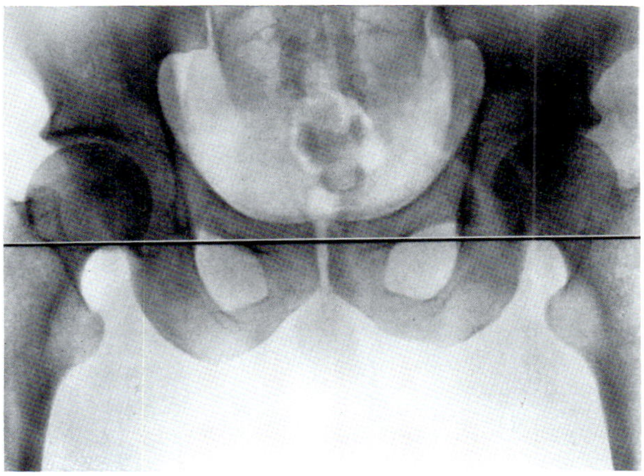

Fig. 439. Normal roentgenogram. Horizontal line showing the level tomographed

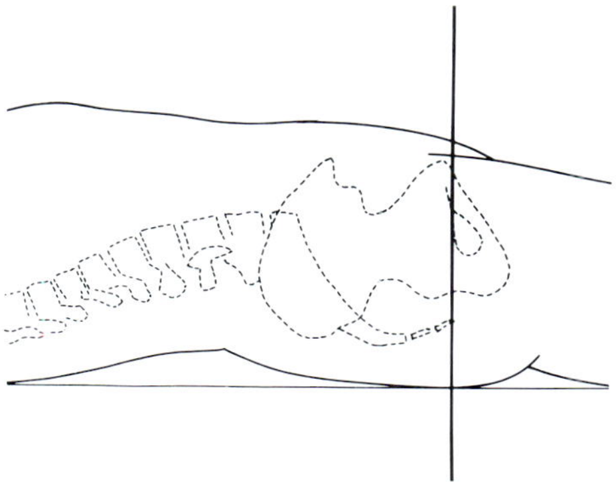

Fig. 440. Schematic drawing of the level tomographed

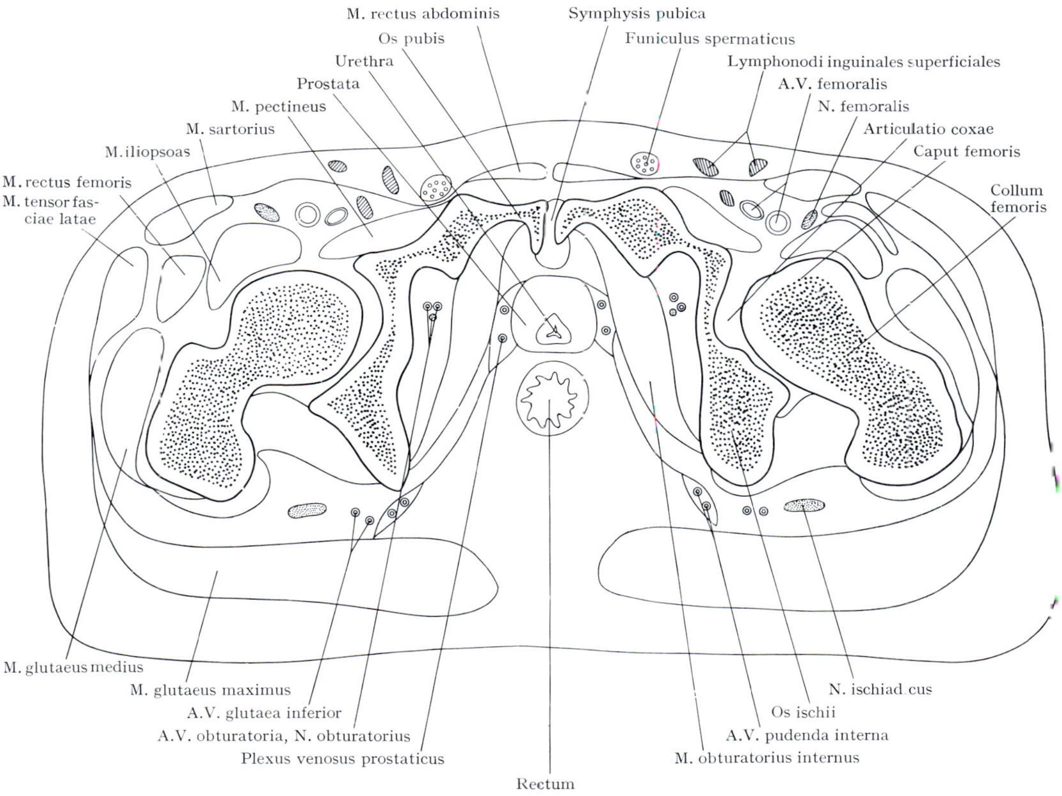

Fig. 441. Anatomical chart

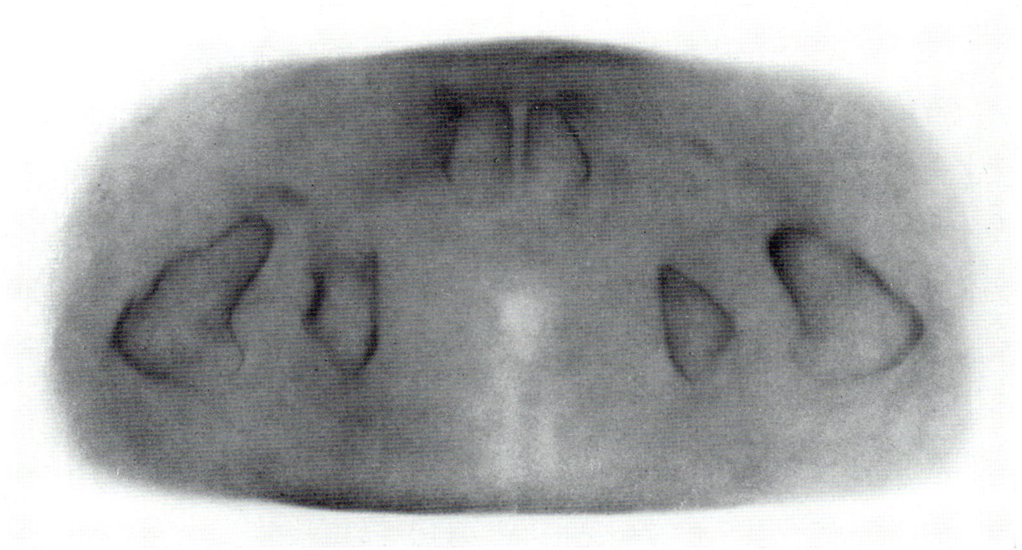

Fig. 442. Axial transverse tomogram

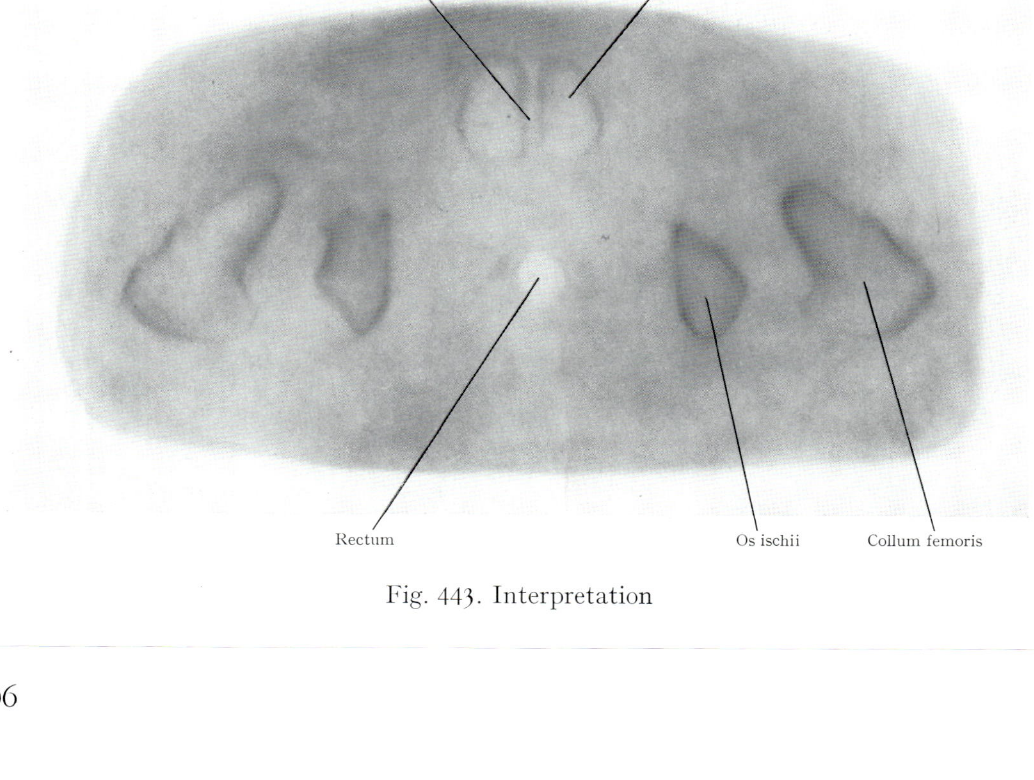

Fig. 443. Interpretation

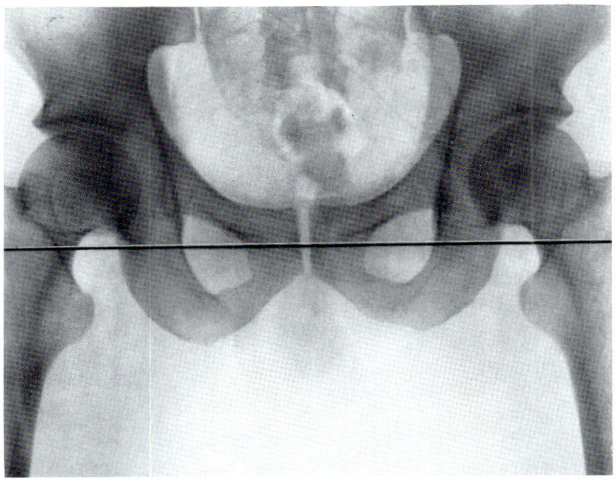

Fig. 444. Normal roentgenogram. Horizontal line showing the level tomographed

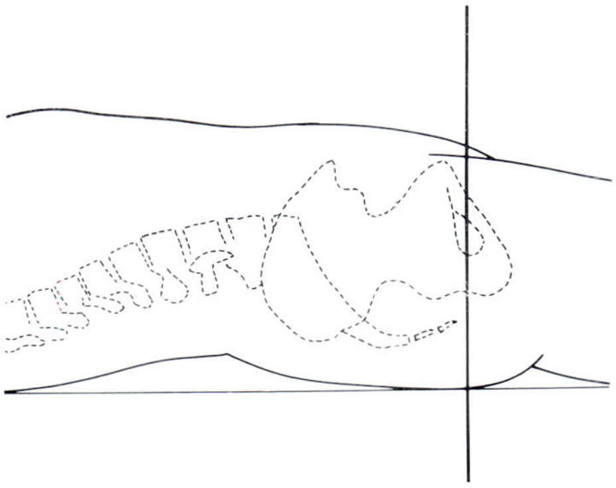

Fig. 445. Schematic illustration of the level tomographed

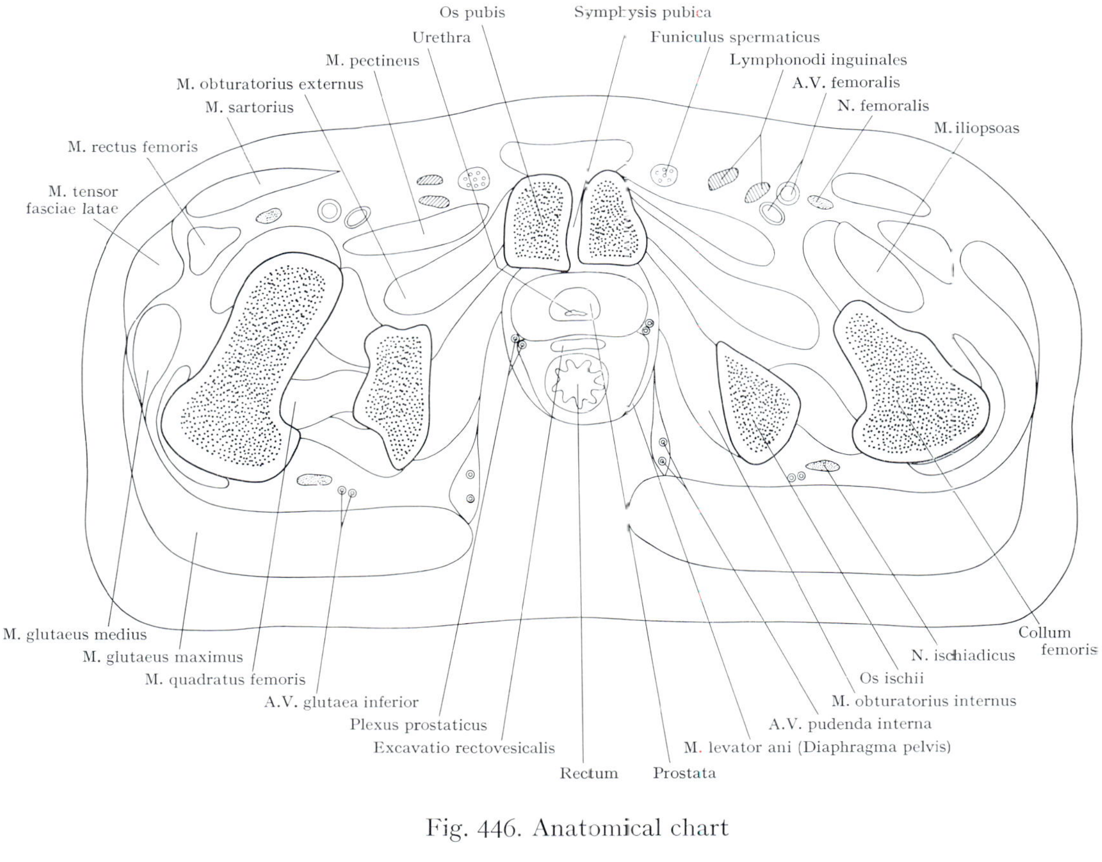

Fig. 446. Anatomical chart

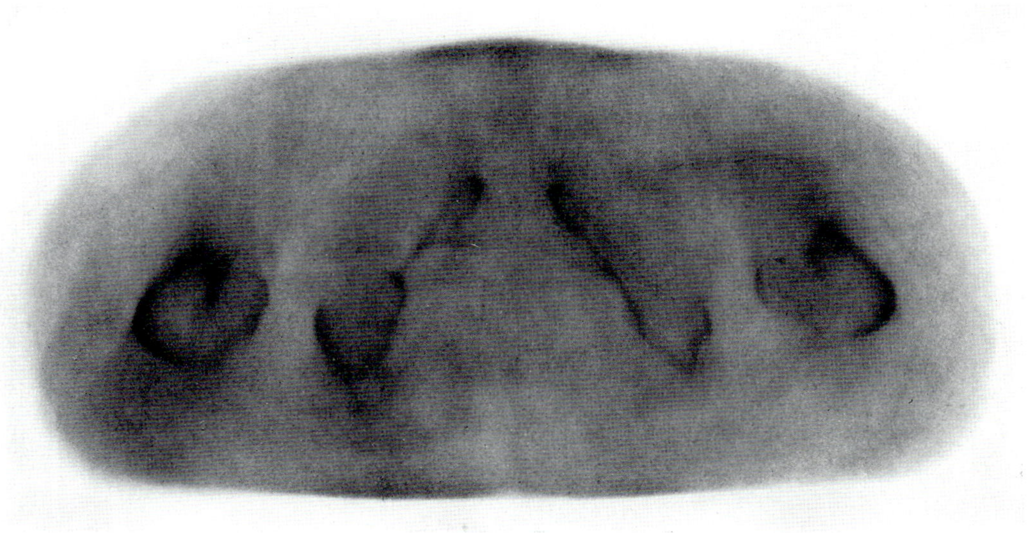

Fig. 447. Axial transverse tomogram

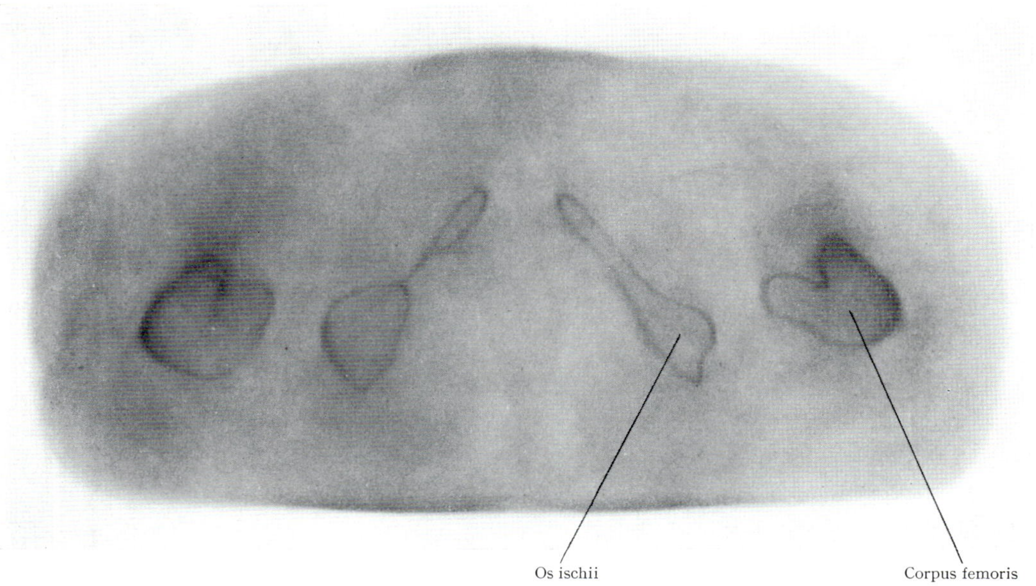

Fig. 448. Interpretation

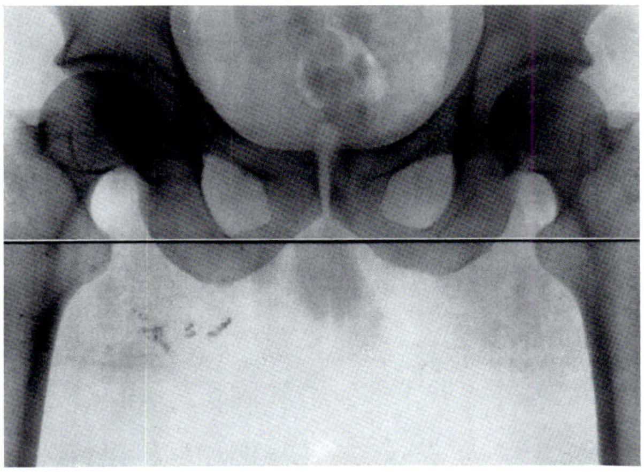

Fig. 449. Normal roentgenogram. Horizontal line showing the level tomographed

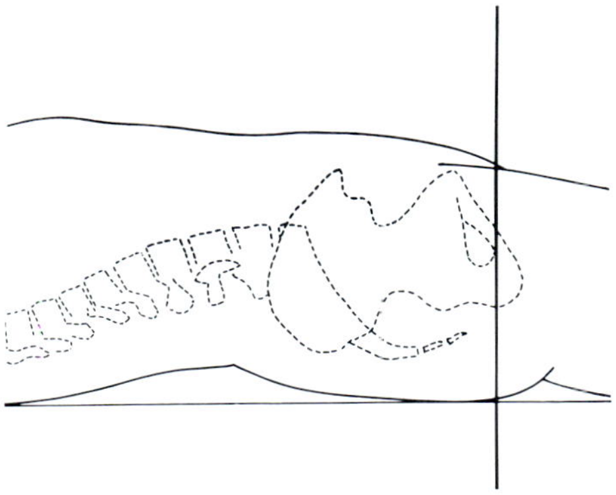

Fig. 450. Schematic drawing of the level tomographed

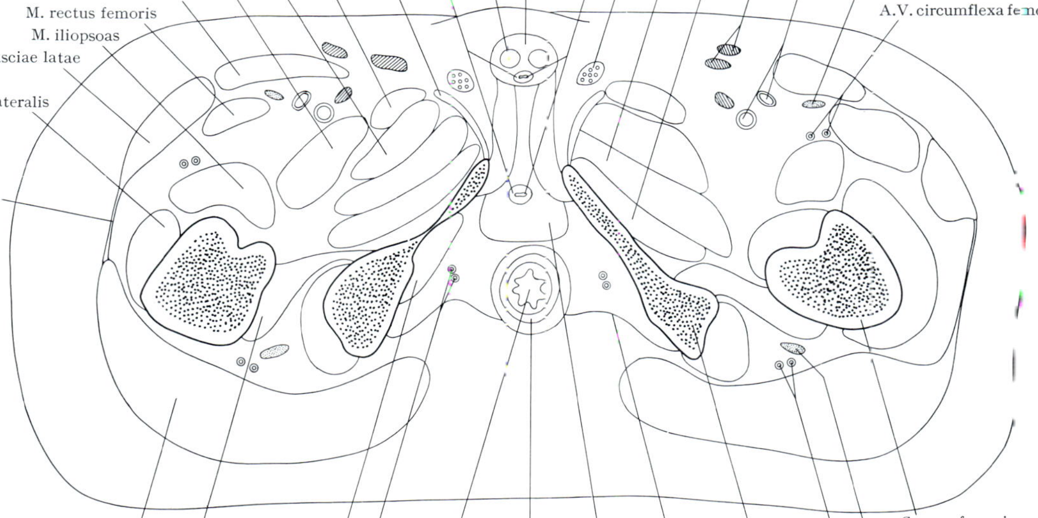

Fig. 451. Anatomical chart

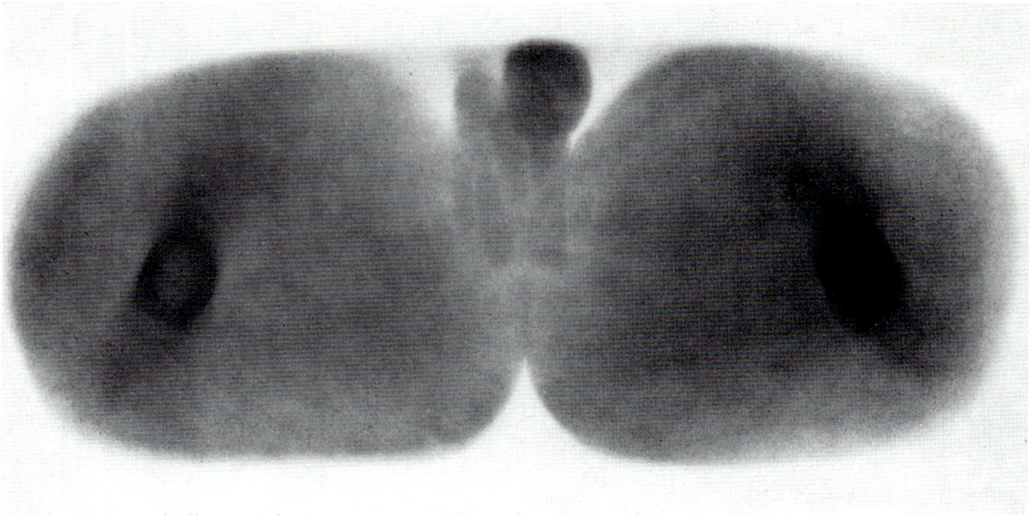

Fig. 452. Axial transverse tomogram

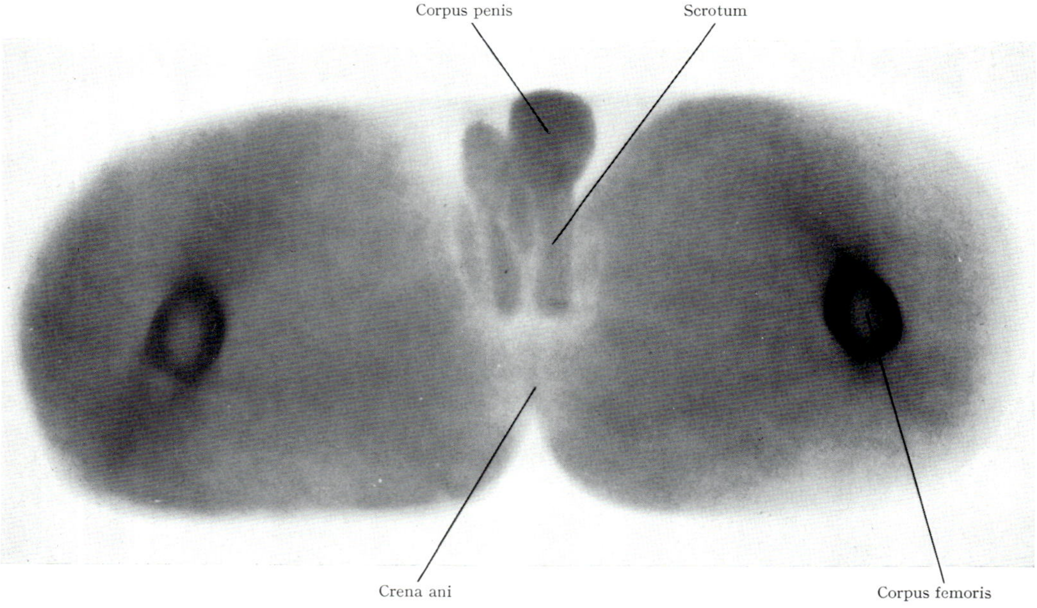

Fig. 453. Interpretation

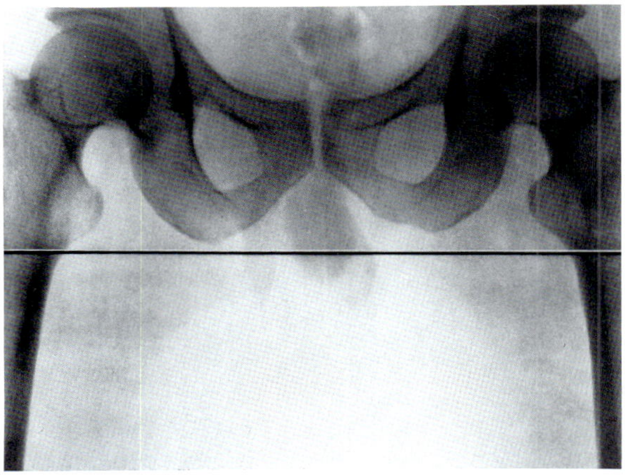

Fig. 454. Normal roentgenogram. Horizontal line showing the level tomographed

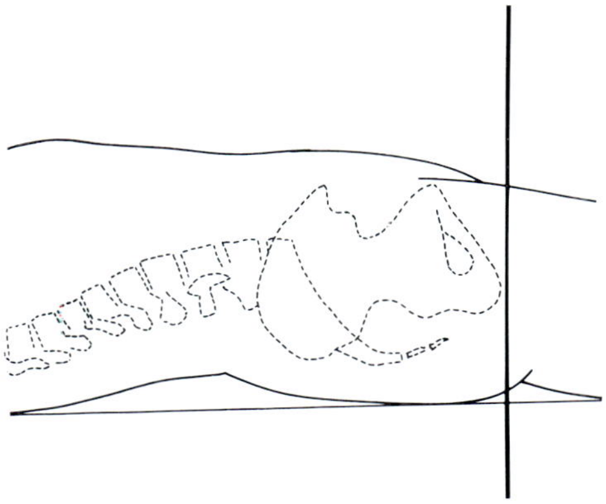

Fig. 455. Schematic drawing of the level tomographed

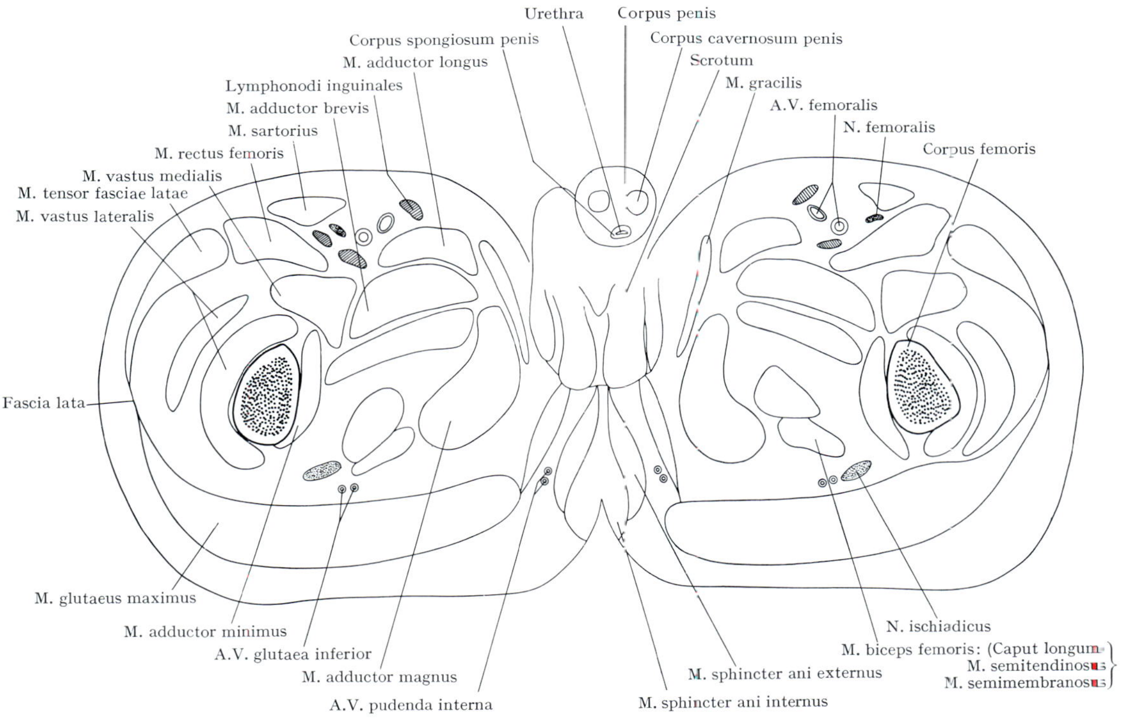

Fig. 456. Anatomical chart

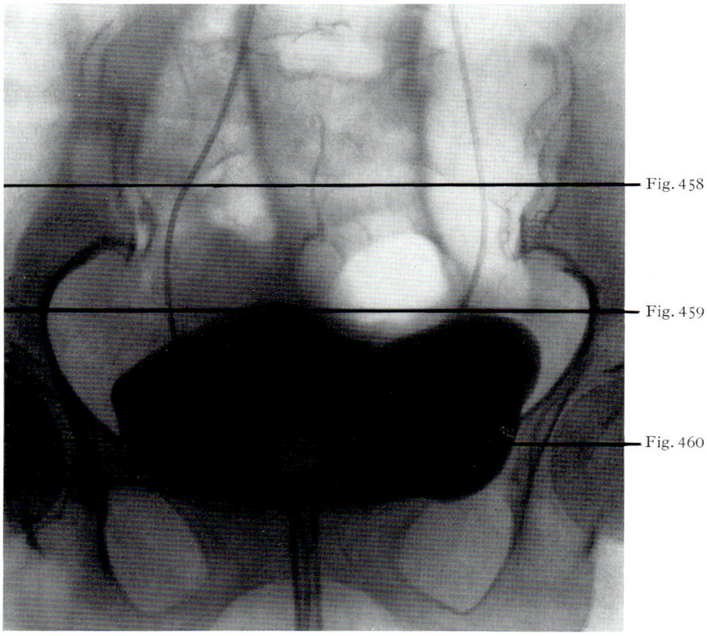

Fig. 457. Normal roentgenogram of the ureter with catheters introduced

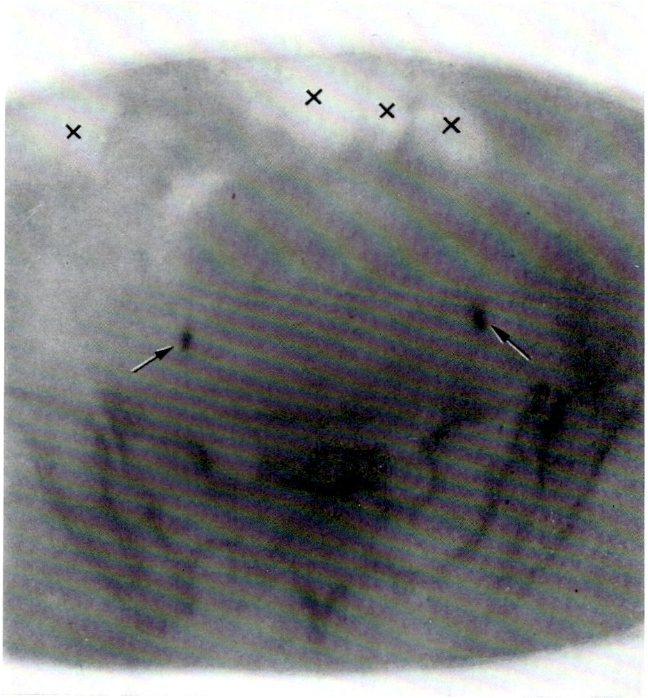

Fig. 458. Axial transverse tomogram of the ureter (↗) (see Figs. 387—391). Colon transversum (×)

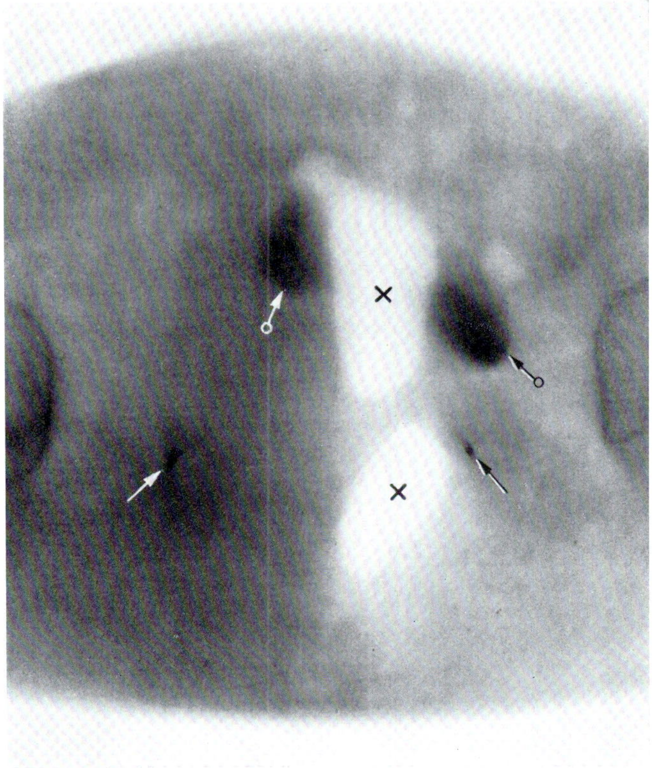

Fig. 459. Axial transverse tomogram of the ureter (↗), colon sigmoideum (×) and Vesica urinaria (↗). Colon sigmoideum imaged at the middle of the urinary bladder (see Figs. 397—401)

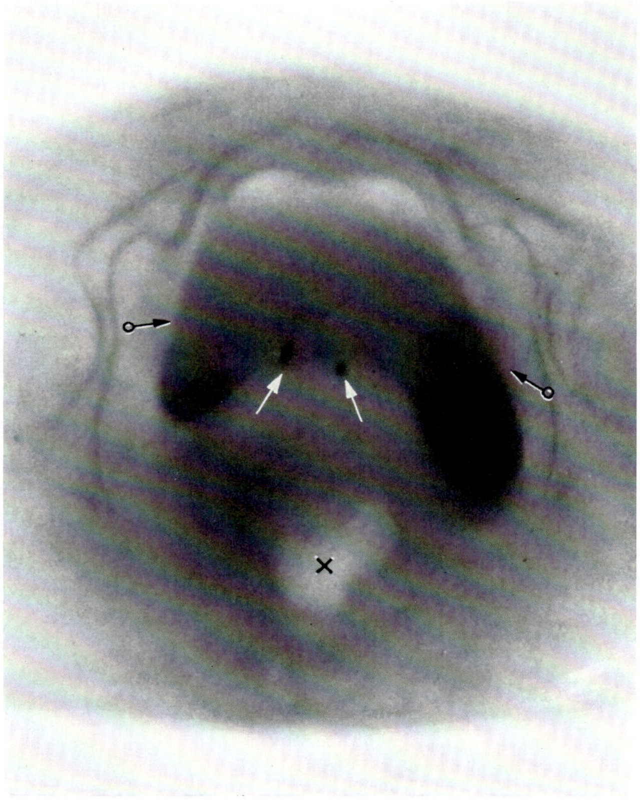

Fig. 460. Axial transverse tomogram. The ureter (↗) is seen in front of the orifice of the urinary bladder. This image can only be produced by axial transverse tomography (see Figs. 407—411, 437—441). Vesica urinaria (↗); Rectum (×)

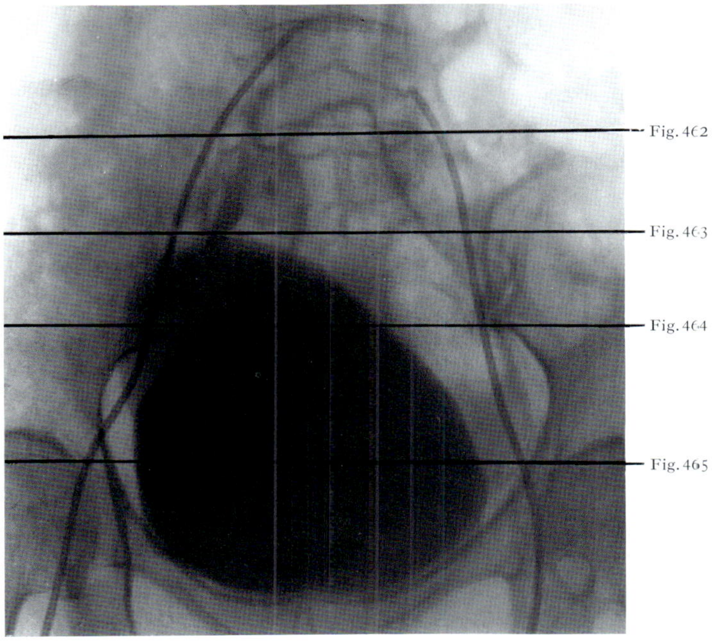

Fig. 461. Normal roentgenogram of the external iliac artery with Oedman-Ledin catheters

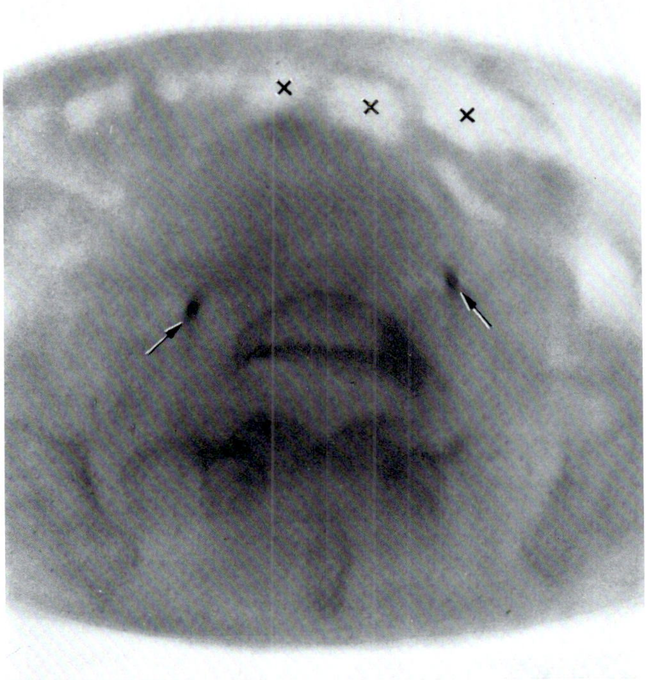

Fig. 462. Axial transverse tomogram of the external iliac artery (↗) (see Figs. 377—381). Colon transversum (×)

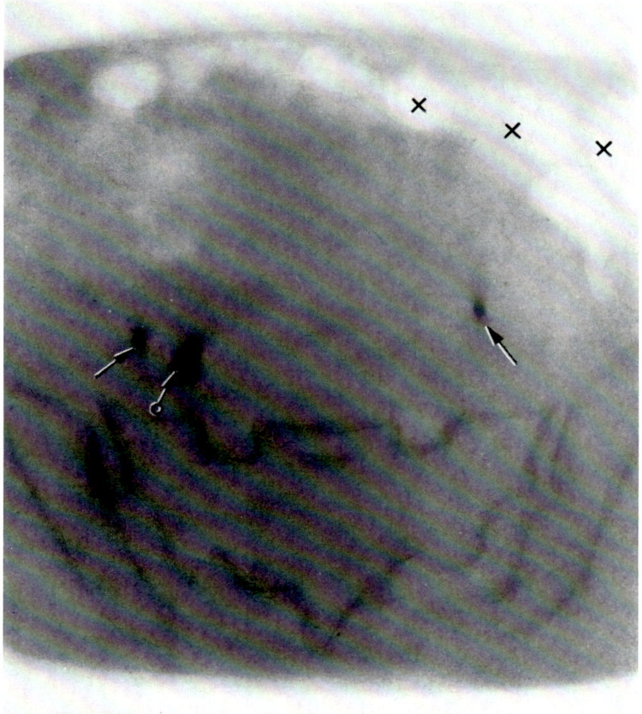

Fig. 463. Axial transverse tomogram of the external iliac artery (↗) (see Figs. 387—391). Colon transversum (×); Ureter dext (↗)

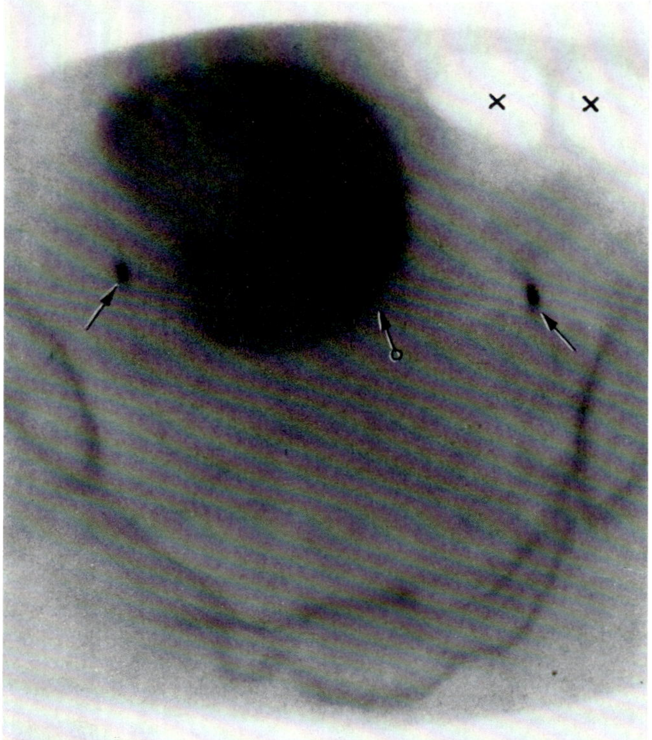

Fig. 464. Axial transverse tomogram of the external iliac artery (↗) (see Figs. 392—401). Colon transversum (×); Vesica urinaria (↗)

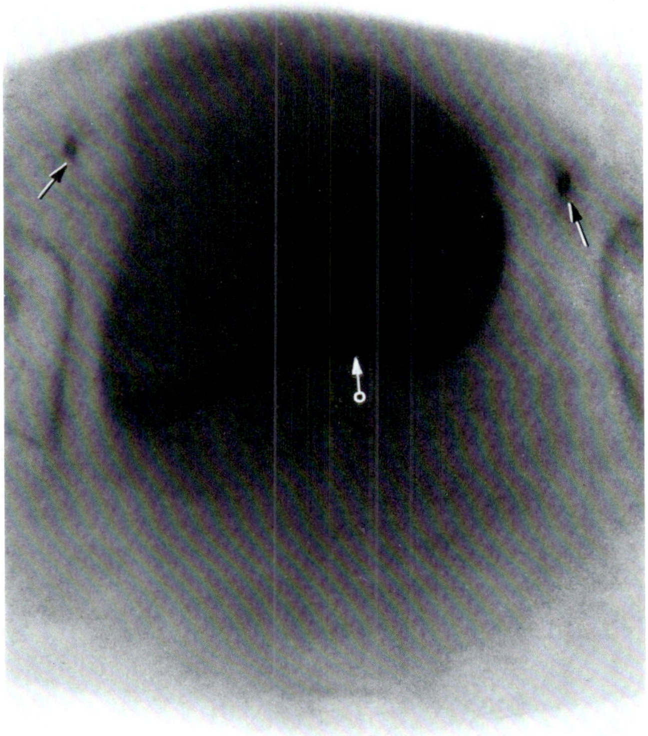

Fig. 465. Axial transverse tomogram of the external iliac artery (↗) (see Figs. 402—406, 432—436). Vesica urinaria (↗)

Arm

Eight axial transverse lympho-tomograms.

Findings visible on the axial transverse tomogram are printed in *italics* in the anatomical chart.

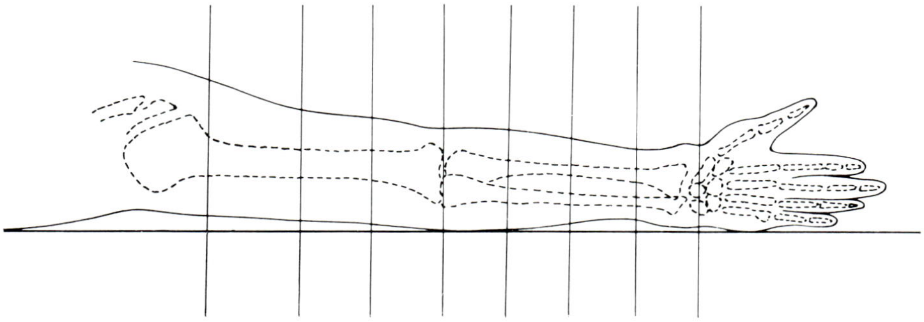

Fig. 466. Schema of tomographed levels

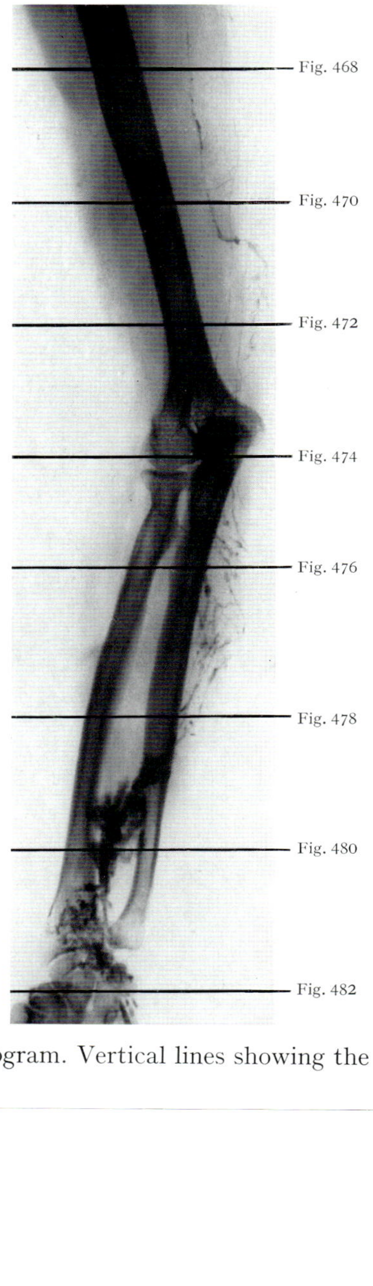

Fig. 467. Normal roentgenogram. Vertical lines showing the levels tomographed

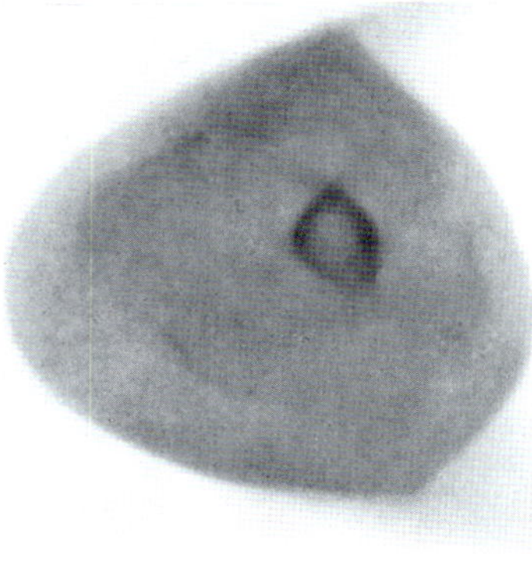

Fig. 468. Axial transverse tomogram

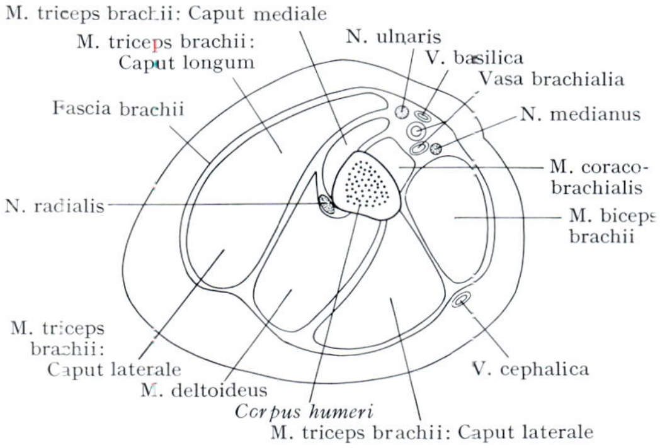

Fig. 469. Anatomical chart

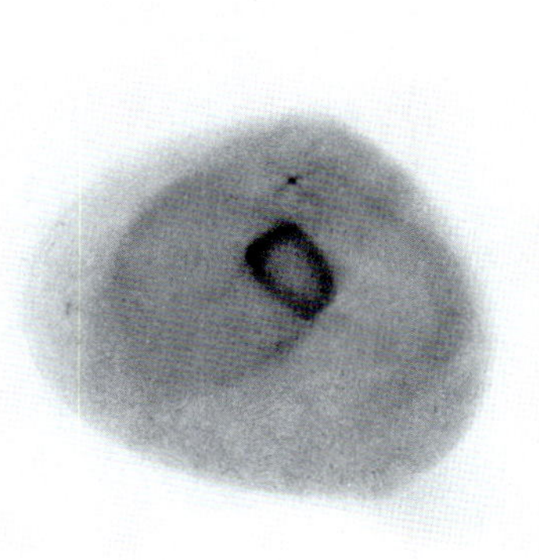

Fig. 470. Axial transverse tomogram

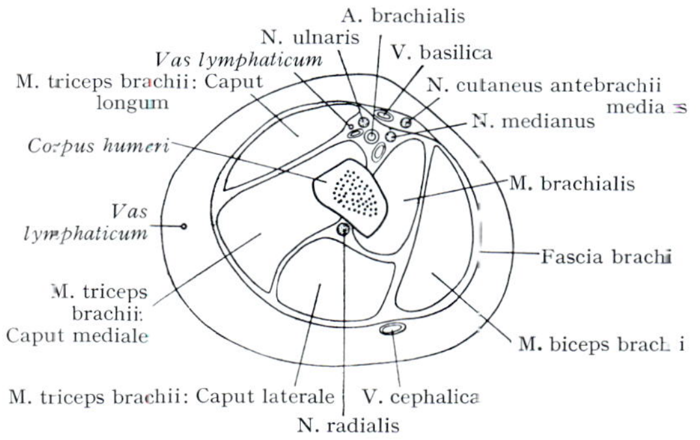

Fig. 471. Anatomical chart

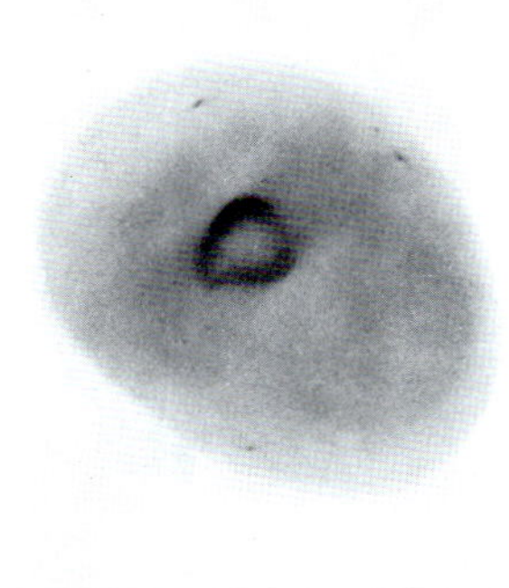

Fig. 472. Axial transverse tomogram

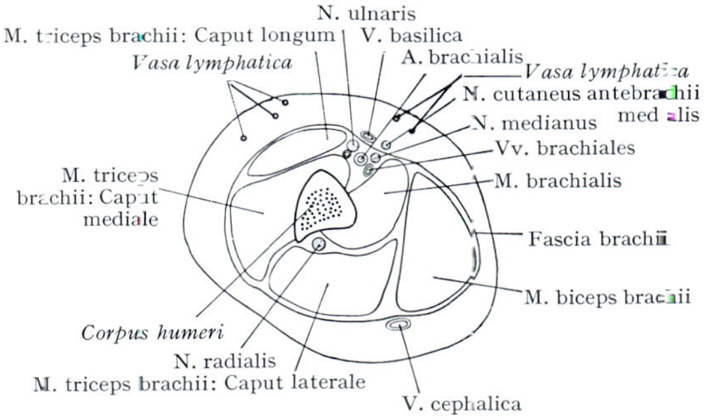

Fig. 473. Anatomical chart

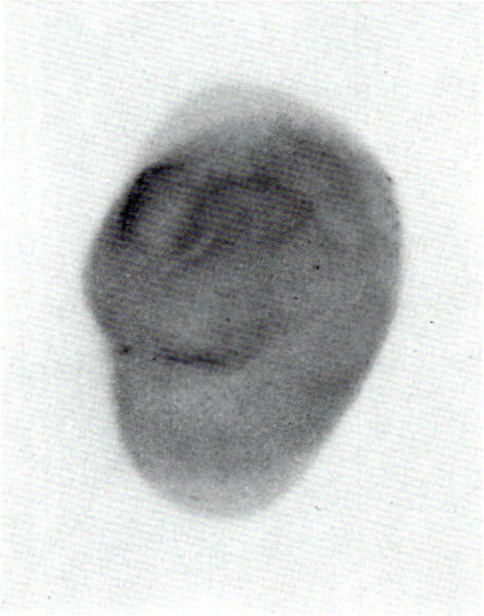

Fig. 474. Axial transverse tomogram

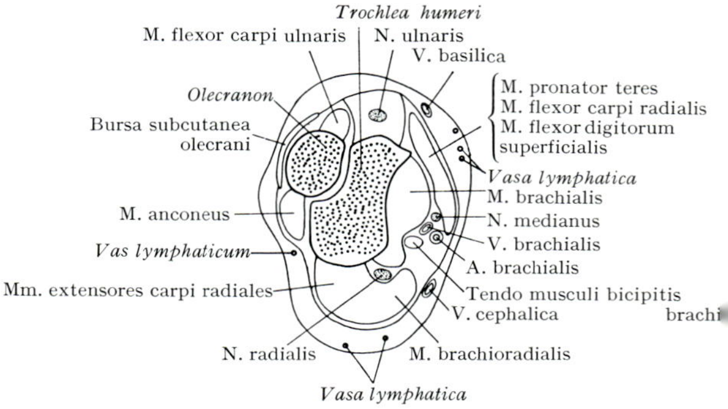

Fig. 475. Anatomical chart

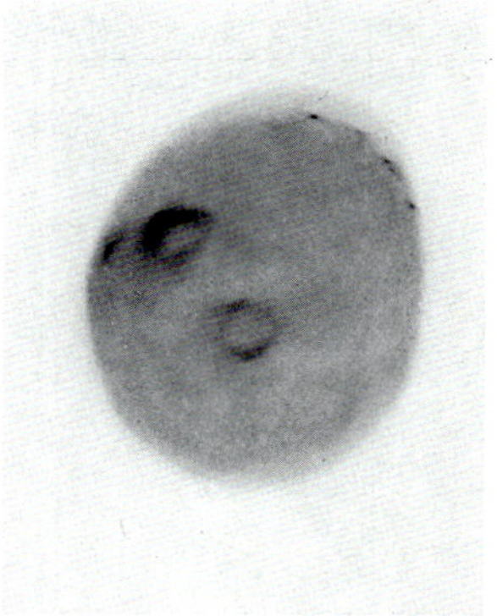

Fig. 476. Axial transverse tomogram

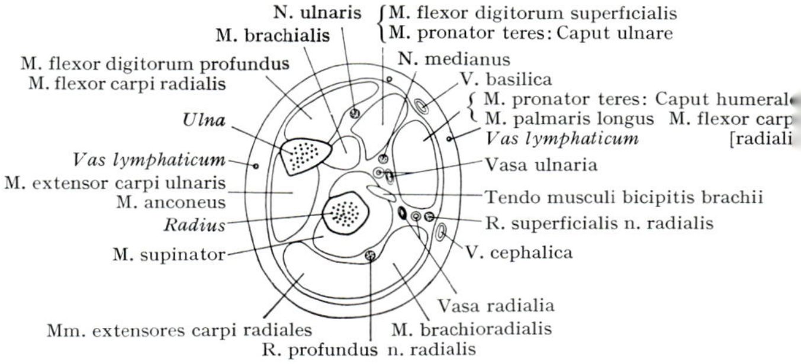

Fig. 477. Anatomical chart

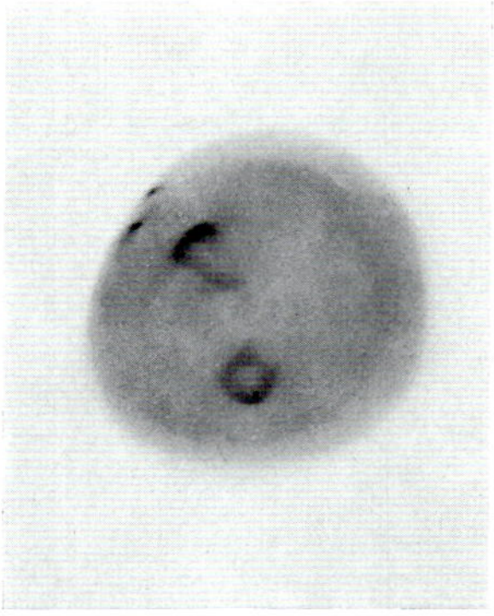

Fig. 478. Axial transverse tomogram

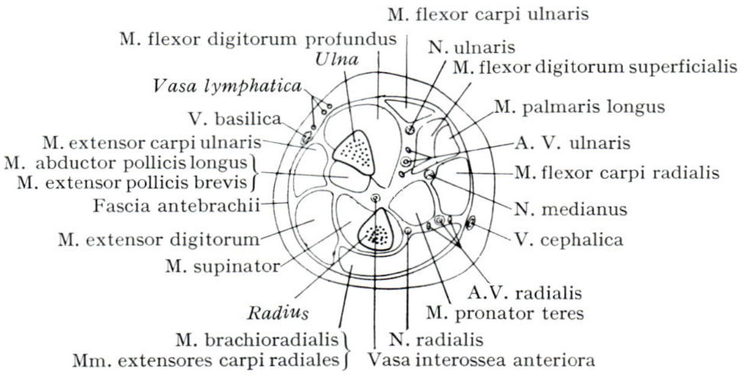

Fig. 479. Anatomical chart

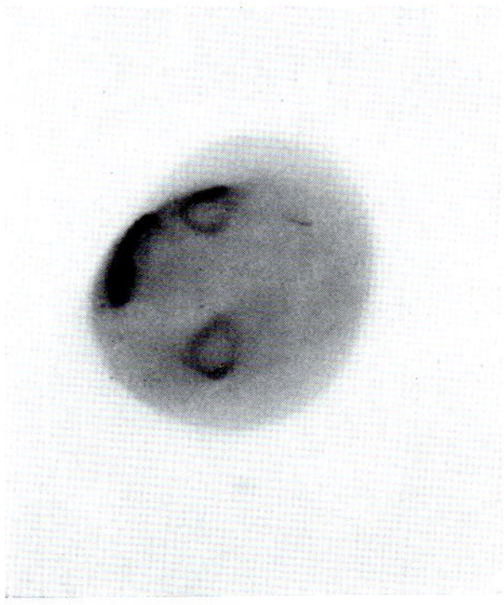

Fig. 480. Axial transverse tomogram

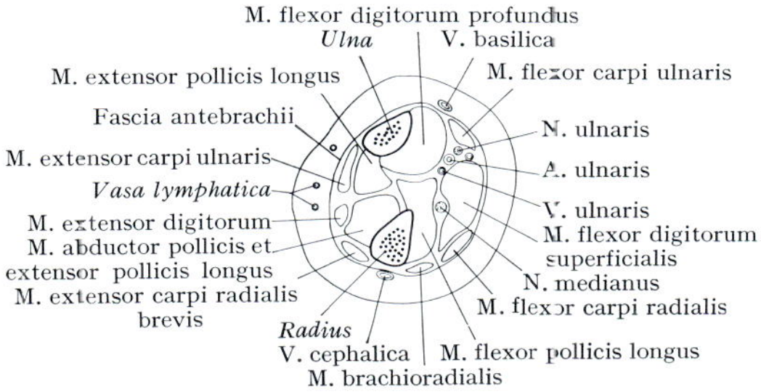

Fig. 481. Anatomical chart

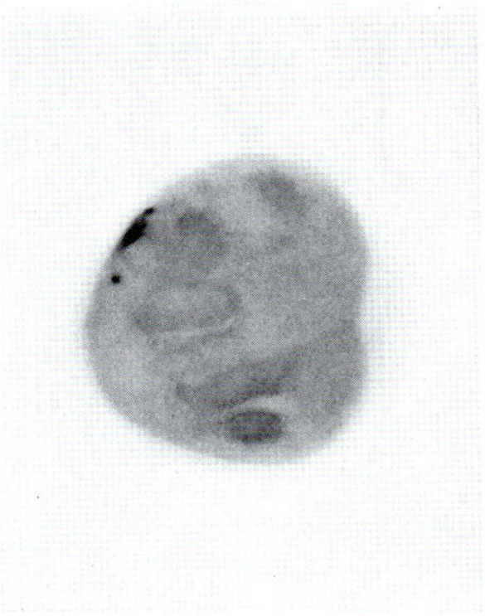

Fig. 482. Axial transverse tomogram

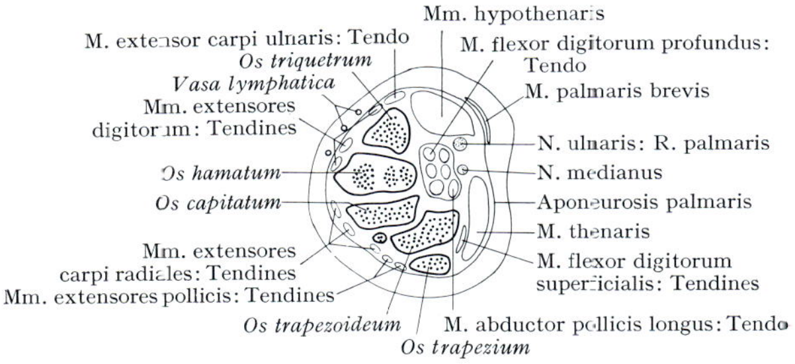

Fig. 483. Anatomical chart

Leg

Seven axial transverse phlebo- and lympho-tomograms.

Findings visible on the axial transverse tomogram are printed in *italics* in the anatomical chart.

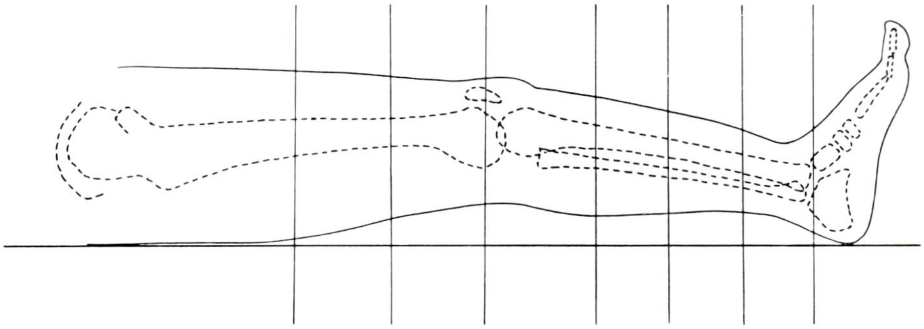

Fig. 484. Schema of tomographed levels

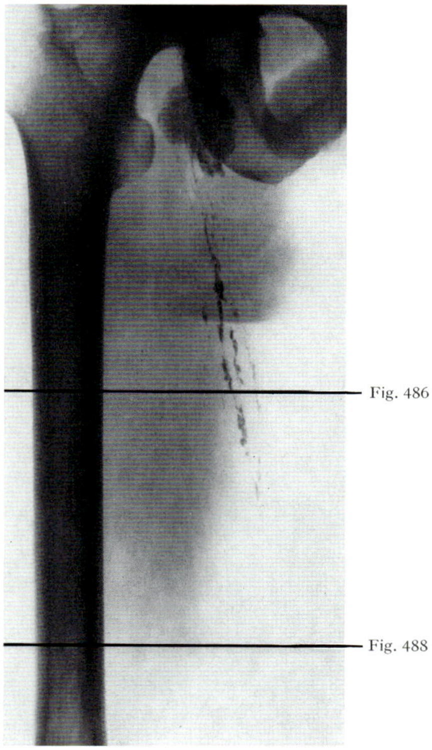

Fig. 485. Normal roentgenogram. Horizontal lines showing the levels tomographed

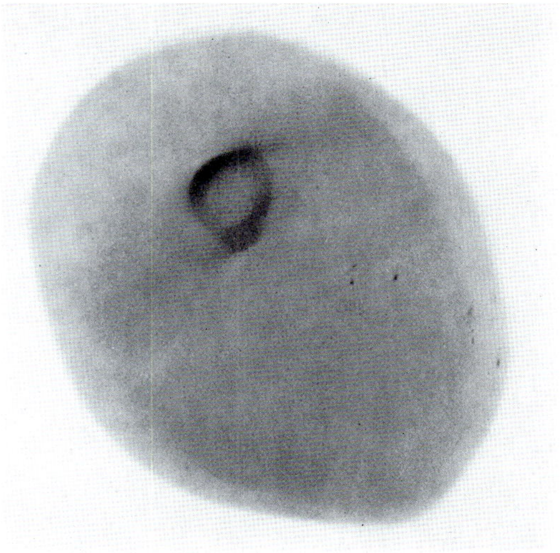

Fig. 486. Axial transverse tomogram

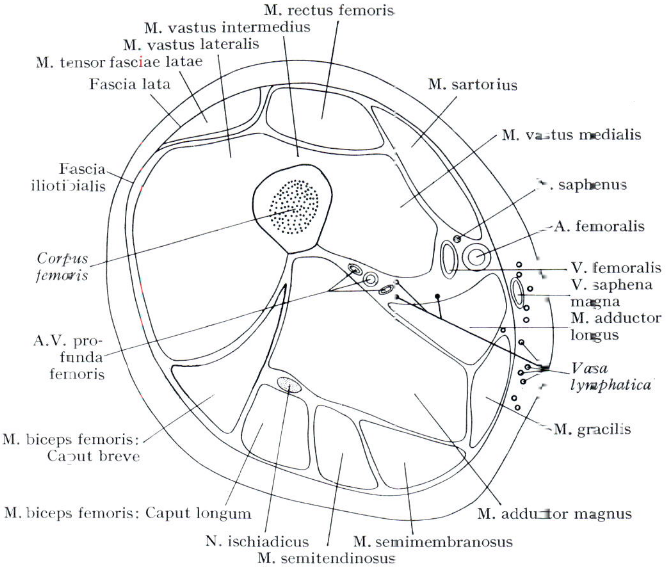

Fig. 487. Anatomical chart

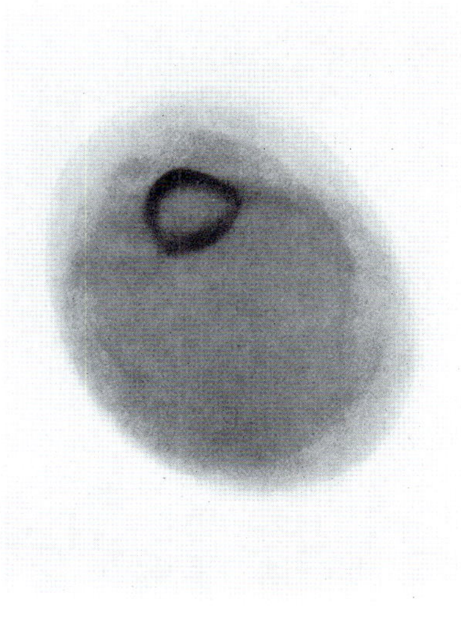

Fig. 488. Axial transverse tomogram

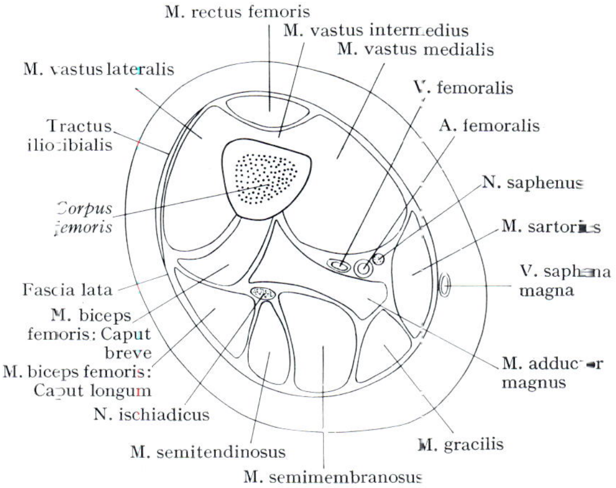

Fig. 489. Anatomical chart

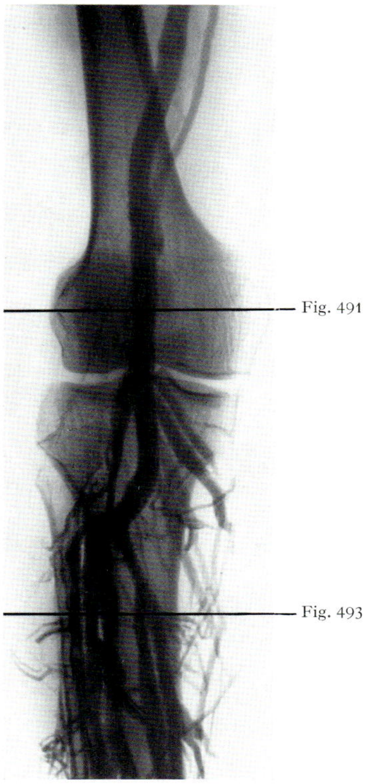

Fig. 490. Normal roentgenogram. Horizontal lines showing the levels tomographed

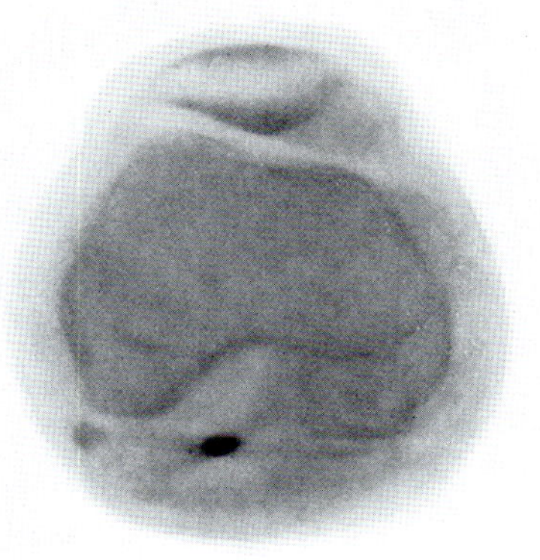

Fig. 491. Axial transverse tomogram

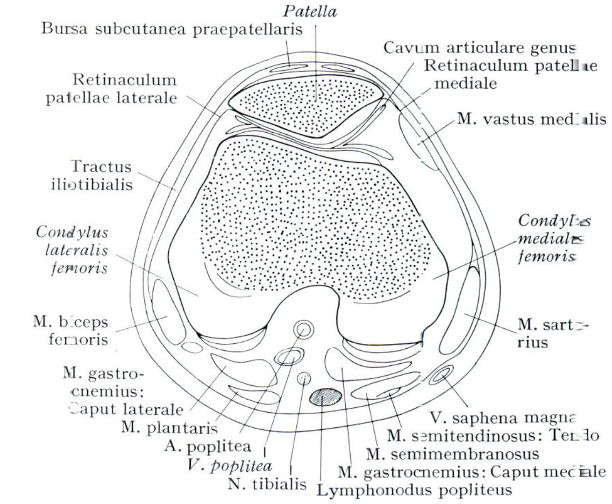

Fig. 492. Anatomical chart

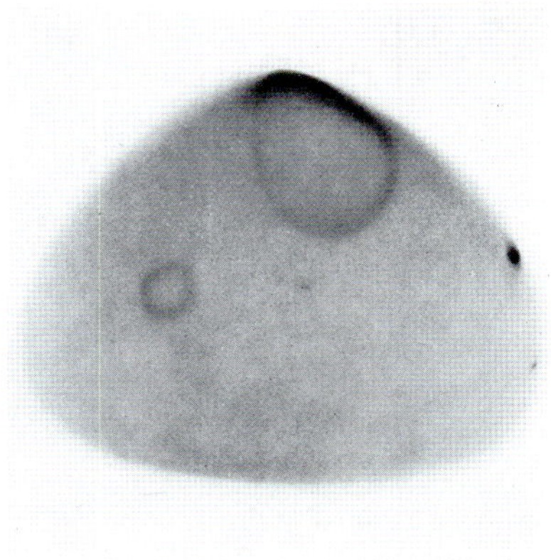

Fig. 493. Axial transverse tomogram

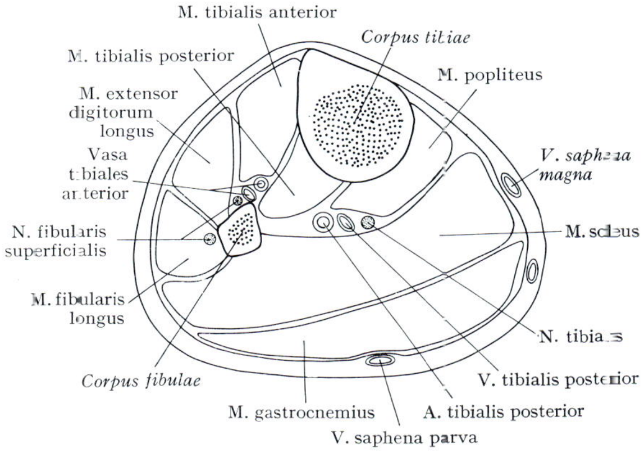

Fig. 494. Anatomical chart

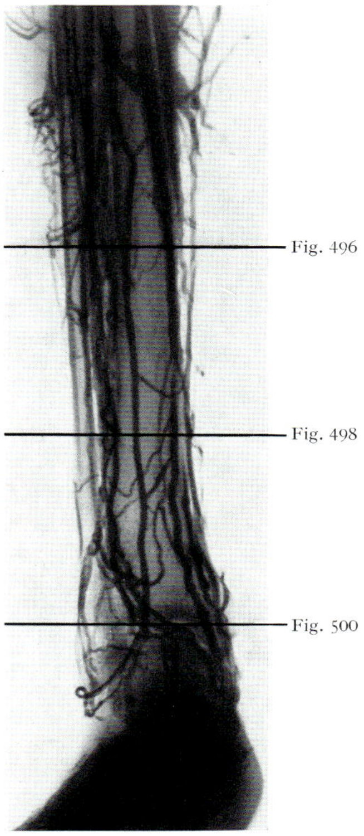

Fig. 495. Normal roentgenogram. Horizontal lines showing the levels tomographed

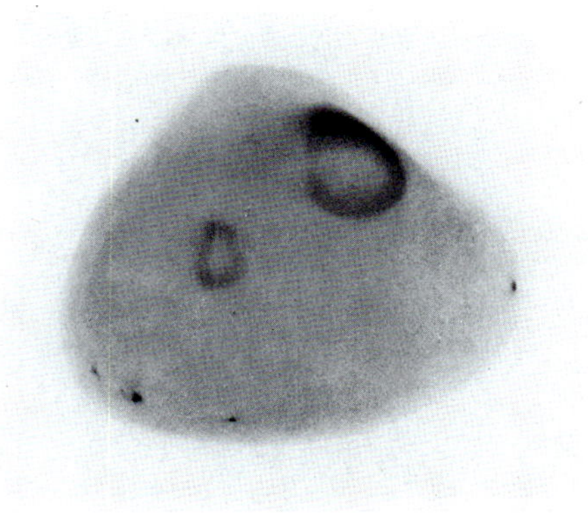

Fig. 496. Axial transverse tomogram

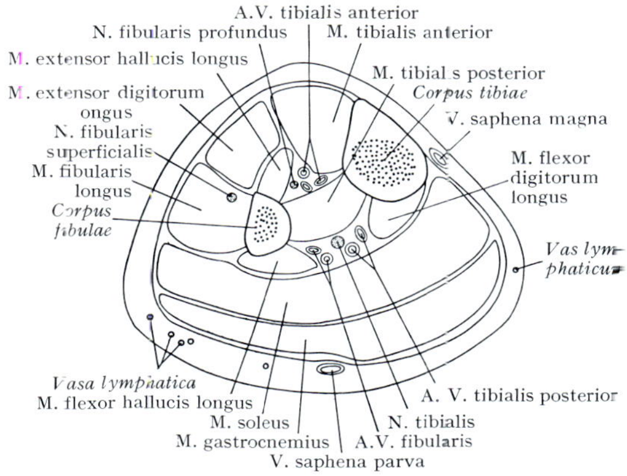

Fig. 497. Anatomical chart

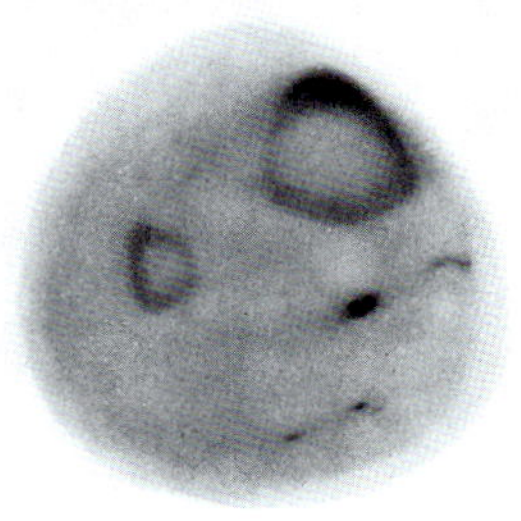

Fig. 498. Axial transverse tomogram

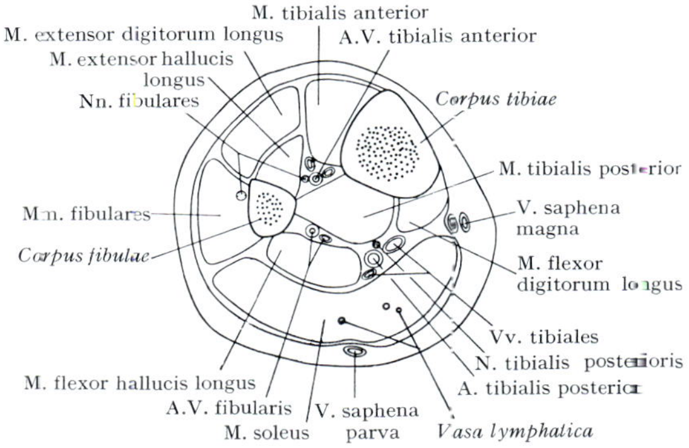

Fig. 499. Anatomical chart

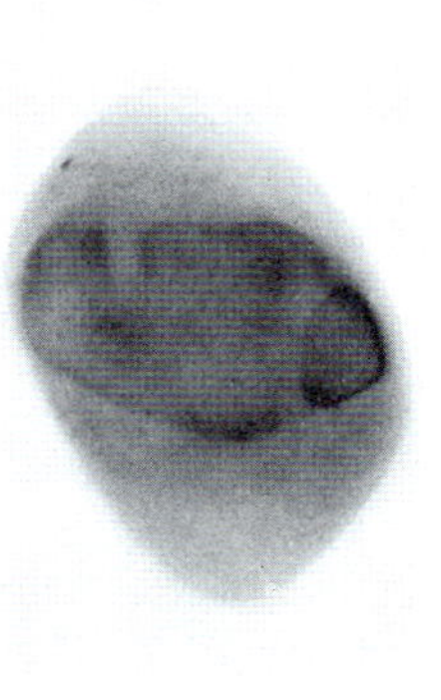

Fig. 500. Axial transverse tomogram

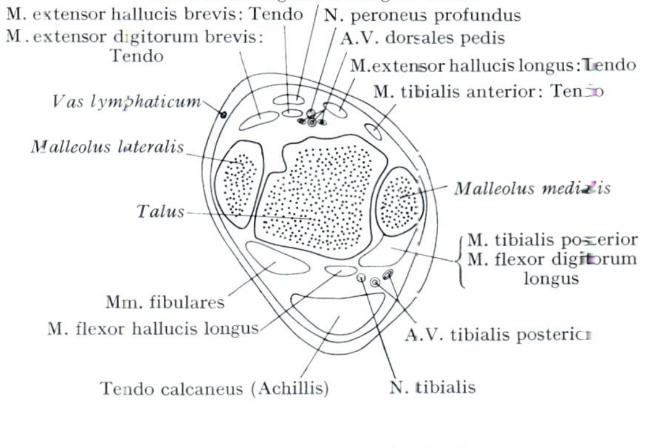

Fig. 501. Anatomical chart

Part 2

Clinical Applications of Axial Transverse Tomography

Introduction

Axial transverse tomography applied to clinical practice, especially to diagnosis, has been reported in a number of papers.

The papers I have to hand are as follows:

For axial transverse encephalotomography, papers have appeared by *di Chiro* (16), *Gebauer* (33, 171), *Sansone* et al. (105) while the papers concerning the head were described by *Hammer* (40).

The neck was studied by *Amisano* (5) and the thyroid was examined with insufflation of air into the neck by *Benedetti* (9) and *Farinet* et al. (22).

Pulmonary tuberculosis was dealt with by *Barenbojm* (8), *Kitabatake* (43), *Oliva* (82), *Roussel* et al. (99), *Sharma* et al. (115), *Shimazaki* (118), *Takahashi* (125) and *Voigt* et al. (163), and diagnosis of the tuberculous cavity in the lung by *Matsuda* (65, 67), *Macarini* (56), and *Suchán* (120). Tumor of the lung is discussed by *Balestra* et al. (7) and *Schaudig* et al. (114).

In the diagnosis of the chest the mediastinum is one of the most interesting topics, as the mediastinum is difficult to diagnose by other diagnostic techniques, such as pneumomediastinography, alone; this followed by axial transverse tomography was reported by *Mattine* et al. (76). Mediastinal lesions were examined by *Monod* et al. (78), *Sanquirico* et al. (102), *Sansone* et al. (103), and *Takamatsu* et al. (142). Diagnosis of heart disease was reported by *Bulgarelli* et al. (11—14), *Gremmel* (38), *Ode* et al. (80) and *Vallebona* (155). Aneurysm as well as aortic disease was dealt with by *Alè* et al. (3), *Pompili* et al. (94), *Lodin* (54), *Oliva* (81) and *Thomas* et al. (145, 146). Thymic disease was described by *de Maestri* et al. (61) and *Pompili* et al. (94). Mediastinal lesions were reported by *Buzzi* (15), *Lodin* (53) and *Martin* et al. (62).

The remaining chest diseases were reported by the following: *Fumagalli* et al. (30), *Gebauer* (35, 171, 172), *Hammer* (40), *Kobayashi* et al. (49), *Lodin* (55), *de Maestri* (60), *Matsuda* (64, 69), *Moldenhauer* (77), *Ono* (85, 86), *Ono* et al. (88), *Passeri* (90), *Rollandi* et al. (96), *Sato* (112), *Sharma* et al. (115), *Takahashi* et al. (135), *Vallebona* (153), *de Vulpian* (164) and *Wilk* (168).

As for the diagnosis of the upper abdomen there are very few papers other than those dealing with the pancreas. The pancreas is visualized when air is insufflated into the retroperitoneal space, as was shown by *Clément* (18), *Giraud* et al. (36, 37), *Levrat* et al. (52), *Macarini* et al. (57), *Sansone* et al. (104, 108, 109) and *Wangermez* et al. (165).

The pelvis was studied by *Sansone* et al. (106, 107) for diagnosis of obstetric conditions by *Ono* (84), and congenital luxation of the hip joint by means of a horizontal type unit by *Hachiya* et al. (39).

Recently the method of axial transverse tomography has tended to be applied to radiotherapeutic planning, as it proves useful also to know the bodily extent perpendicular to the body axis.

Nevertheless, axial transverse tomography is not so widely applied to clinical practice as had been expected. One of the reasons could be that interpreters usually have a poor knowledge of the topographical relationship of the organs and tissues arranged in the axial transverse cross section of the body. Moreover, the defect that the existing axial transverse tomograph provides only an indiscernible contour of the axial transverse cross section, due to overexposure at the contour of the body, would make it difficult to apply this method to the planning of radiation therapy. Further, the existing unit of erect type is applied mainly to chest disease but would be difficult to apply to all parts of the body.

Before proceeding to the clinical application of axial transverse tomography either to diagnosis or to therapy, a thorough knowledge of the topographical anatomy of the axial transverse cross section should be obtained, because the establishment of correct roentgen diagnosis and its application to surgical and radiological treatment may be difficult if this knowledge is lacking. This is why this book contains so many normal anatomical illustrations of axial transverse cross section.

In *part two* utilization of axial transverse tomography for diagnostic and therapeutic purposes will be discussed, as the readers are now considered to have obtained from *part one* a sufficient capacity for interpreting normal axial transverse tomograms. The pathological findings of diseased cases are considered to be only deviations from normal cases. With a knowledge of the pathological anatomy as well as of the findings of the axial transverse tomogram of the normal person, the interpretation of the tomographic image of the patient will not be difficult for readers.

I. Application to Diagnosis

Interpretation of findings for the diagnosis of all types of diseases appearing on the axial transverse tomograms will not be described here in order to make the book as simple as possible. It will be dealt with mainly from the theoretical and clinical points of view explaining why and in what points axial transverse tomography is superior to existing methods of roentgenological examination, such as normal roentgenography, conventional tomography and others.

1. Features of Axial Transverse Tomography

Axial transverse tomography is defined as two-dimensional comprehension of the axial transverse cross section of the human body in roentgenological examination. There are two features.

The first is to know the extent of disease in axial transverse cross section by means of a one- shot procedure of roentgenography, and the second is to establish the diagnosis of the disease in one layer of the body by removing shadows of overlapping organs and tissues.

For examining a lesion in the body, normal roentgenography is the most popular type of roentgen examination. In normal roentgenography, conducted by roentgen tube A, however, the three-dimensional body structureis projected on to the two-dimensional roentgen film A′, where the concept of depth in the body, dimension X, is lost (Fig. 502).

In order to know the three-dimensional structure of the body, roentgenography conducted by roentgen rays from two directions, A and B, is widely practised.

Findings on a normal roentgenogram A consist of overlapping images of everything contained in the pyramid AA′ with its top at focal spot A and its base at roentgen film A′. As in the normal roentgenogram A′ the dimension X of the pyramid is lost, the actual construction of the body is not revealed by the roentgen image. In addition to that, the lesions L overlapped by the other tissues T, lacking contrast, would not be discernible and so their existence would be missed. When a normal roentgenogram B is taken in order to avoid these drawbacks, the findings of the pyramid BB′ are also examined now. Much more information is obtained thus than from one single normal roentgenogram AA′. The roentgenogram B′ newly reveals lesion L free from overlap with tissue T, which in the case of normal roentgenography A alone would be missed.

However, even when these two roentgenograms A′ and B′ are examined together, the body is still misrepresented as a square pillar rather than a cylinder.

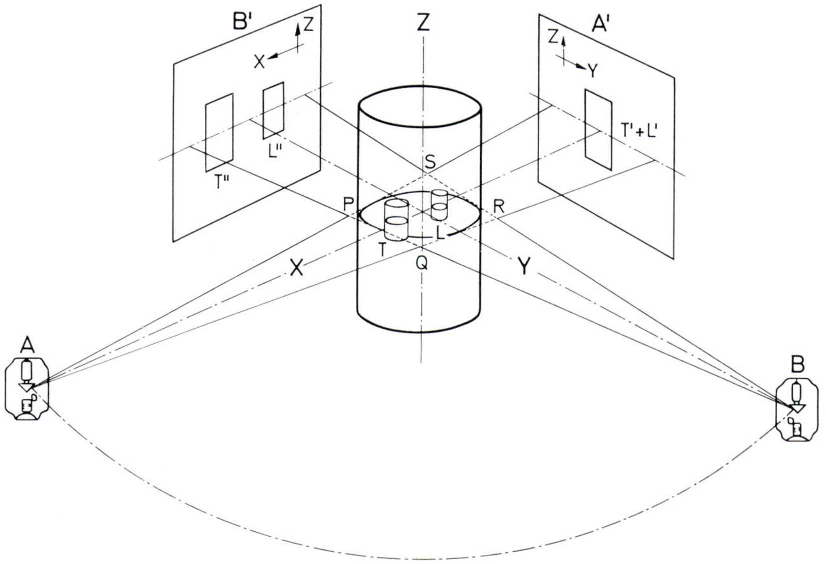

Fig. 502. Schematic drawing of normal roentgenography conducted with two projections. Limited knowledge of three-dimensional structure of the body is obtained. A, B: Roentgen tube. A′, B′: Film. On the film A′ the dimension X is not imaged. T and L are not imaged on film A′, but imaged on film B′. Comparative study of film A′ and B′ does not provide the correct knowledge of the cylinder but misleading knowledge of the square pillar having the rectangular cross-section PQRS

In spite of this fact, it has been generally considered beyond question that a three-dimensional knowledge of the body is obtained if saggital and lateral roentgenograms are taken and examined together.

The femur, for instance, is not regarded as a square pillar, but as a cylinder, when two such roentgenograms are taken and examined.

This is only due to our anatomical knowledge, learned beforehand. As a matter of fact, such a conclusion is theoretically incorrect or, at least, unfounded.

Further, the diagnosis of disease falls outside the normal anatomical field. Lesions take on abnormal position, shape and size in the body and this cannot be concluded from our knowledge of normal anatomy. From this point of view, roentgenograms taken from two directions have essentially weak points for correct diagnosis.

Indeed, roentgenograms taken from many different directions provide more information than those taken from two directions, but the disadvantage still remains that the conclusion obtained from these procedures deviates from the actual construction of the body. Moreover, interpretation becomes a much more troublesome and time-consuming procedure, because the three-dimensional construction of the body is concluded only by integration of these two-dimensional roentgen images.

Even by such an effort, however, the axial transverse cross-section of the body is by no means obtained (Fig. 503).

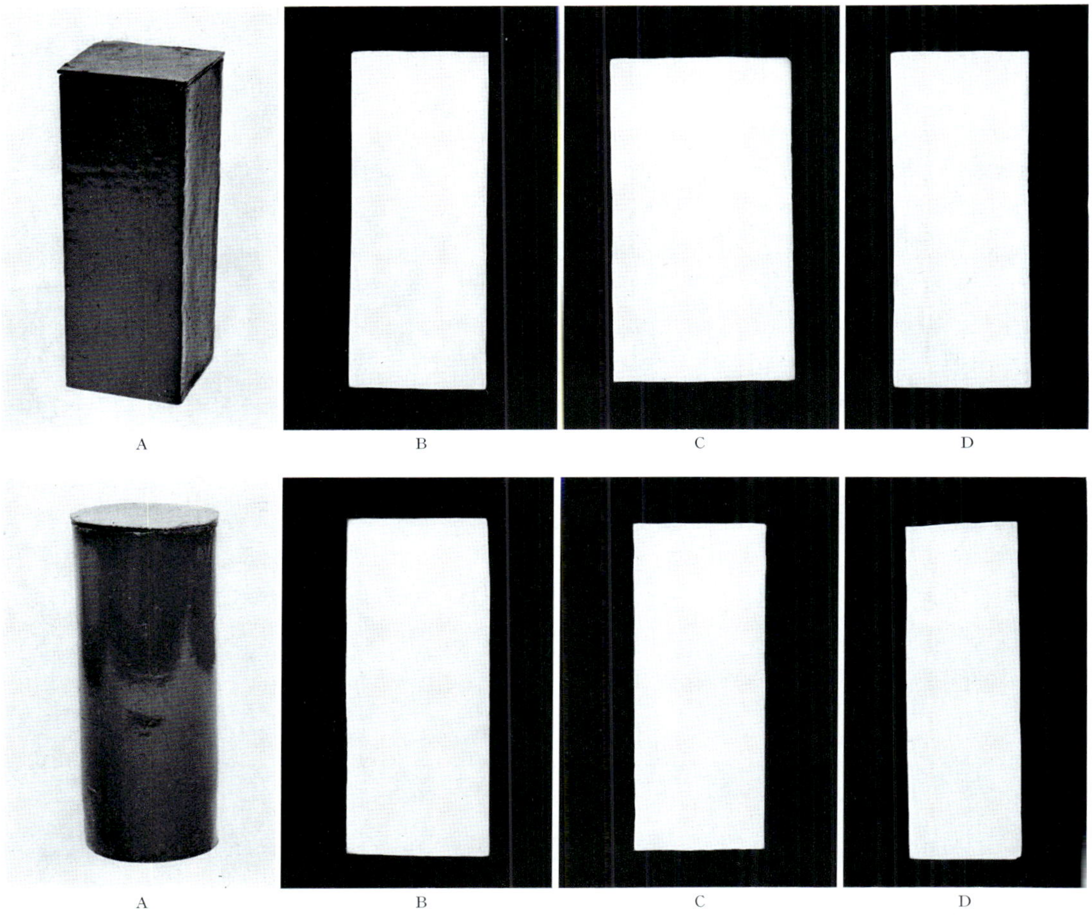

Fig. 503. Three-dimensional knowledge not obtainable by normal roentgenography Top: Normal photo of a square pillar (A), normal roentgenography in PA view (B), in oblique view (C) and in lateral view (D). Bottom: Normal photo of an elliptic cylinder (A), normal roentgenography in PA view (B), in oblique view (C) and in lateral view (D).
Correct identification of pillar and cylinder is difficult

Axial transverse tomography is thus superior to the examination of normal roentgenograms taken from many directions, in that the dimensions of X and Y can be obtained accurately and concretely with a simple one-shot procedure

There is another roentgenographic method which provides the information of the dimension of depth and permits the detection of new foci. By means of multisection radiography it may become possible for us to know the three-dimensional structure of the body. Actually, however, multisection radiography is not usually used for such a purpose, because the body structure is not clearly seen because of disturbance by obstructive shadows, especially when the linear tomograph is used. Recently, multidirectional tomography, which is characterised by creating fewer obstructive shadows than linear tomography, has been applied to clinical roentgenology and it is hoped that it can be used for examining the three-dimensional structure of the body. Even by means of either of these conventional forms of tomography, however, the procedure for obtaining information about the axial transverse cross section of the body is still indirect. If an axial transverse tomogram is taken, the axial transverse figure is obtained with a one-shot exposure. This tomogram shows negligible obstructive shadows, if an appropriate arrangement is made of the unit and the range of rotation of roentgen tube. This is the special feature of this type of tomography. Conventional tomography is thus not considered adequate to supply the knowledge of axial transverse cross section or of the three-dimensional structure of the body (*Takahashi* et al. (136)).

Nevertheless, axial transverse tomography is similar to the usual tomography in the principle of image formation in a single layer of the body. It is also able to detect a new focus overlapped by other organs. This tomography is carried out by circular movement of the X-ray tube resulting in the occurrence of fewer obstructive shadows than in the usual linear tomography. For convenience, its features are given in Table 2.

Table 2. *Diagnostic features of several types of roentgenography for establishment of diagnosis*

	Normal roentgenography	Normal roentgenographs taken from two directions	Normal roentgenography and conventional tomography	Normal roentgenography and axial transverse tomography
Detection of lesions	+	++	+++	+++
Comprehension of axial transverse layer	—	+ (indirectly)	+ (indirectly)	+++
Three-dimensional comprehension of the body	—	++	++ or +++	+++

— difficult; + good; ++ better; +++ excellent.

2. Establishment of Diagnosis for Clinical Cases

As the lesions are imaged on the normal roentgenogram, with overlap of shadows of various tissues and organs in the body, the level of the body to be transversely tomographed is determined by observation of the normal roentgenogram. The level to be cross-sectioned is selected and marked in ink on the corresponding portion of the patient's skin. The patient is laid on the roentgenographic table of the horizontal type unit. Normal roentgenography in which the wire representing the level to be tomographed is imaged on the roentgenogram is conducted as described on p. 6.

If there is no gross difference between the location of the expected level and that actually tomographed, axial transverse tomography is then carried out. Otherwise, the position of the patient is adjusted and axial transverse tomography is conducted. Such readjustment will be simple and precise, if an image intensifier or roentgen television is placed under the tomographic table and examined.

At clinical interpretation the findings appearing on the axial transverse tomograms of the patient are compared with those of the normal persons illustrated in the Atlas.

For this, first of all the axial transverse tomogram of the patient is taken in the same position as that of the normal person of the Atlas. When taking the tomogram of a cancer of the maxillary sinus, for instance, the patient is laid supine on the tomographic table, either with his orbitomeatal line or with his acanthiomeatal line vertical, and the axial transverse tomogram is taken.

The standards for positioning are the orbitomeatal line or acanthiomeatal line for the head; the level of the spine for the neck, the chest and the upper abdomen; the pubic bone or pelvic cavity for the lower abdomen. Only when such a procedure of positioning is made can the findings of the axial transverse tomogram be referred to those of the Atlas and the interpretation carried out easily and correctly.

Although with the standard level the positioning of the patient is made the same as that of the normal person of the Atlas, it will be found at times that the figure of the axial transverse tomogram of the patient does not coincide with that of the Atlas. This is frequently the case in diagnosis of the viscera

In such a case the Atlas is searched for suitable illustrations of the similar part of the body to the figure of the tomogram.

For interpretation of hilum of the lung, for instance, the level tomographed is shown as a transverse line on the normal roentgenogram. The illustration of the Atlas in which the hilum is shown should be adopted. It is advisable not to refer only to the spine as a guide.

For interpretation it is also essential first of all to refer to the original normal roentgenogram. Abnormalities in findings seen or suspected on the normal roentgenogram, which reveals it just on the image of level tomographed, are usually shown on the axial transverse tomogram.

By comparing the normal roentgenogram with the tomogram, the correct diagnosis will be established.

The level of the normal roentgenogram is thus essential for determining the need for tomography, performance of correct positioning and as a guide for interpretation. Without reference to the normal roentgenogram taken with the patient laid on the tomographic table and the Atlas, the application of axial transverse tomography to clinical practice will be limited.

Now, in order to explain how this type of tomography contributes to clinical practice, cases will be shown below.

There is a fear, however, that the number of illustrations could run up to tremendous amount, as this type of radiography has the unique feature of being exclusively capable of imaging axial transverse cross sections of lesions in the body. Yet the space assigned is limited.

Thus, cases are shown here in a rather limited number of presentations, but with examples of every part of the body. The main reasons for this are, first: the illustrations of normal persons which will contribute to the diagnosis are already supplied in the Atlas and, second: no book containing cases of every part of the body has been published before.

In our description we have tried especially to show the unique features of axial transverse tomography in contributing to diagnosis better than or as well as conventional tomography for detecting new lesions, or contributing better to diagnosis than normal roentgenography or conventional tomography, in that axial transverse tomography makes clear with a one-shot procedure the size, shape and location of the lesions in axial transverse cross section of the body.

Cases will be shown with the diagnosis and the history of the patient. Prior to the description of the findings of the axial transverse tomogram concerned, the normal roentgenograms or tomograms will be interpreted.

Diagnosis: Cancer of the right maxillary sinus.

Case: T. O., age 65, female.

History: The patient complains of slight but gradually increasing swelling of the face on the right side and rhinorrhea. Exophthalmus developed in the right side recently.

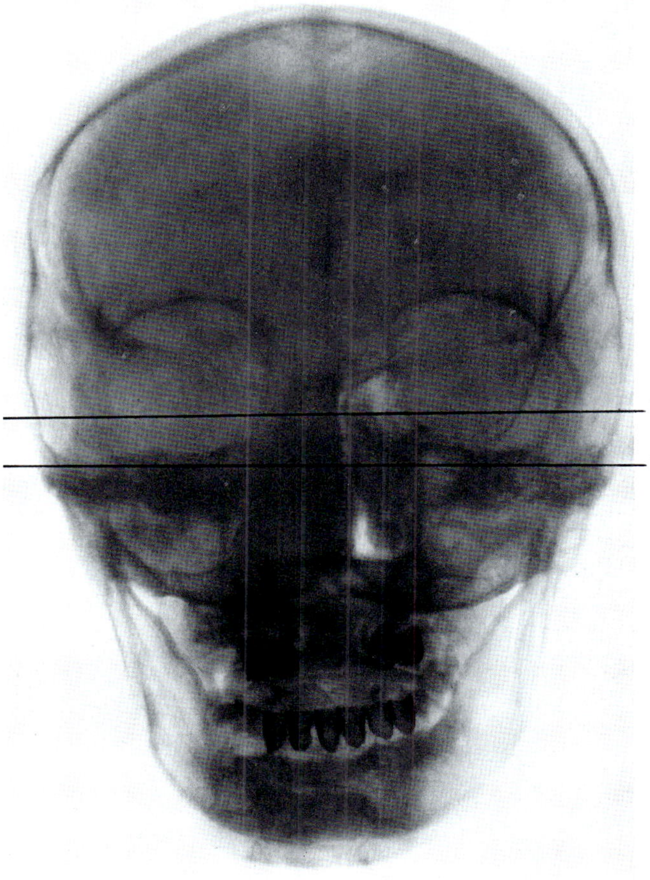

Fig. 504. Normal roentgenogram. Horizontal line showing the level tomographed. There is homogeneous density in the right inferior nasal cavity and ethmoid sinus. The lateral wall of the right maxillary sinus is slightly destroyed

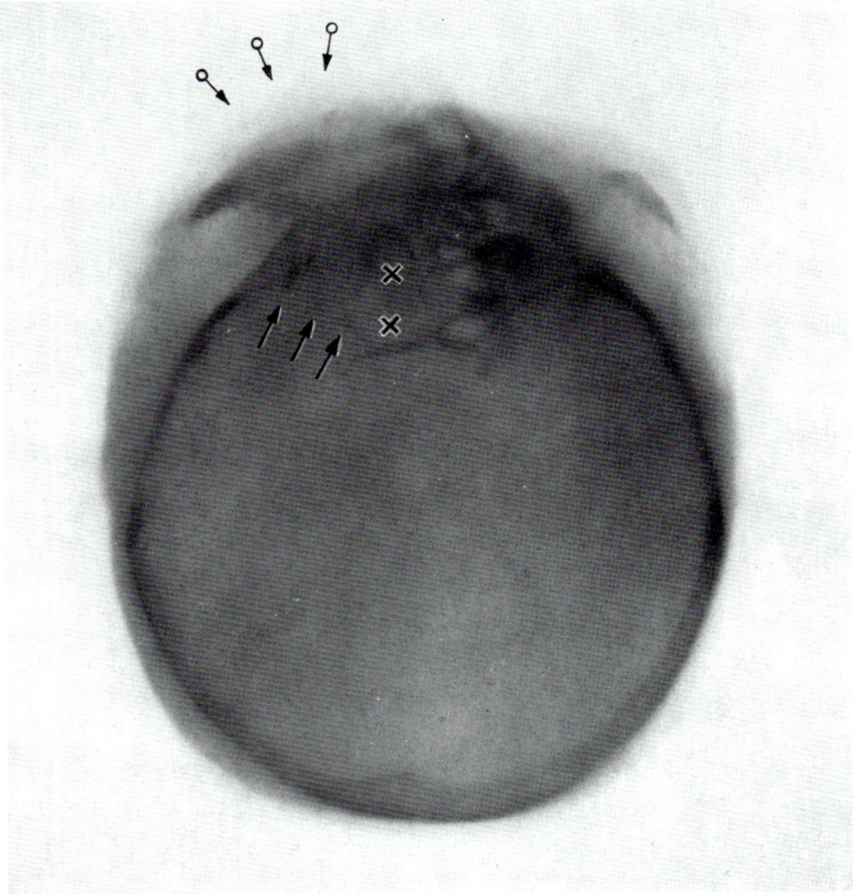

Fig. 505. Axial transverse tomogram. Refer to the normal Figs. 61—65, p. 38. There is soft tissue swelling (↗) on the right lateral aspect of the face. The anterior and posterior ethmoid sinuses are occupied by a soft tissue mass (×). The ala major of the sphenoid bone shows destruction (↗)

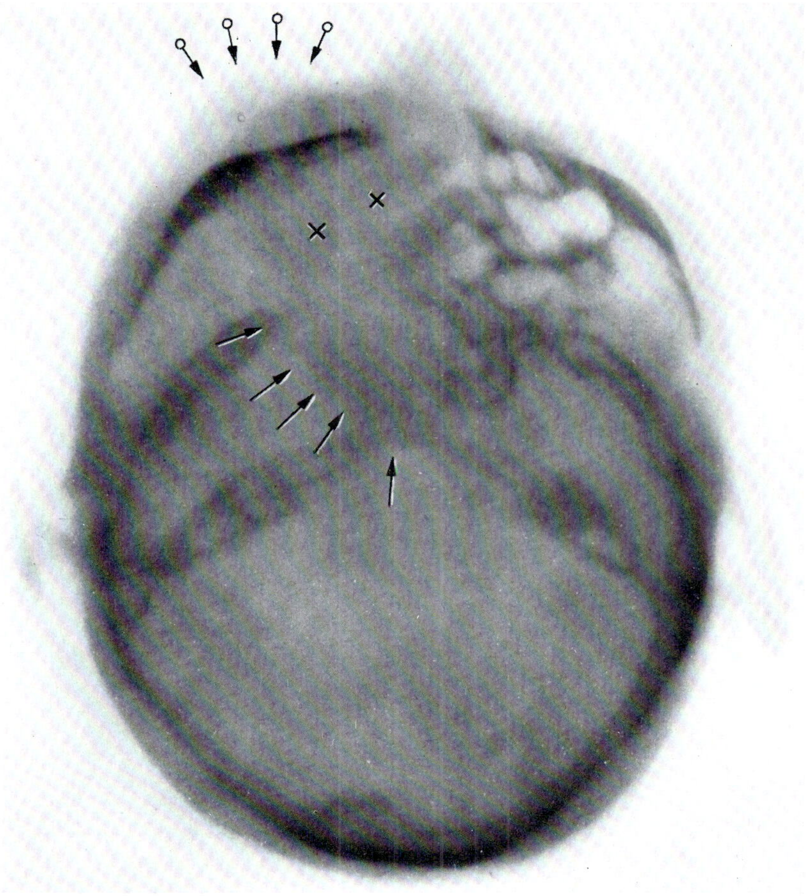

Fig. 506. Axial transverse tomogram. Refer to the normal Figs. 71—75, p. 42. There is soft tissue swelling (↗) noted on the anterior and lateral aspect of the maxillary sinus. The maxillary sinus and nasal cavity on the right side are hazy but no translucency is noted (×). The posterior wall of the maxillary sinus as well as processus coronoideus are indistinctly seen (↗). The anterior wall of the maxillary sinus is partially destroyed

Diagnosis: Metastatic cancer of the mandible.

Case: M. S., age 30, male.

History: After the removal of the cancer from the base of the tongue 3 years ago a tumor mass the size of a pigeon's egg appeared in the chin.

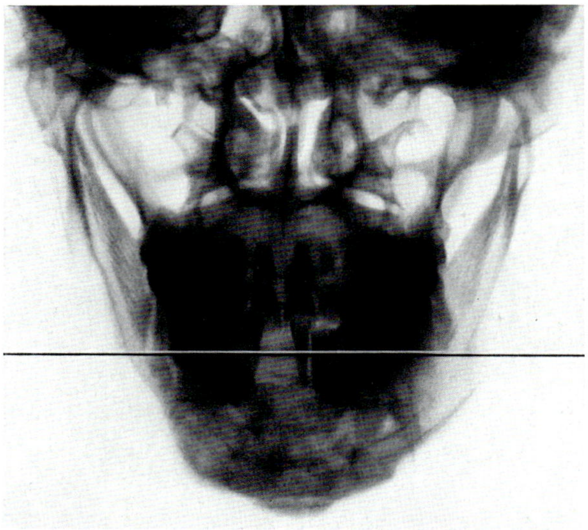

Fig. 507. Normal roentgenogram. Horizontal line showing the level tomographed. Irregular bony defect associated with absence of the incisor in the mandible is suspected. These findings are not easily seen due to superimposition of the cervical spine

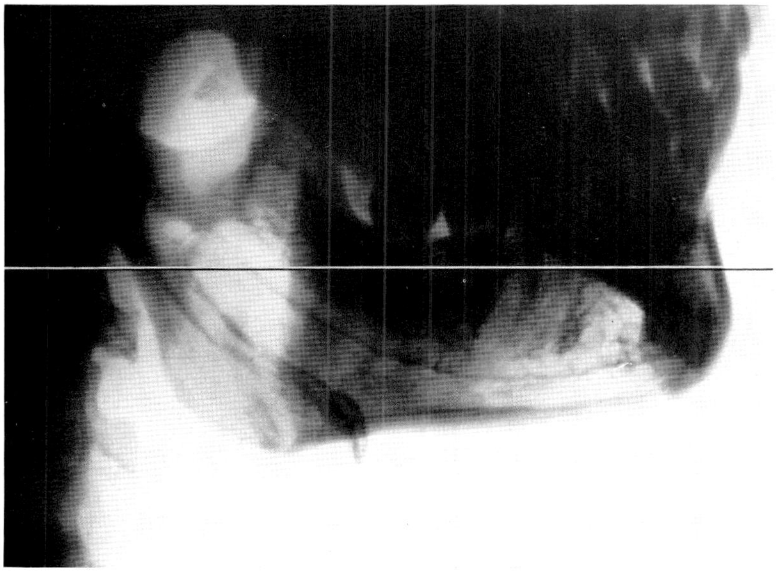

Fig. 508. Normal roentgenogram. Horizontal line showing the level tomographed. In the oblique view, there is a small defect in the anterior portion of the mandible. In the lateral view of the mandible, no evidence of bony defect is noted

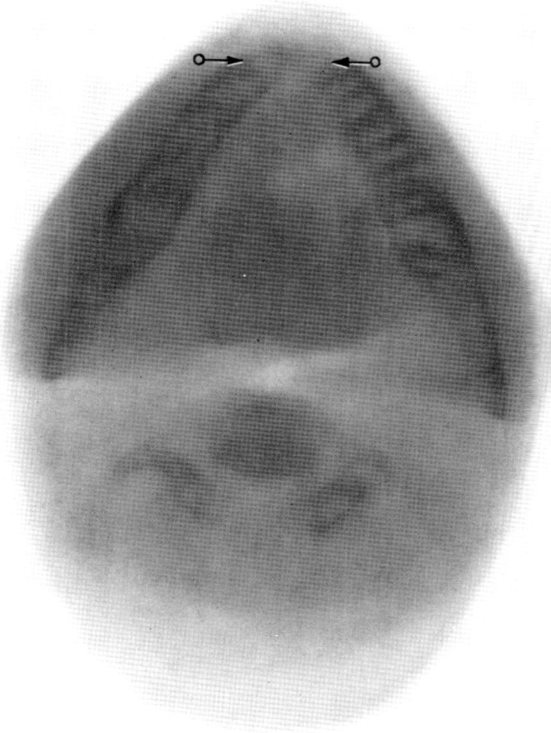

Fig. 509. Axial transverse tomogram. See Figs. 101—105, p. 56, for normal axial transverse tomogram of this level. Axial transverse tomogram shows a defect (↗) measuring 20 mm in length in the midportion of the mandibular body. No other abnormality is seen

Diagnosis: Suspected myositis ossificans.

Case: S. H., age 54, male.

History: Numbness of the extremities and difficulty in walking for 7 to 8 years.

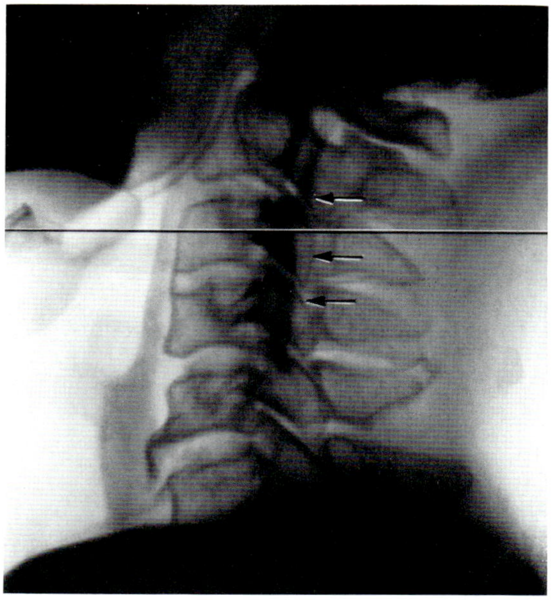

Fig. 510. Normal roentgenogram. Horizontal line showing the level tomographed. The lateral view of the cervical spine shows a tape-like calcific density (↗) superimposed on the laminae of the second, third and fourth cervical vertebrae. There is a calcific plaque of 7 × 10 mm in size in the soft tissues in the posterior aspect of the spine (ligamentum nuchae)

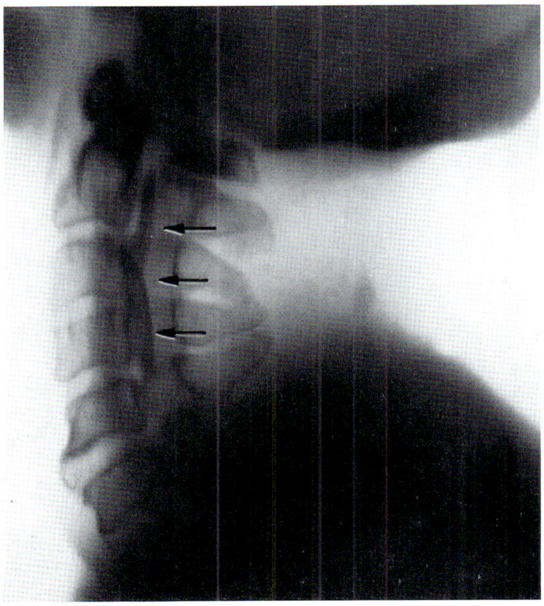

Fig. 511. Conventional tomogram. The lateral view reveals a tape-like calcific density (↗) along the posterior aspect of the vertebral bodies of C_2, C_3, C_4, C_5

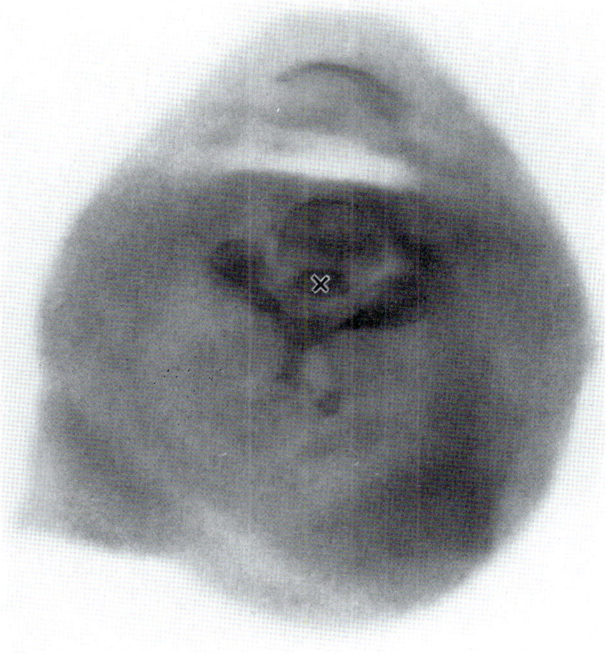

Fig. 512. Axial transverse tomogram. See Figs. 121—125, p. 64, for normal axial transverse tomogram at this level. In the normal neck no calcification is noted in the spine space. The axial transverse tomogram shows the cross-section of the vertebral body, spinal process and other structures of the spine. There is an oval-shaped calcific thickening (×) in the cervical spinal canal which in view of its position and shape is considered to be calcified posterior longitudinal ligament

Diagnosis: Tumor of the left thyroideal lobe

Case: K. S., age 36, female

History: Swelling of the neck and hoarseness for two years. The tumor of the left thyroideal lobe region is noted.

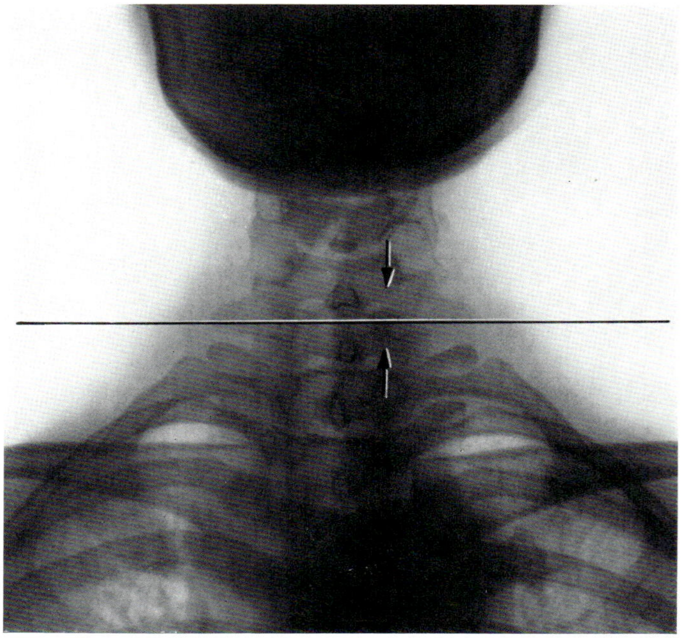

Fig. 513. Normal roentgenogram. Horizontal line showing the level tomographed. The cervical trachea is deviated to the right. A calcified body (↗), one cm in diameter, is seen to be superimposed upon the seventh cervical vertebral body on the left

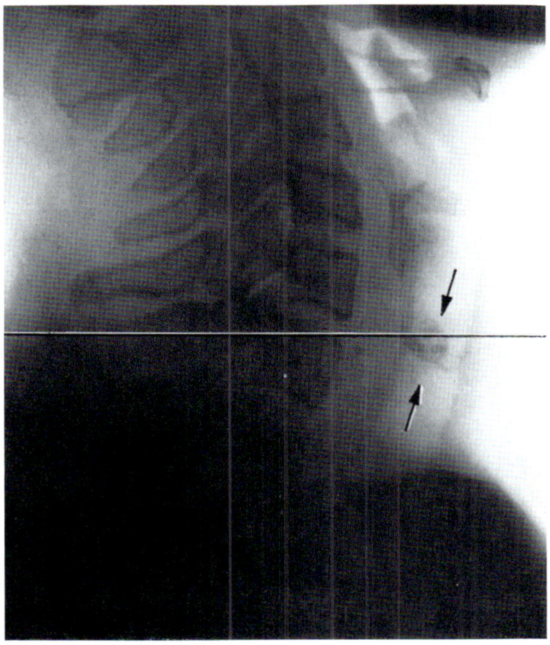

Fig. 514. Normal roentgenogram. Horizontal line showing the level tomographed. Lateral view of the neck shows the body (↗) superimposed on the trachea

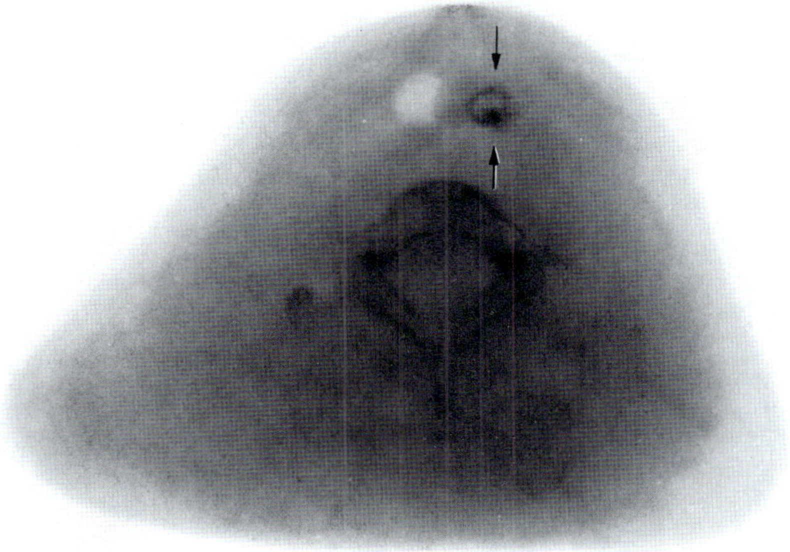

Fig. 515. Axial transverse tomogram. See Figs. 141—145, p. 72 for normal axial transverse tomogram at this level. A light swelling of soft tissue is seen in the left anterior neck. The trachea, whose left side wall is compressed by the tumor, is deviated to the right. A ring shadow with irregular contour of high density is seen in the tumor (↗). In view of the position, the calcification seems to be in the struma

Diagnosis:	Tuberculous cavity of the lung.
Case:	K. T., age 28, male.
History:	For 18 months productive cough and fatigue. For the last 10 months he has been treated with an antituberculous agent.

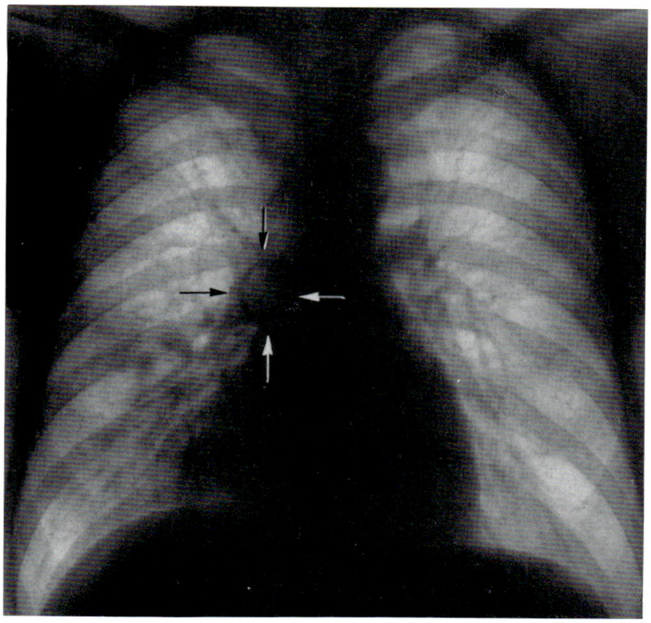

Fig. 516. Normal roentgenogram taken 10 months ago reveals the cavity (↗) of 3.0 × 2.5 cm in size at the hilum

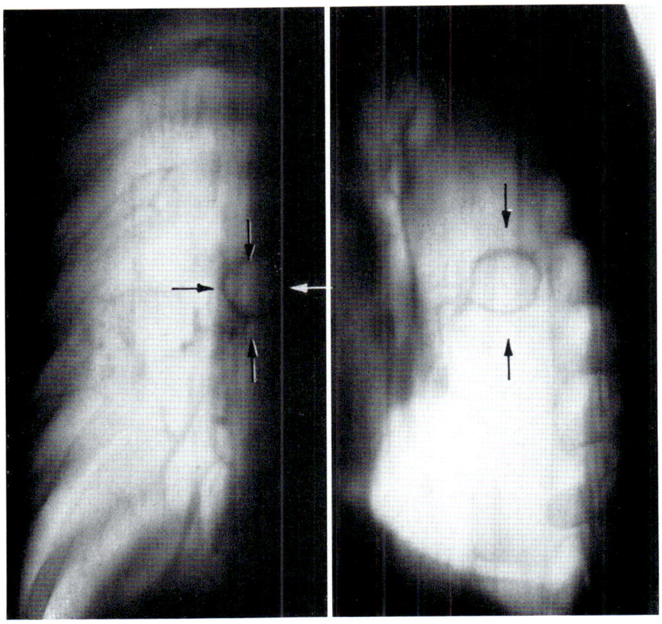

A B

Fig. 517A and B. Conventional tomograms taken at that time show clearly the location and size of the cavity (↗) in a.p. and lateral view

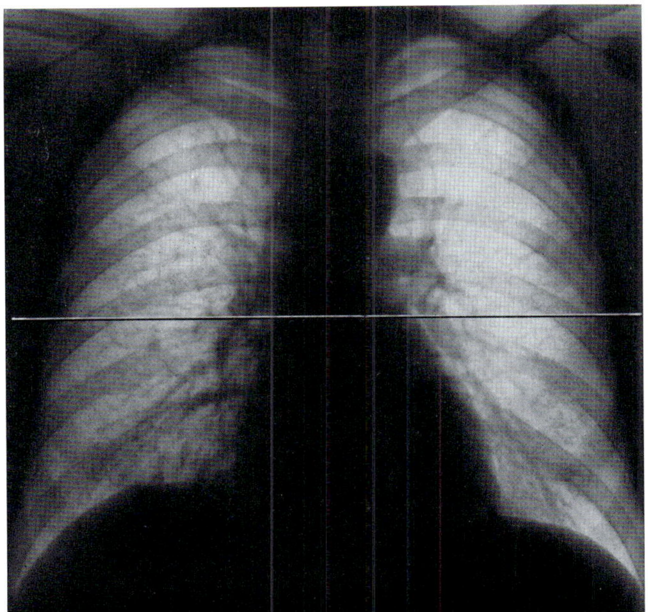

Fig. 518. In the normal roentgenogram taken very recently, nodular lesions are seen to be scattered in the right lower lung field. No evidence of cavity. Horizontal line showing the level tomographed

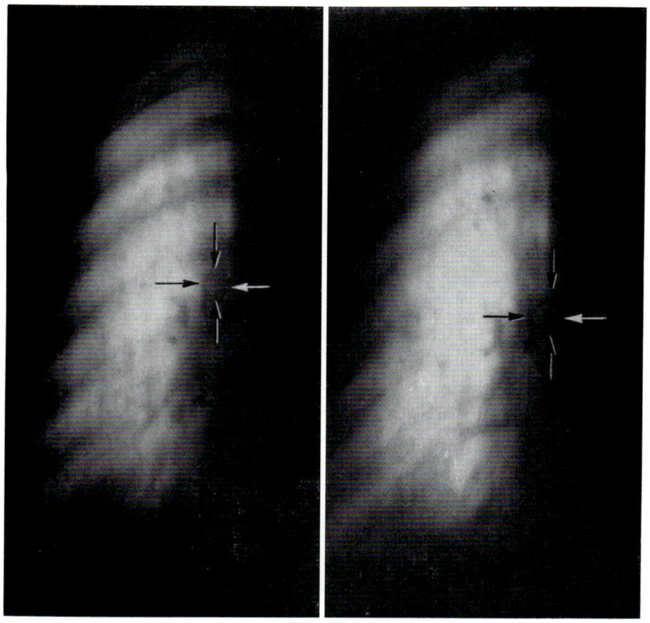

A B

Fig. 519A and B. The conventional tomogram at 5 cm level from posterior chest wall, A, reveals a small thin-walled cavity (↗) medially measuring 8 mm in diameter, while at 6 cm, B, the cavity is 12 mm in diameter

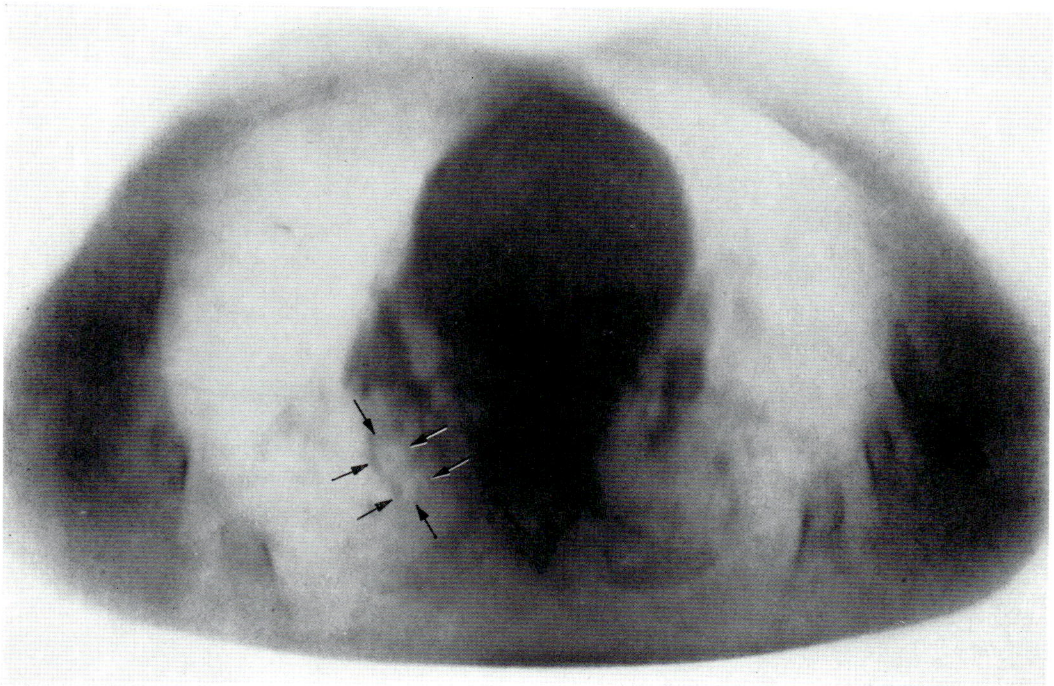

Diagnosis:	Foreign body.
Case:	T. K., age 35, male.
History:	The patient swallowed a nail three months ago accidentally. Right chest pain, cough and expectoration were noted recently.

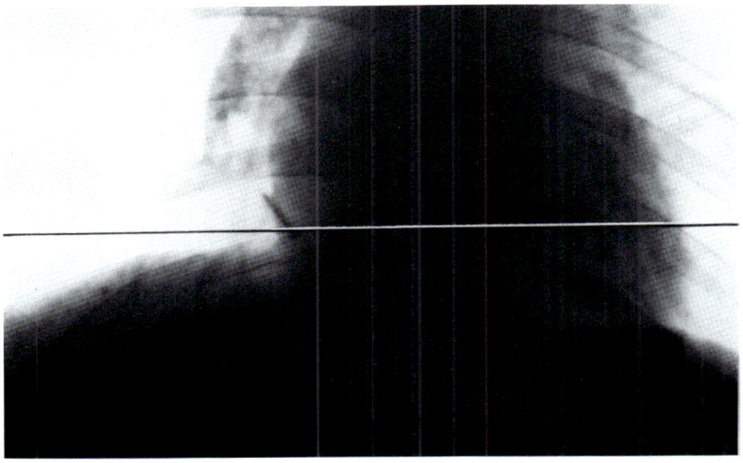

Fig. 521. Normal roentgenogram. Horizontal line showing the level tomographed. In the a.p. view a small nail is seen at the right base medially superimposed on the shadow of the heart

Fig. 520. Axial transverse tomogram. See the normal Figs. 223—227, p. 108. A dumb-bell-shaped radiolucent shadow (↗) is seen in the area of pulmonary infiltration in the right posterior lung field. The location of the cavity coincides with the cavity of the normal roentgenogram taken before chemotherapy and with that of the conventional tomogram taken at the same time as this examination. The anterior part of the cavity is 15 mm in diameter, while the posterior part is 10 mm in diameter. The cavitation is surrounded by the infiltration, and is seen at the postero-median region of the right lung field

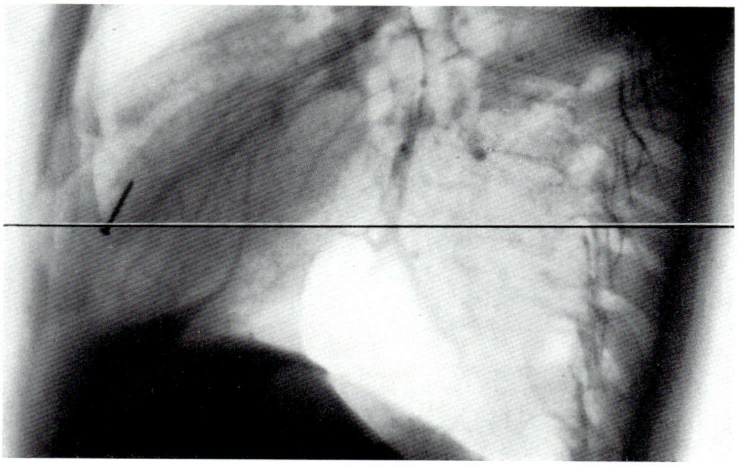

Fig. 522. In the lateral view, the nail is located anteriorly, but still superimposed on the heart. If only these two roentgenograms are used for examination, the nail might be concluded to be in the heart muscle

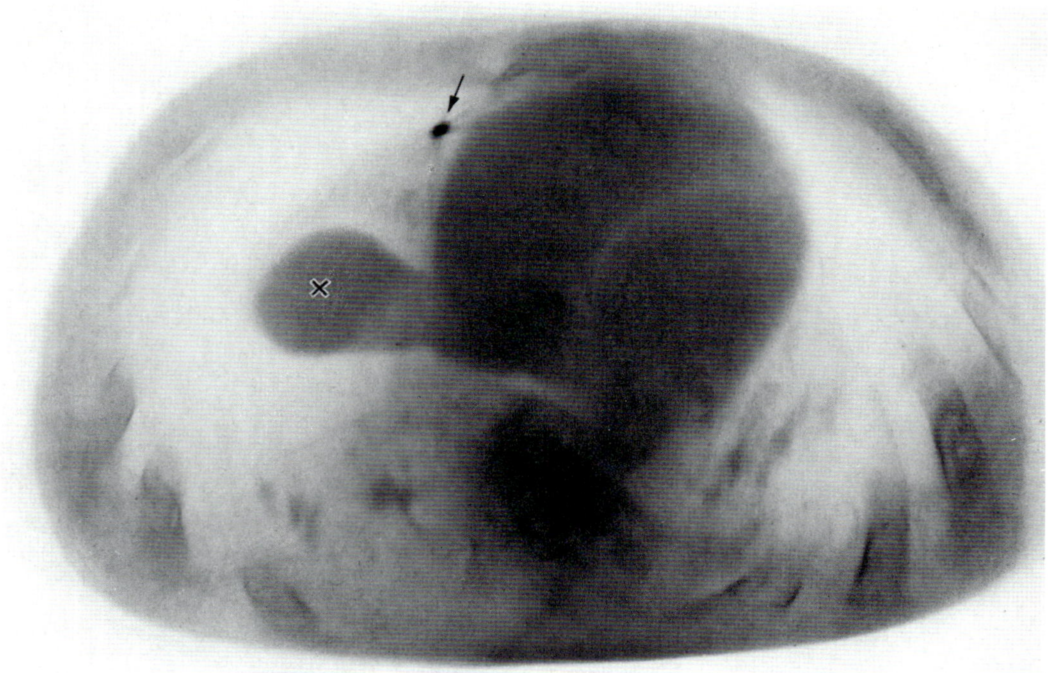

Fig. 523. Axial transverse tomogram. See Figs. 248—252, p. 118, for normal axial transverse tomogram at this level. It is clear from the axial transverse tomogram that the nail (↗) is located definitely in the lung. After establishment of the diagnosis, transbronchial removal of the nail was tried but failed. The foreign body was removed by thoracotomy. Diaphragm (×)

Diagnosis: Malignant lymphoma.

Case: M. A., age 42, male.

History: The patient complains of general fatigue and swelling of the lymph nodes in the various parts of the body.

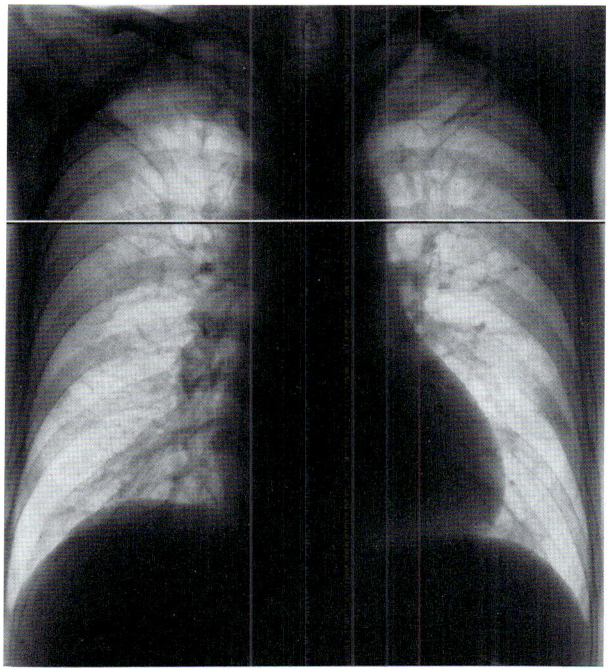

Fig. 524. Normal roentgenogram. Horizontal line showing the level tomographed. The p.a. view reveals slight widening of the superior mediastinum on the right side but nothing on the left. Both lung fields are clear

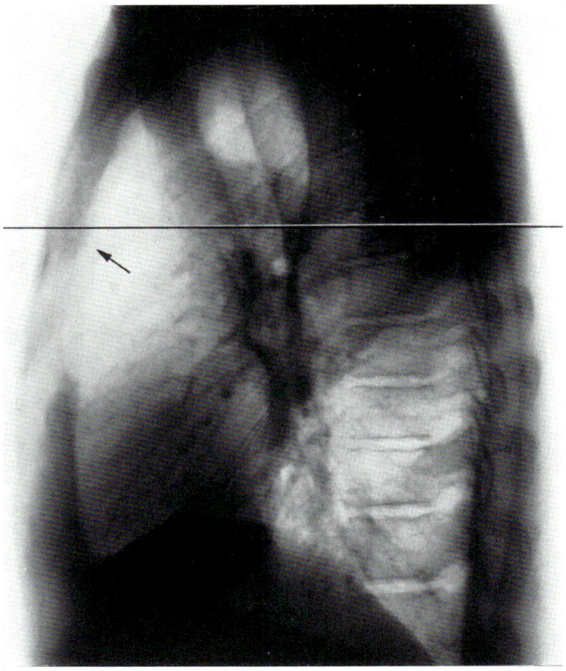

Fig. 525. Normal roentgenogram. Horizontal line showing the level tomographed. Lateral view of the chest, a soft tissue mass (↗) is suspected substernally, measuring about 5 cm in length and 0.5 cm in width

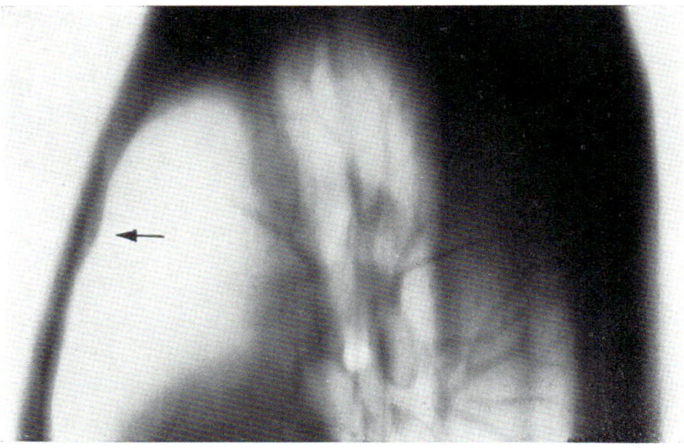

Fig. 526. Conventional tomogram. When the conventional lateral tomogram of this part of the chest is taken (2 cm left of median), a homogeneous, thin crescent-shaped shadow (↗) is seen substernally

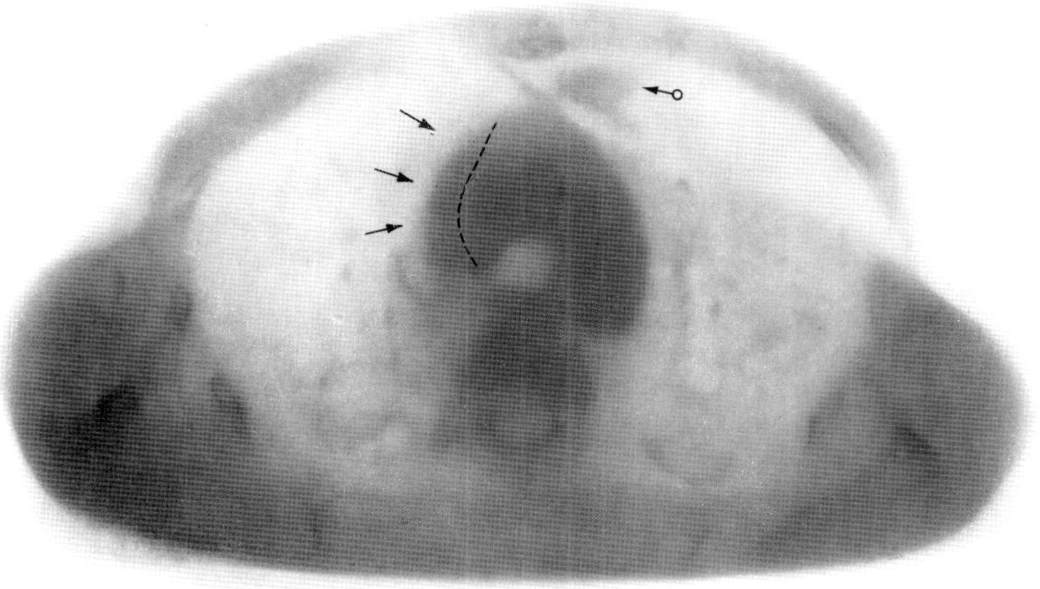

Fig. 527. Axial transverse tomogram. See Figs. 193—202, p. 96, for normal axial transverse tomogram at this level. There is a triangular opacity (↗) substernally on the left side, just anterior to the aortic arch, which is not seen on the normal roentgenogram. The increasing area of homogeneous shadow (↗) adjacent to the ascending aorta is manifested by broadening of its width which corresponds to the shadow noted on the normal roentgenogram

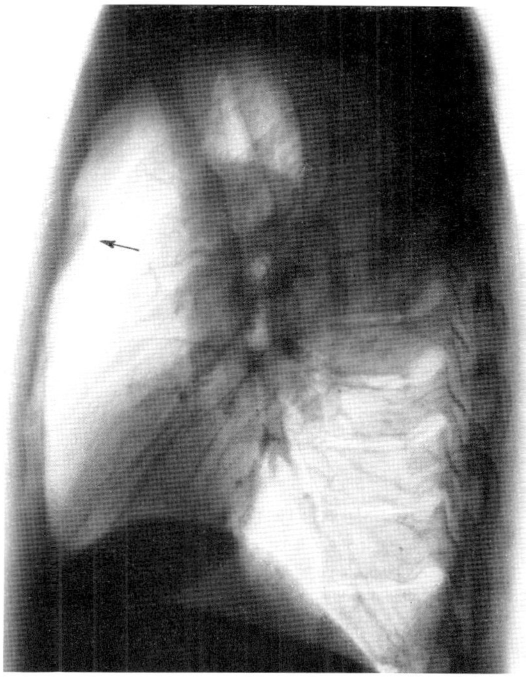

Fig. 528. Normal roentgenogram taken 3 months later reveals the marked crescent-shaped homogeneous shadow (↗) which is considered to be due to the swelling of the lymph nodes along the internal mammary artery

Diagnosis: Mediastinal tumor.

Case: M. K., age 52, male.

History: Lower body paralysis of 2 years' duration. Hoarseness and dyspnea of one year's duration. One year ago a chest X-ray study revealed a mediastinal tumor which disappeared after ^{60}Co teletherapy.

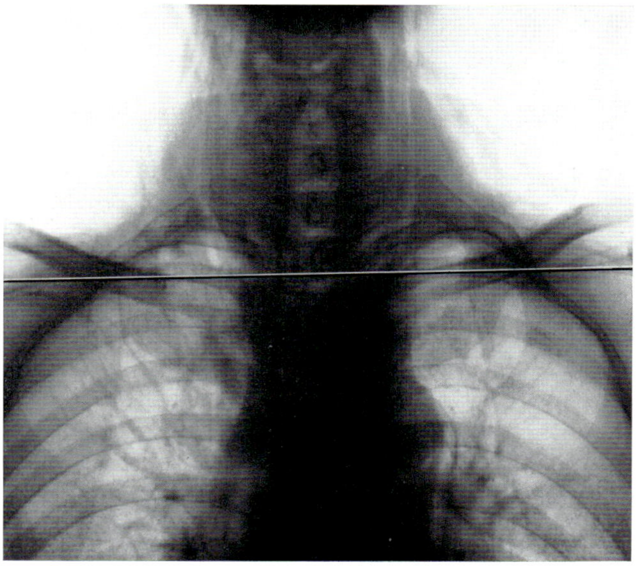

Fig. 529. Normal roentgenogram. Horizontal line showing the level tomographed. The p.a. view of the chest reveals nothing remarkable. A small calcification in the right pulmonary apex but with right clavicle superimposed. Insufflated air is imaged in the mediastinum and in the neck

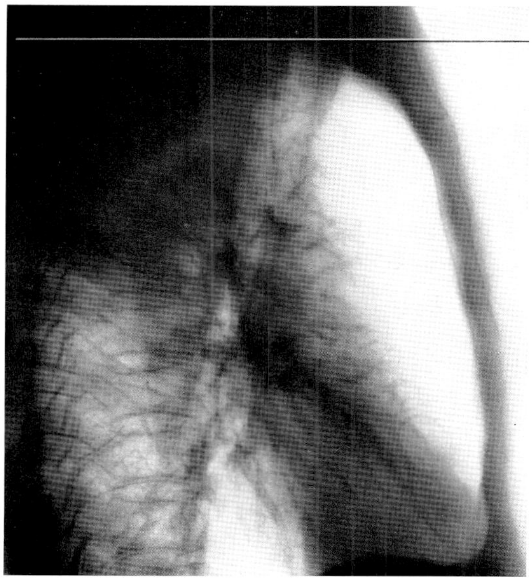

Fig. 530. Normal roentgenogram. Horizontal line showing the level tomographed. A soft tissue mass is suspected in the superior mediastinum posteriorly in the lateral view

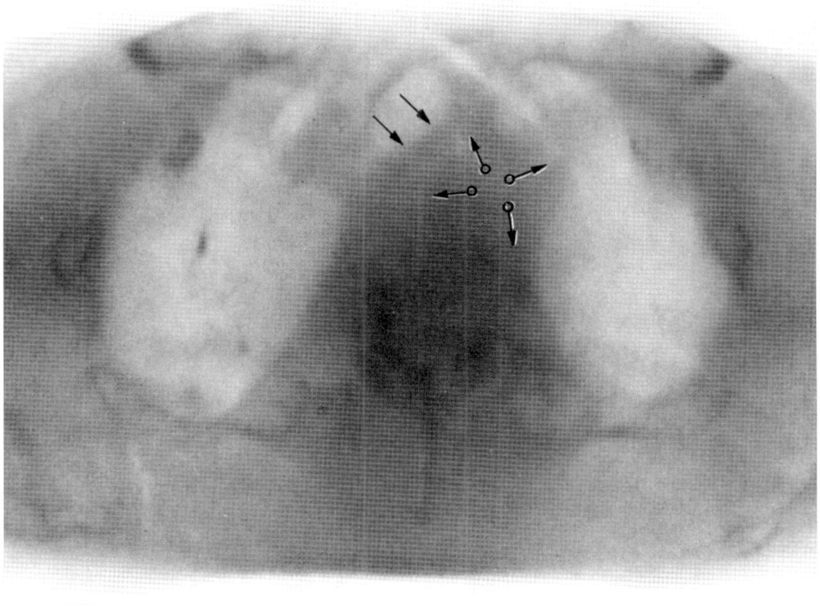

Fig. 531. Axial transverse tomogram. See Figs. 168—172, p. 86, for normal axial transverse tomogram at this level. A soft tissue mass about 3 × 3 cm is seen in the superior mediastinum on the left side, compressing the trachea slightly anteriorly to the right (↗). The cross-section of the trachea is not circular but semilunar. Increase of shadow (↗) at the anterior mediastinum especially sinistrally. Small opaque spot in the right lung field is the shadow of calcification seen on the pulmonary apex of the normal roentgenogram

Diagnosis: Sarcoidosis.

Case: K. K., age 10, male.

History: Fever and cough of two months' duration.

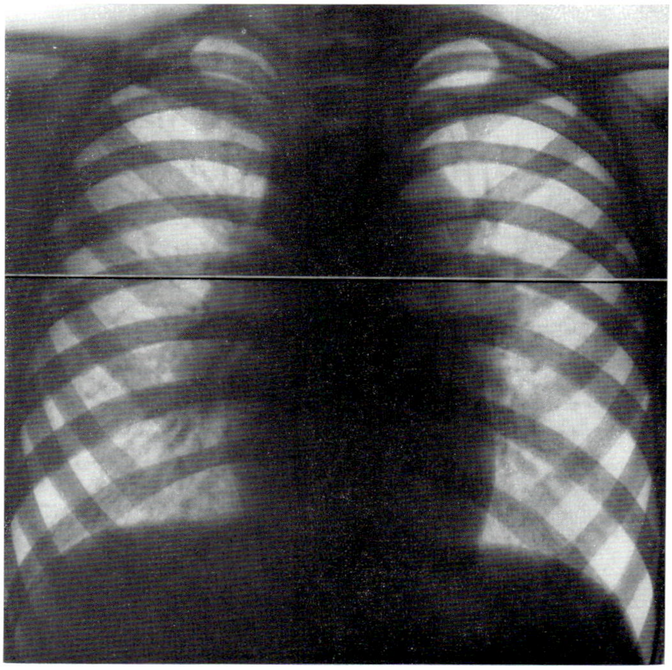

Fig. 532. Normal roentgenogram. Horizontal line showing the level tomographed. Bilateral hilar adenopathy with enlargement of mediastinal shadow. The lung fields are clear

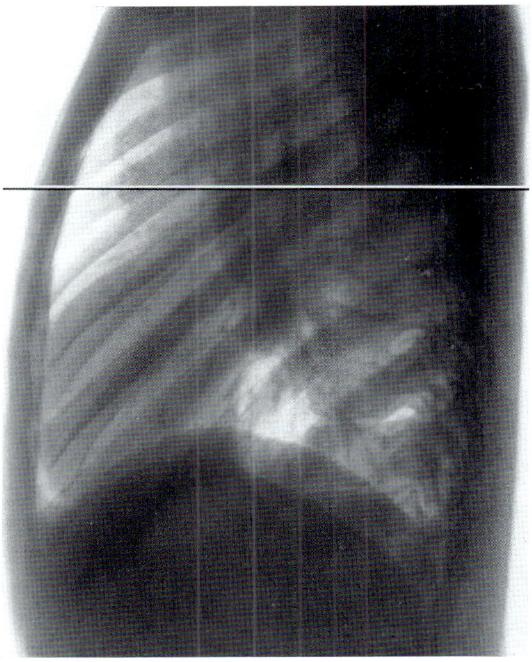

Fig. 533. Normal roentgenogram. Horizontal line showing the level tomographed. Lateral view shows similar findings to Fig. 532

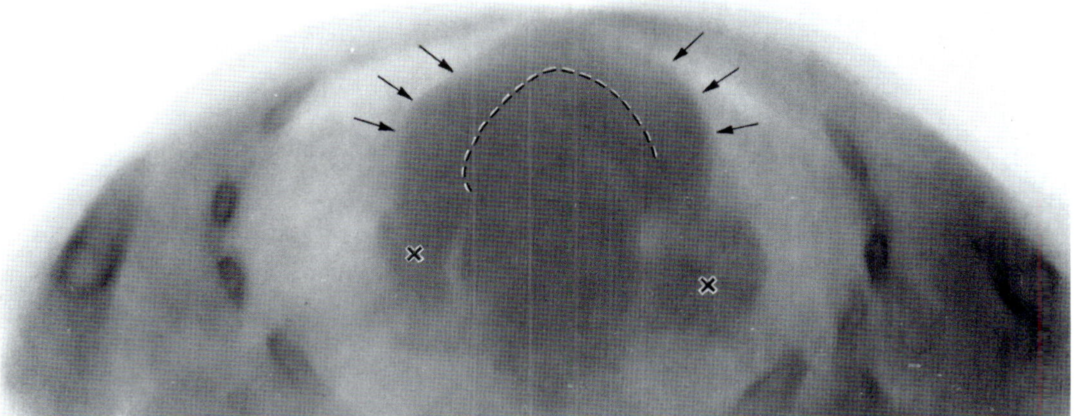

Fig. 534. Axial transverse tomogram. See Figs. 218—222, p. 106, for normal axial transverse tomogram at this level. The axial transverse tomogram reveals a remarkable mediastinal lymphadenopathy. The bronchopulmonary lymph nodes (×) are also markedly enlarged along both sides of the bronchus. The shadow of the anterior mediastinum increases in width, suggesting a marked swelling of the anterior mediastinal lymph nodes (↗)

Diagnosis: Vanishing tumor.

Case: T. M., age 53, female.

History: The patient, who has a history of cured cancer of the uterus, noted low backaches and coughs.

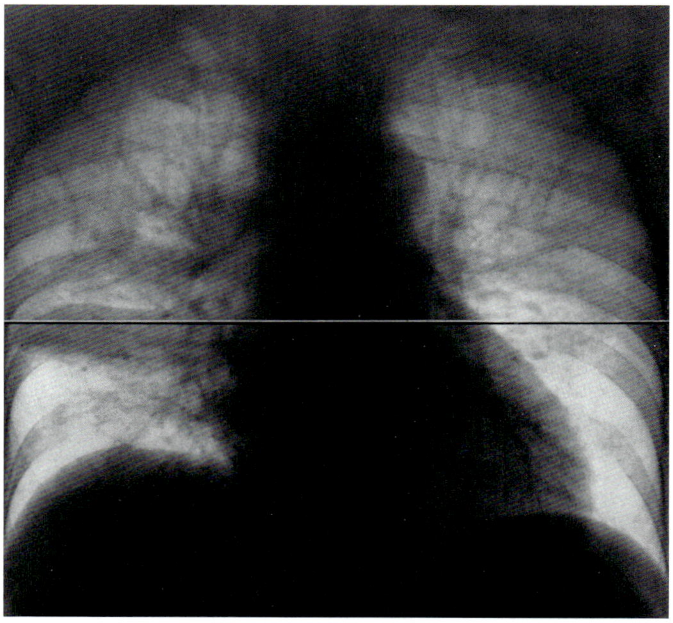

Fig. 535. Normal roentgenogram. Horizontal line showing the level tomographed. In the p.a. view there is an ellipsoid homogeneous shadow in the right horizontal fissure

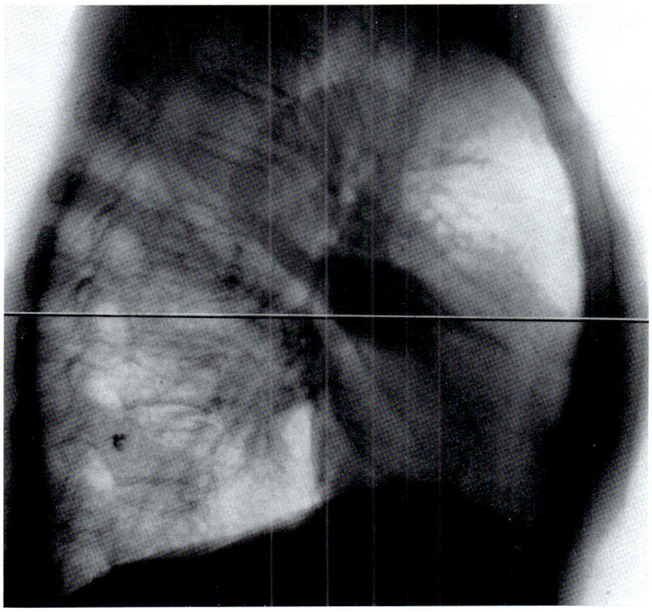

Fig. 536. Normal roentgenogram. Horizontal line showing the level tomographed. The lateral view reveals a round homogeneous shadow with three wings spreading over the main and horizontal fissures

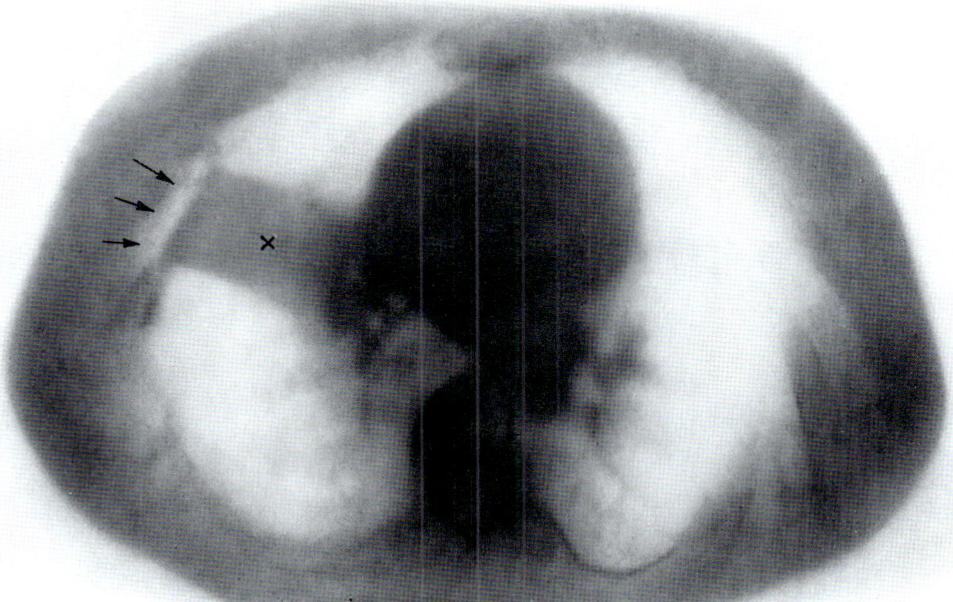

Fig. 537. Axial transverse tomogram. See Figs. 223—227, p. 108, for normal axial transverse tomogram at this level. The axial transverse tomogram reveals a rectangular homogeneous opacity (×) in the middle lobe of the right lung slightly anteriorly. A slit-like radiolucency (↗) is noted between the opacity and the lateral chest wall, revealing the curved downward turn of the horizontal fissure

Diagnosis: Aneurysm of the thoracic aorta.

Case: S. T., age 56, male.

History: Dyspnea, palpitation and difficulty in swallowing of two months' duration.

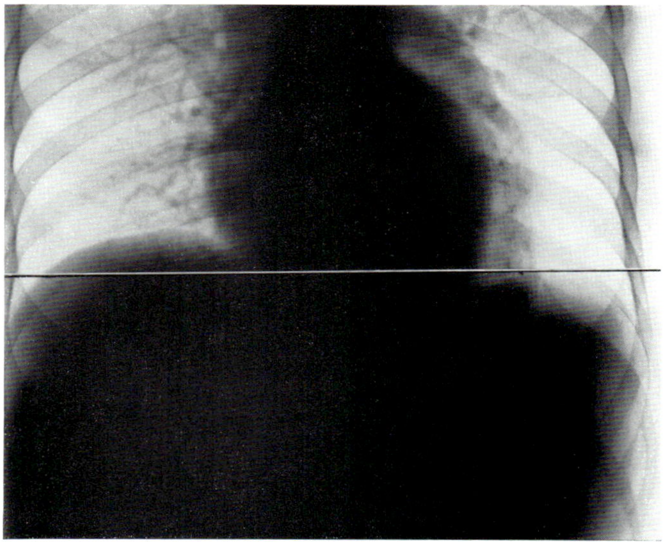

Fig. 538. Normal roentgenogram. Horizontal line showing the level tomographed. Supine a.p. view shows a homogeneous band-like shadow along the left margin of the shadow of the heart

Fig. 540. Axial transverse tomogram. See Figs. 258—267, p. 122, for normal axial transverse tomogram at this level. There is a large aneurysmal dilation (×) of the aorta, about 7 cm in diameter, with semicircular calcification left laterally (↗). The widening of the aorta causes moderate displacement of the fornix of the stomach (S) toward the anterior

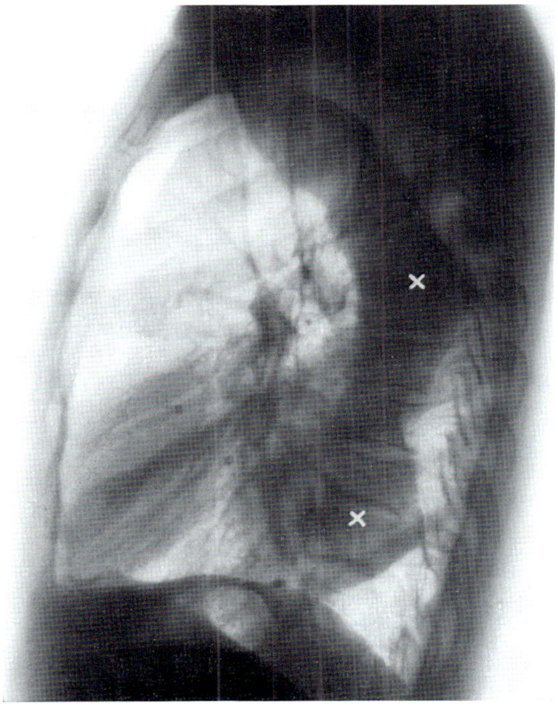

Fig. 539. The lateral view of the chest reveals at least two aneurysmal dilatations (×) of the descending thoracic aorta with calcification of the wall

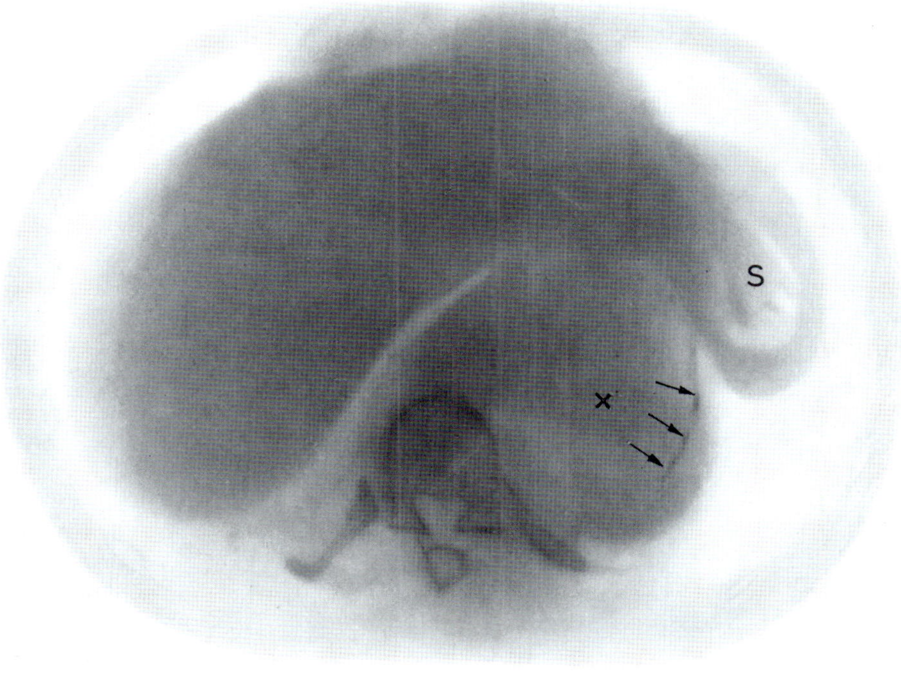

Diagnosis:	Metastatic cancer of the pleura.
Case:	A. N., age 32, male.
History:	About one year ago, a tumor the size of a fist was removed surgically from the right anterior mediastinum.

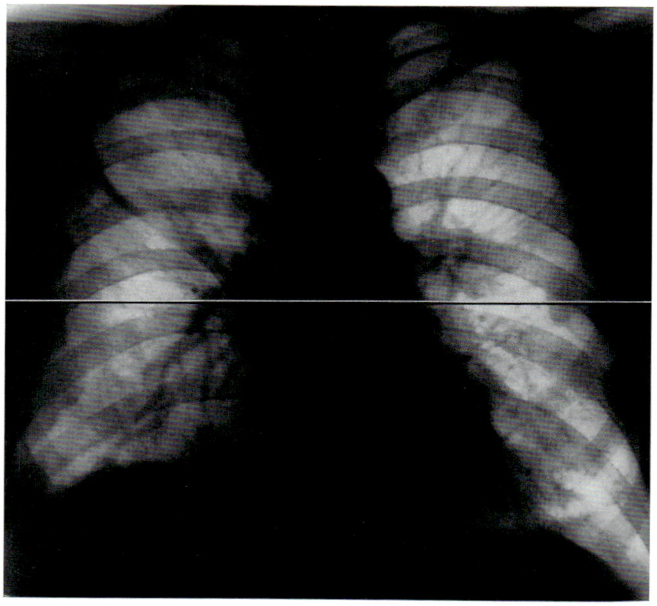

Fig. 541. Normal roentgenogram. Horizontal line showing the level tomographed. The p.a. view reveals bilateral multiple round and crescent-shaped homogeneous shadows in the lateral margins of the lung field

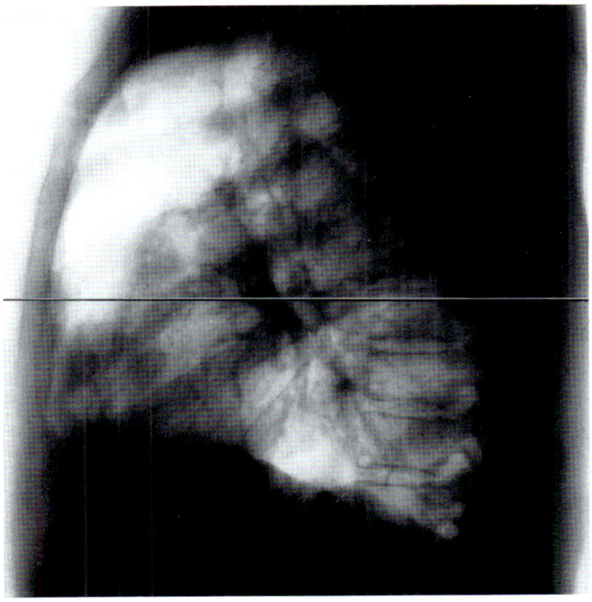

Fig. 542. Normal roentgenogram. Horizontal line showing the level tomographed. In the lateral view the findings are similar to the above. The increased shadows at the hilum are noted

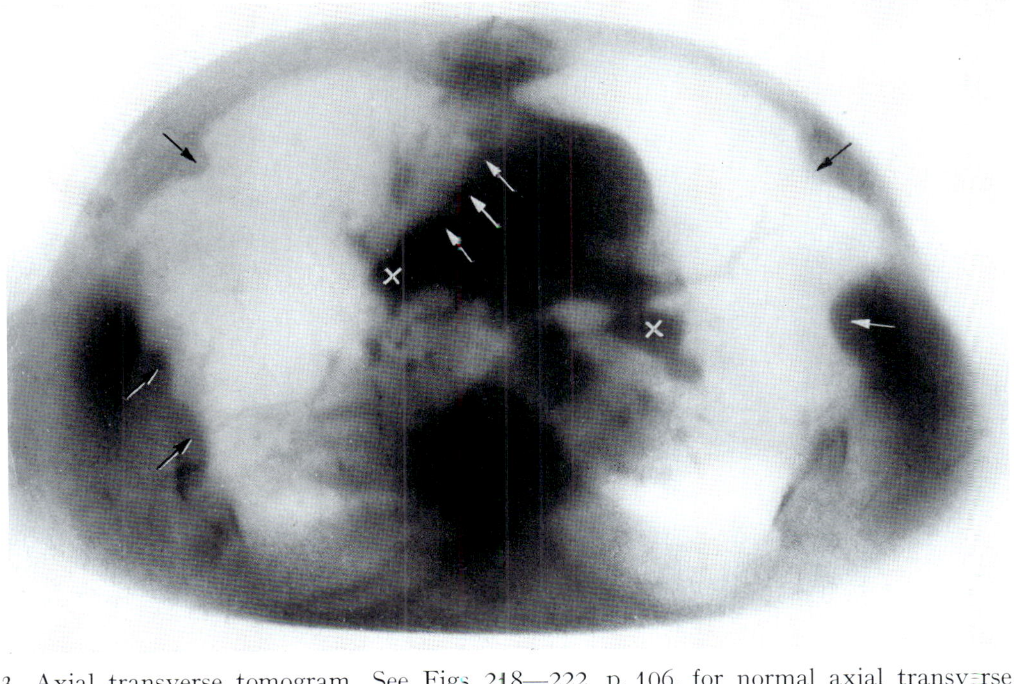

Fig. 543. Axial transverse tomogram. See Figs. 218—222, p. 106, for normal axial transverse tomogram at this level. There are multiple crescent-shaped tumors of homogeneous density (↗) on the pleural surface, protruding bilaterally into the lung field. In both hilar regions there are round opacities (×) of various sizes, 2 on the right and 3 on the left. The findings represent pleural, metastasis and hilar lymph node involvement. These changes are also seen in the contour of the anterior mediastinum which is imaged exclusively on the axial transverse tomogram. No evidence of lesions in the lung

Diagnosis: Cold abscess of the anterior chest wall.

Case: M. K., age 51, male.

History: Swelling of the right anterior chest wall was noted five years ago. The swelling started growing in size one year ago. Pain and tenderness.

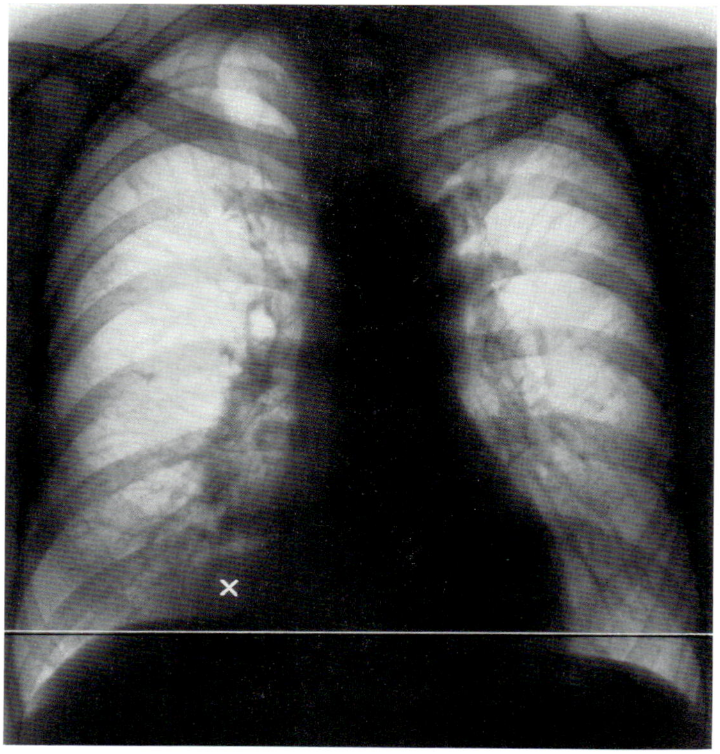

Fig. 544. Normal roentgenogram. Horizontal line showing the level tomographed. Some abnormal shadow (×) is seen at the right cardiophrenic angle in the p.a. view. Fibronodular and bilateral apical pleural thickening is seen in the left superior lung field, suggestive of old tuberculous changes

Fig. 546. Axial transverse tomogram. See Figs. 253—257, p. 120, for normal axial transverse tomogram of this level. There is a large soft tissue mass of homogeneous density on the right breast anteriorly. The mass (↗) is protruding anteriorly through the chest wall and is about 8 cm in diameter. The posterior part of the mass (×) is in contact with the right hemidiaphragm and the heart. The calcification in the central part of the mass probably represents a calcified cartilaginous rib

Fig. 545. Normal roentgenogram. Horizontal line showing the level tomographed. In the lateral view, a dumb-bell-shaped soft tissue shadow (×) is noted substernally

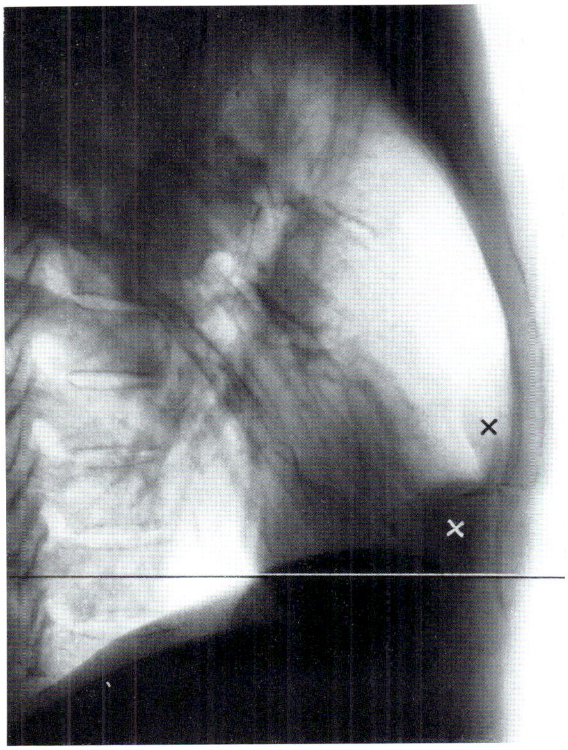

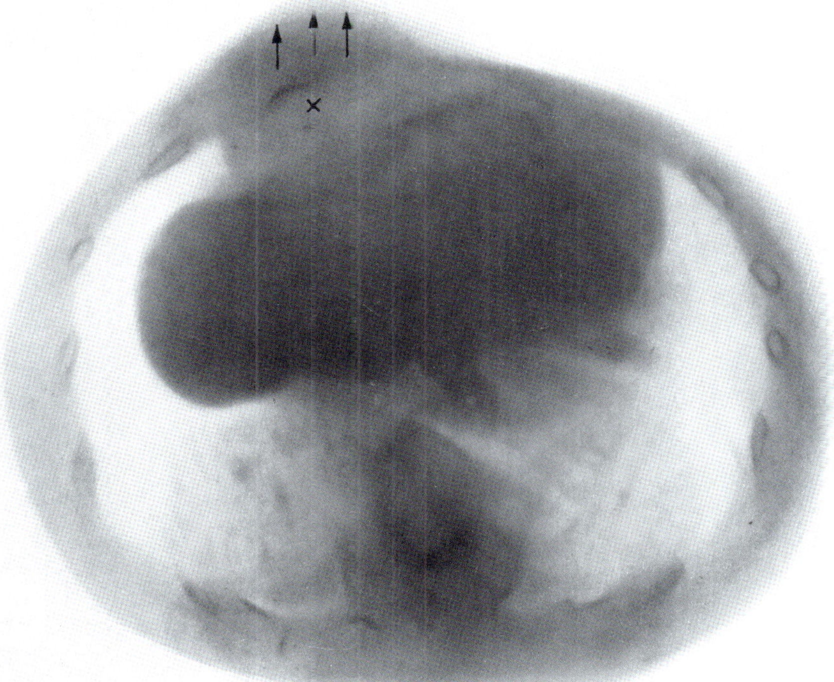

Diagnosis:	Cancer of the pancreas.
Case:	T. S., age 65, female.
History:	Abdominal pain in the left upper abdomen and backaches with anorexia and loss of weight of 6 months' duration. Recently a hard mass was noted in the left hypochondrium.

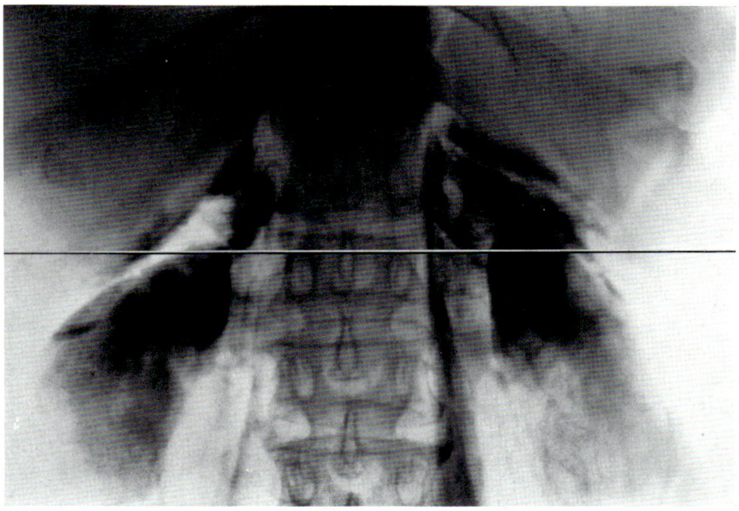

Fig. 547. Normal roentgenogram. Horizontal line showing the level tomographed. The psoas muscle bilaterally well delineated due to retroperitoneal air insufflation. Neither the a.p. nor the lateral view of the normal roentgenogram reveals and identifies a mass which could be a suspected pancreas tumor

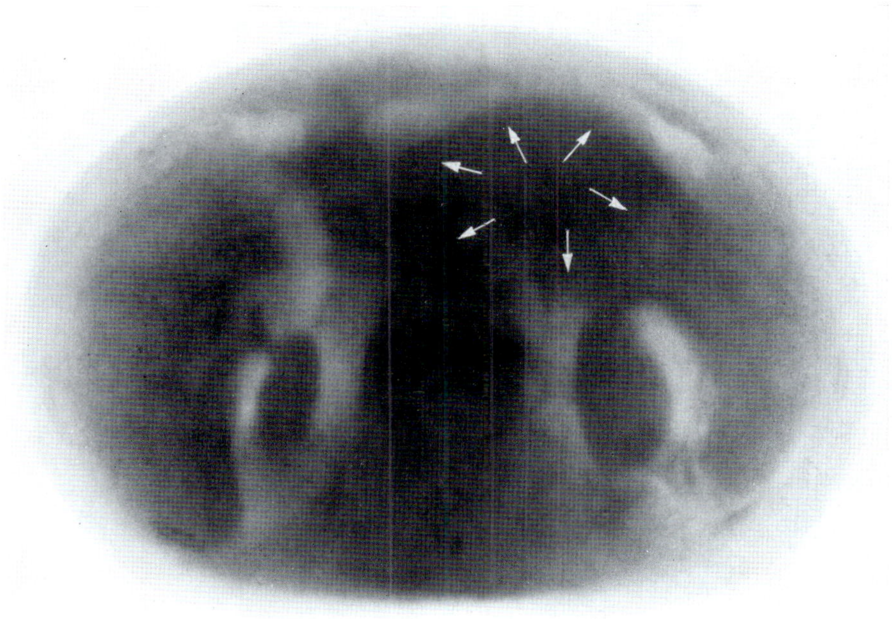

Fig. 548. Axial transverse tomogram. See Figs. 311—315, p. 150, for normal view at this level. There is a large homogeneous opacity (↗) due to compression occupying the position from the vertebral body to the narrowed pylorus. The opacity is surrounded by air sinistrally at the front of the left kidney and dextrally at the right of the vertebral body

Diagnosis: Left suprarenal cyst.

Case: M. N., age 38, female.

History: Epigastric discomfort of two years' duration.

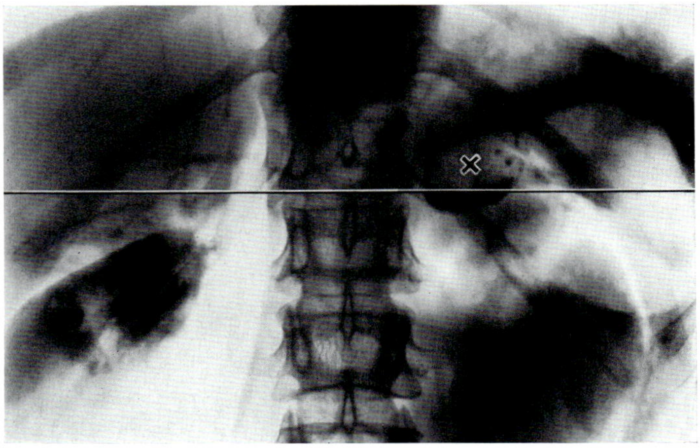

Fig. 549. Normal roentgenogram. Horizontal line showing the level tomographed. In the p.a. view an egg-shaped calcific thickening (×) of thumb-head size is seen on the left side of the 12th thoracic vertebra

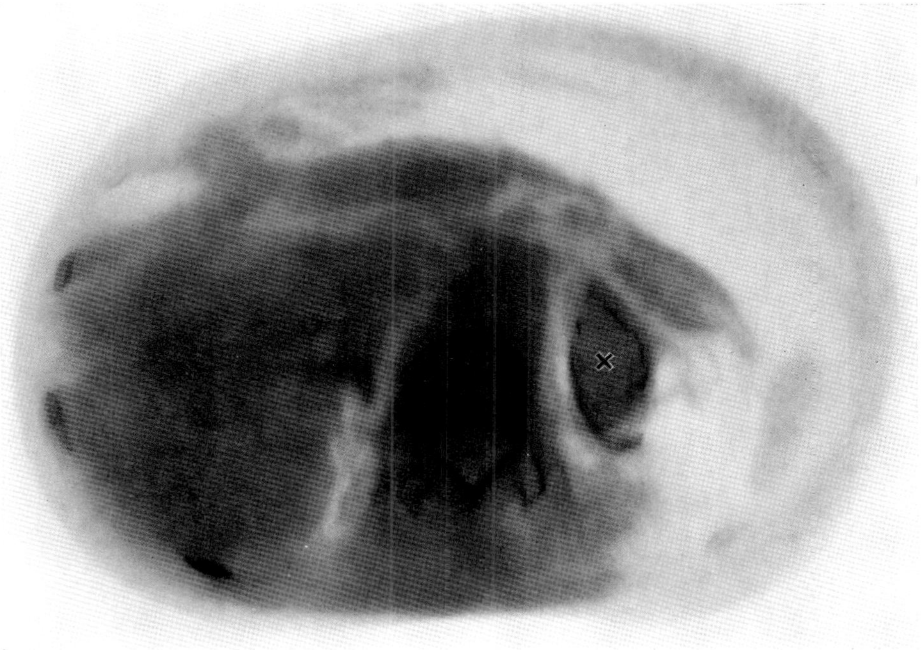

Fig. 550. Axial transverse tomogram. See Figs. 301—305, p. 146, for normal view at this level. An oval soft tissue mass (×) with thin calcific plaque is seen on the outer wall in the left retroperitoneal cavity which is projected just to the left of the vertebral body. In view of its location, it was concluded it could only be a suprarenal tumor. After surgical operation it was histologically proved to be a suprarenal cyst

Diagnosis: Thorotrast liver.

Case: S. T., age 56, male.

History: About 30 years ago the patient was examined for coronary thrombosis by arteriography, using thorotrast contrast medium. Recently the patient developed bilateral pleural effusion and liver enlargement. The liver scintigram shows a moderate sized defect in the region of left lobe.

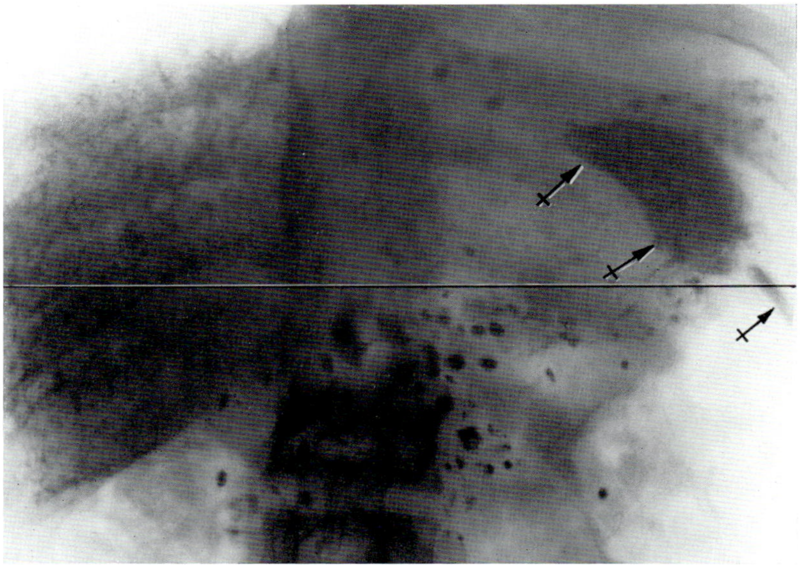

Fig. 551. Normal roentgenogram. Horizontal line showing the level tomographed. The antero-posterior view of the upper abdomen shows diffuse deposition of the thorotrast in the liver in a reticular pattern. The spleen (↗) is smaller than normal with thorotrast deposits. Multiple deposits are noted in the mesenteric lymph nodes

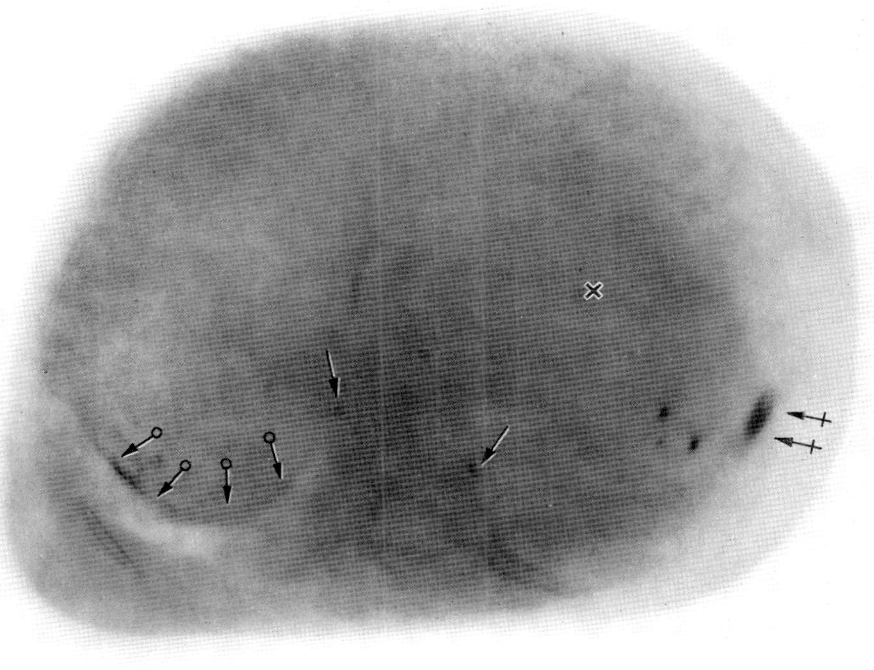

Fig. 552. Axial transverse tomogram. See normal Figs. 296—300, p. 144. A curvilinear density is seen in the posterior margin of the right lobe of the liver (o↗), and a few calcific densities in the anterior aspect of the vertebral body due to thorotrast deposits in the mesenteric (×) and retroperitoneal lymph nodes (↗). There is an oval calcific density in the left lateral aspect of the abdomen due to a lower tip of the spleen (x↗) with thorotrast deposit

Diagnosis:	Tuberculous calcification of the mesenteric lymph nodes.
Case:	K. A., age 52, male.
History:	He suffered from the tuberculosis of the lung about 25 years ago. Backaches for 2 years.

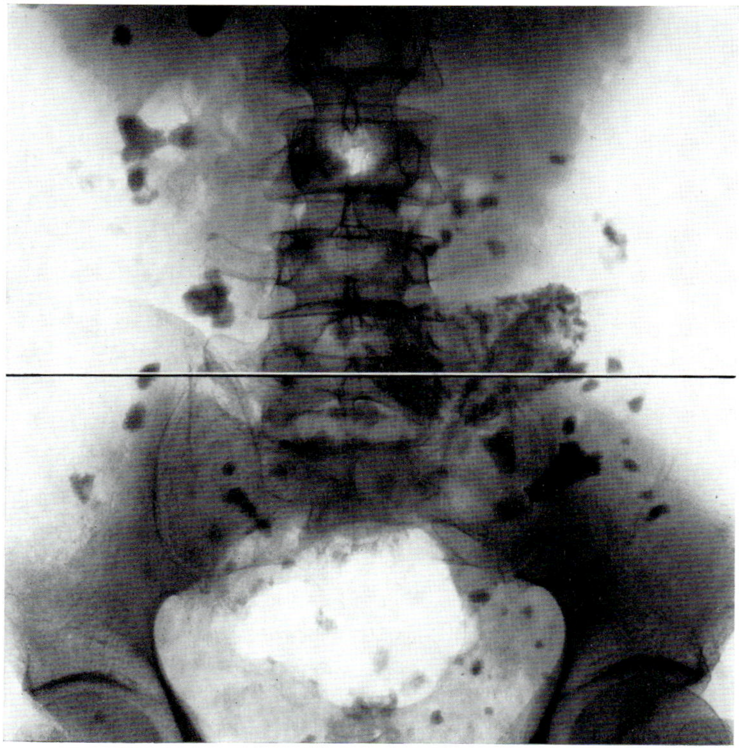

Fig. 553. Normal roentgenogram. Horizontal line showing the level tomographed. Multiple calcified bodies of various sizes are seen in the abdomen in the p.a. view

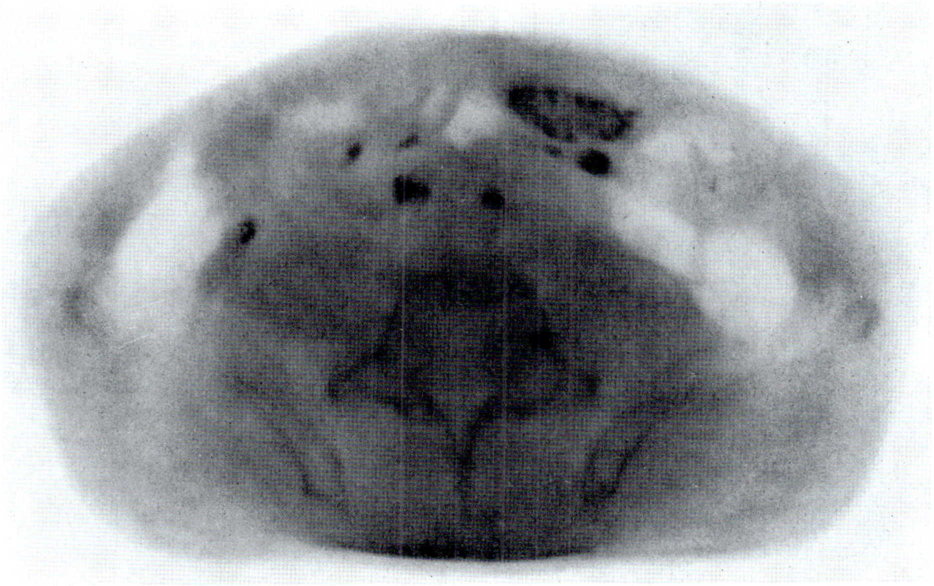

Fig. 554. Axial transverse tomogram. See Figs. 377—381, p. 180, for normal view at this level. The location of the calcified bodies is limited to the anatomical position of the mesenterium and is distinguishable from intestinal gas patterns

Diagnosis: Myoma uteri.

Case: S. Y., age 42, female.

History: A large pelvic mass was found incidentally. The patient had not complained.

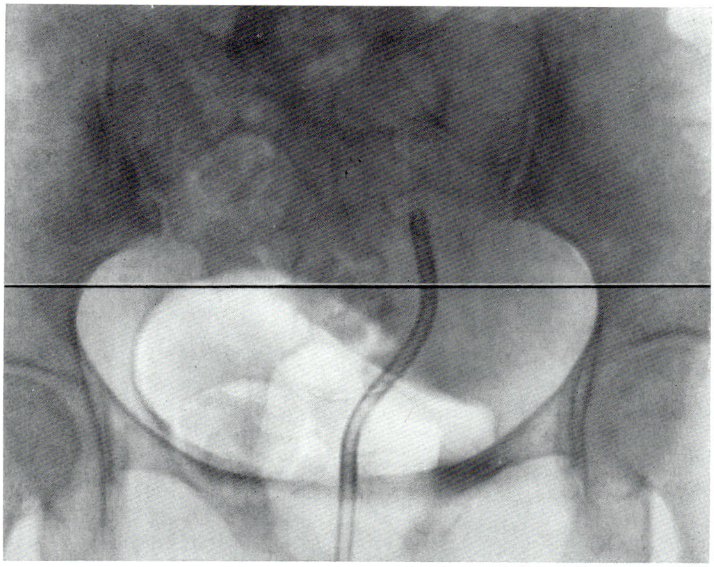

Fig. 555. Normal roentgenogram. Horizontal line showing the level tomographed. The a.p. view of the pelvis with a radiopaque catheter introduced into the uterine cavity through the vagina, air insufflation of the bladder and insertion of the radiotranslucent mass into the vagina reveals the presence of a large homogeneous density in the left pelvis which compresses the superior bladder wall

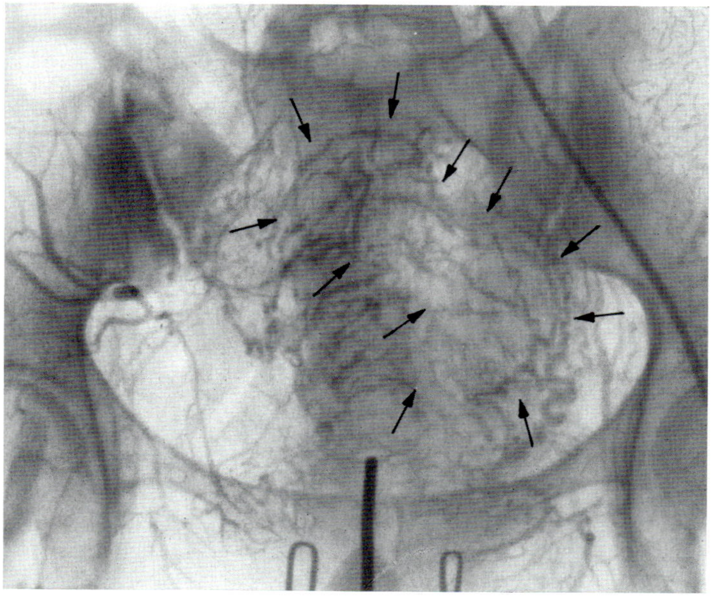

Fig. 556. Angiogram of the pelvis shows the location and the size of the tumor (↗)

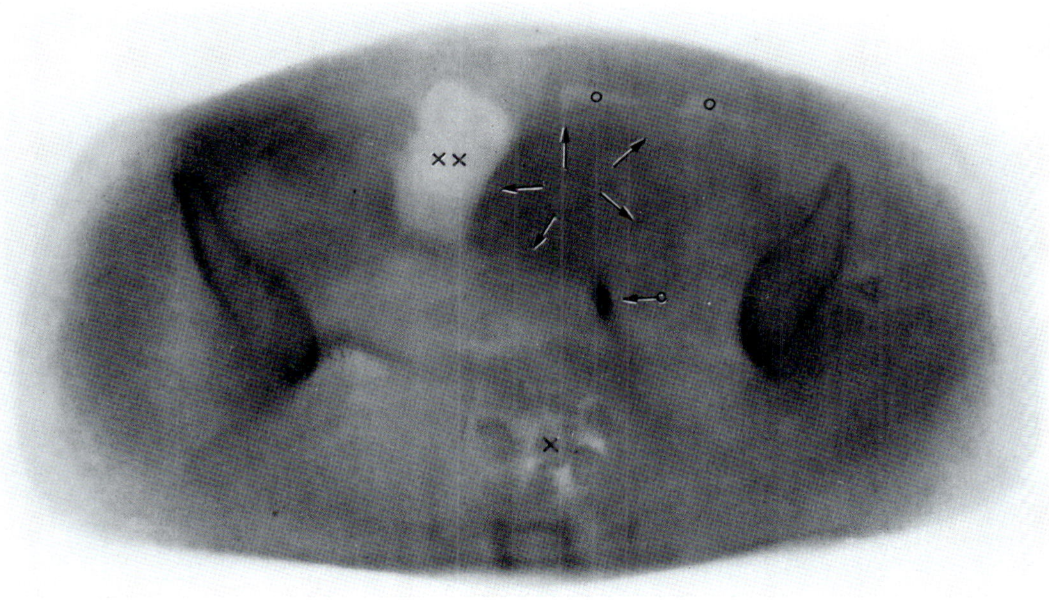

Fig. 557. Axial transverse tomogram. See Figs. 397—401, p. 188, for normal axial transverse tomogram at this level. The cross-section of the catheter (↗) imaged at the center of the tomogram reveals the position of the uterine cavity in the pelvis. Just behind this shadow, there is imaged the rectum (×) filled with feces in heaps mixed with a small amount of gas. At the anterior aspect of the catheter a large homogeneous shadow (↗) of 6 × 7 cm in size is noted suggesting the tumor mass of the anterior wall of the uterus. The left wall of the bladder (××) is compressed and deformed by this shadow. The narrow translucent zone between the tumor shadow and the abdominal skin is concluded to be the small intestine (o) by interpreting the finding of the normal roentgenogram

Diagnosis: Fracture of the left iliac bone.

Case: H. N., age 29, male.

History: Three months ago a heavy iron pillar fell on him and he sustained a bruise on his left hip.

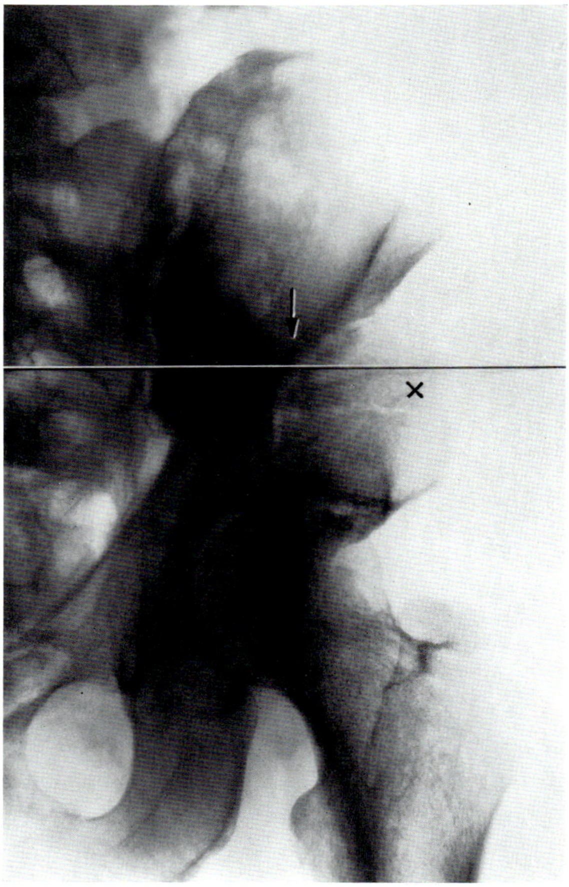

Fig. 558. Normal roentgenogram. Horizontal line showing the level tomographed. Extensive fracture (×) of the left iliac bone. A spindle-shaped opacity (↗) of 1.5 × 0.3 cm in size is seen at the center of the fracture

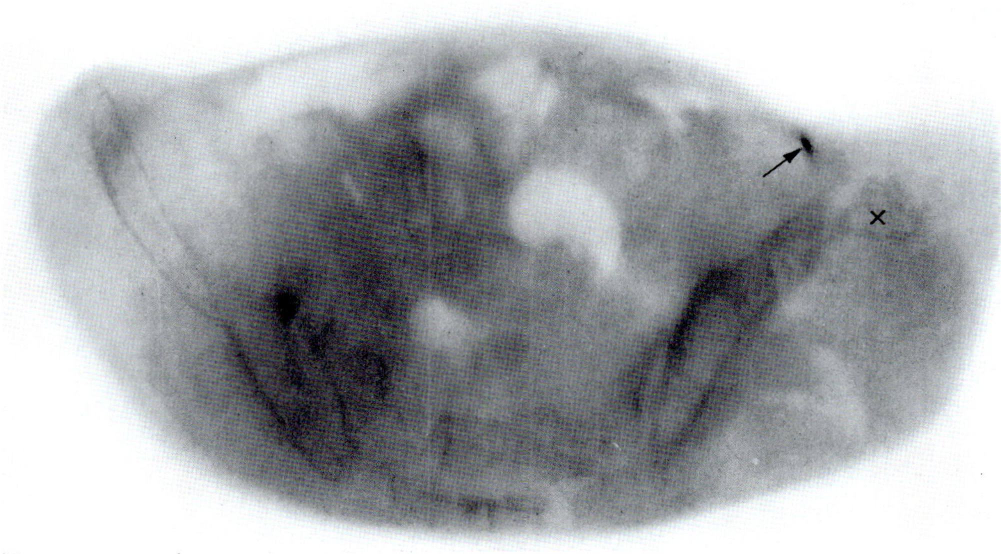

Fig. 559. Axial transverse tomogram. Refer to Figs. 387—391, p. 184. The axial transverse tomogram taken at the level of the opacity reveals the fractured part of the anterior iliac bone (×). The opacity (↗) is located 1 cm below the skin. That is the foreign body which has been pressed into the lower abdomen at the time of the accident

Diagnosis: Thickening of the periosteum.

Case: Ch. I., age 26, female.

History: The patient complains of pain in the right ankle, aggravated by walking. Neurologically negative.

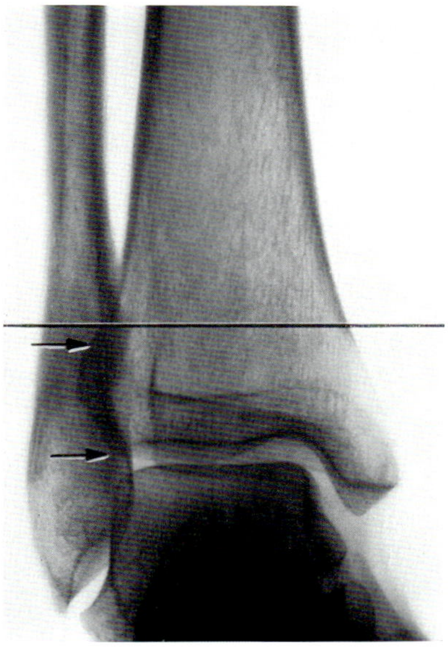

Fig. 560

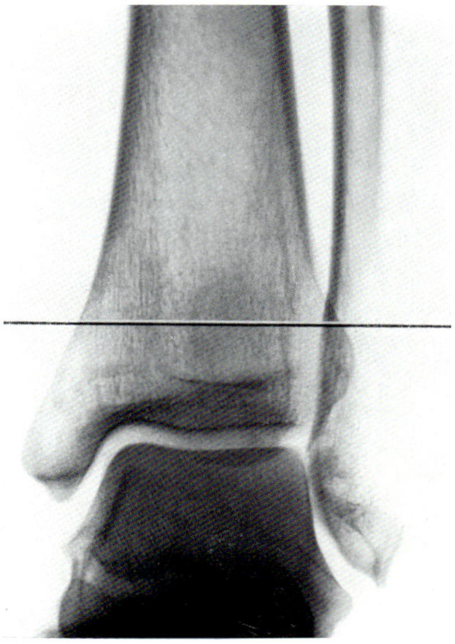

Fig. 561

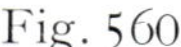

Fig. 560. Normal roentgenogram. Horizontal line showing the level tomographed. Right lower leg shows slight thickening (↗) of the periosteum in the distal portion of the fibula about 3 cm in length

Fig. 561. Normal roentgenogram. Horizontal line showing the level tomographed. Healthy fibula; there is an apparent difference in the thickness of the periosteum compared with Fig. 560

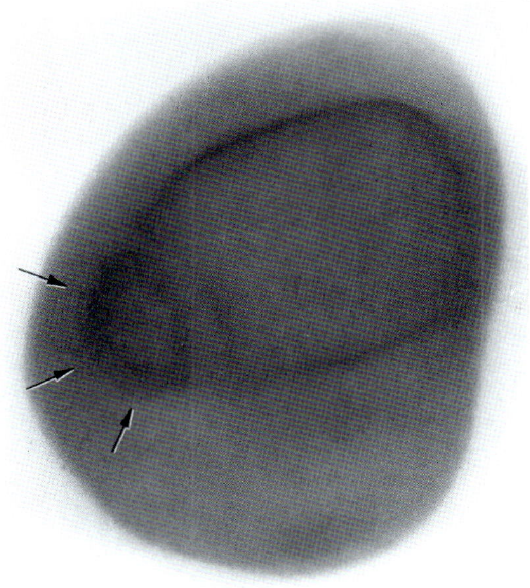

Fig. 562

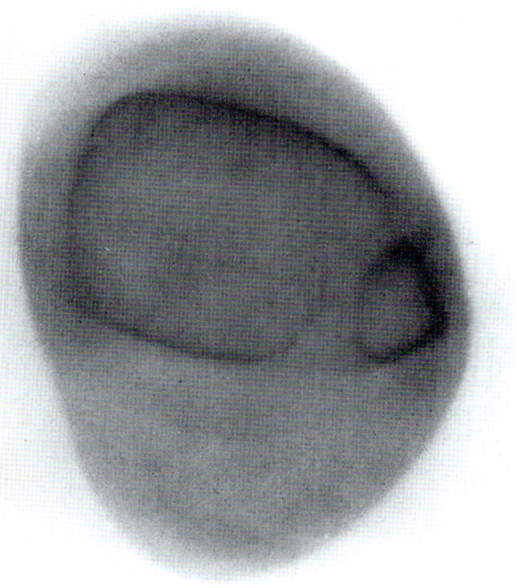

Fig. 563

Fig. 562. Axial transverse tomogram. The right fibula shows thickening of the periosteum with slight irregular marginal outline (↗). This is clearly demonstrated on the axial transverse tomogram and it is apparent in the difference in thickness of the periosteum when compared with that of the healthy fibula on the axial transverse tomogram

Fig. 563. Axial transverse tomogram of the left leg. Normal

Diagnosis: Fibrosarcoma.

Case: Y. T., age 52, female.

History: For two years she has complained of gradually increasing swelling in her right knee.

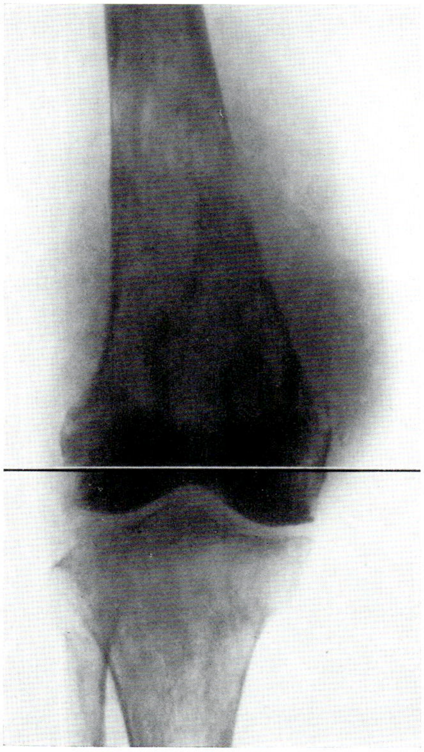

Fig. 564

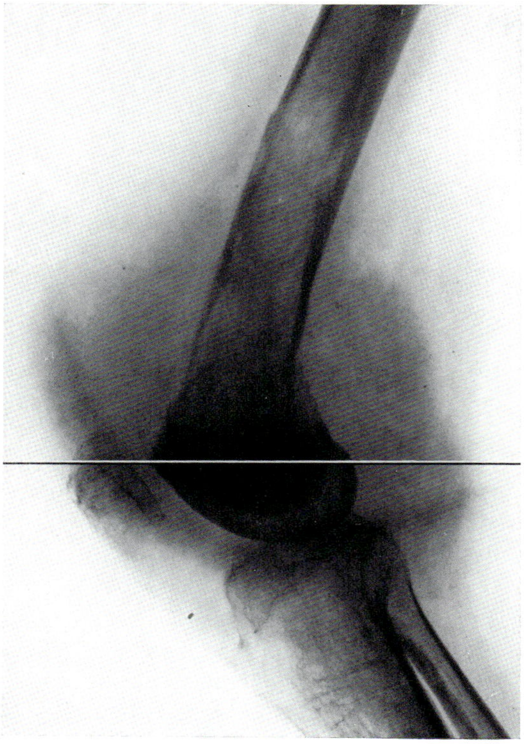

Fig. 565

Fig. 564. Normal roentgenogram in the a.p. view. Horizontal line showing the level tomographed. There is bone destruction involving the lower third of the femur, approximately 10 cm in length. The articular surface of the femur shows moderate increase of bone density, but the joint space is well preserved

Fig. 565. Normal roentgenogram in the lateral view. There is moderate soft tissue swelling at the level of the lower third of the femur described above, mainly in the right anterior aspect

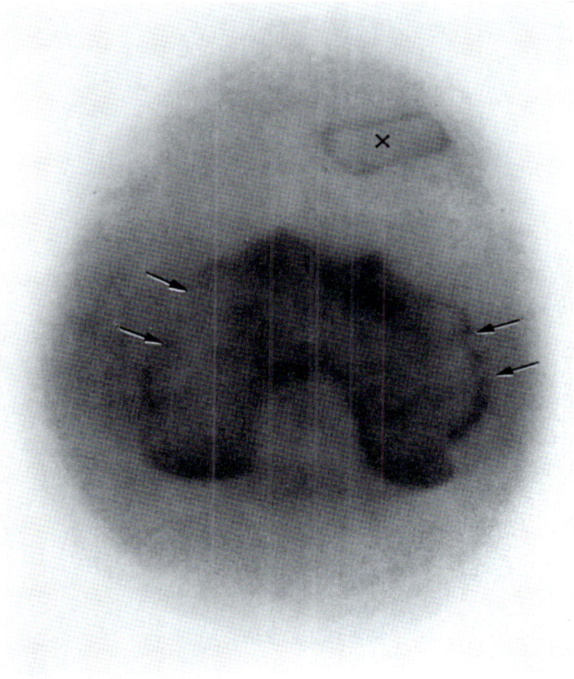

Fig. 566. Axial transverse tomogram. As compared with the normal (Figs. 490—492, p. 228), marked swelling of the anterior and posterior part of the soft tissue in the leg is seen. The patella (×) is shifted to the left and is atrophic. Both sides of the median and lateral condyle (↗) of the femur are destroyed with partial hyperosteosis

II. Application to Pretherapeutic Procedure

For the treatment of disease by means of either irradiation or surgical operation, three-dimensional knowledge of the lesion in the body obtained before the operation will make the procedure easy as well as correct. It will be explained below how and why axial transverse tomography is useful.

1. Radiation Therapy

A basic problem in radiation therapy is to give dense and homogeneous radiation to the tumor alone, while delivering the minimum possible dose to the surrounding normal tissues. This area of high dose is termed by *Takahashi* (175) *beam focus*.

In order to coincide the beam focus with the region to be treated, the first step should be to make the location, size and shape of the region clearly known and determined and to plan the most appropriate technique to produce the beam focus to cover the region to be irradiated. After the consideration of this planning, the actual procedures of the correct positioning of the patient on the treatment table and the correct determination of the direction and the size of radiation beam are performed. Finally, confirmation is needed as to whether this planned treatment has been properly carried out or not. The systematic work for applying the rotation technique to radiation therapy was described by *Takahashi* (175).

Application of axial transverse tomography to the determination of the region to be treated was dealt with by *Pierquin* (93), *Roswit* et al. (98), *Vallebona* (159) and *Watanabe* et al. (166). Its application to the radiation planning was discussed by *Fleischer* et al. (23), *Frain* et al. (28), *Jucker* et al. (46), *Onuma* (89), *Pierquin* et al. (92), *Roswit* et al. (97), *Sannazzari* et al. (101), *Takahashi* et al. (140), *Vallebona* (160) and others, because of its essential value for treatment planning. For positioning of the patient in radiation therapy, *Matsuda* et al. (71) and *Takahashi* et al. (137) described the usefulness of axial transverse tomography. For confirming whether or not correct irradiation was carried out, the contribution of axial transverse tomography was described by *Egan* et al. (21), *Sakuma* et al. (100) and *Takahashi* (141). Actually, however, these procedures have not been much used in the field of radiation therapy up to the present time.

One of the reasons may be that the tomography was usually performed with the unit of the erect type, while the radiotherapy is carried out with the patient in the lying posture. It is the natural conclusion that axial transverse tomography taken by the unit of the erect type is of less value for

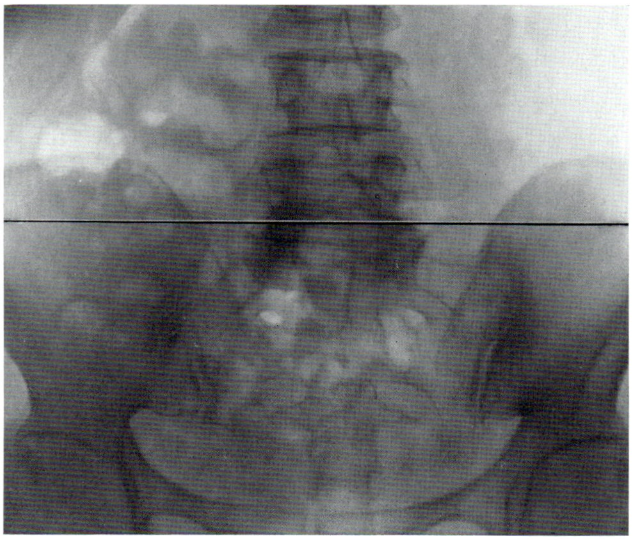

A

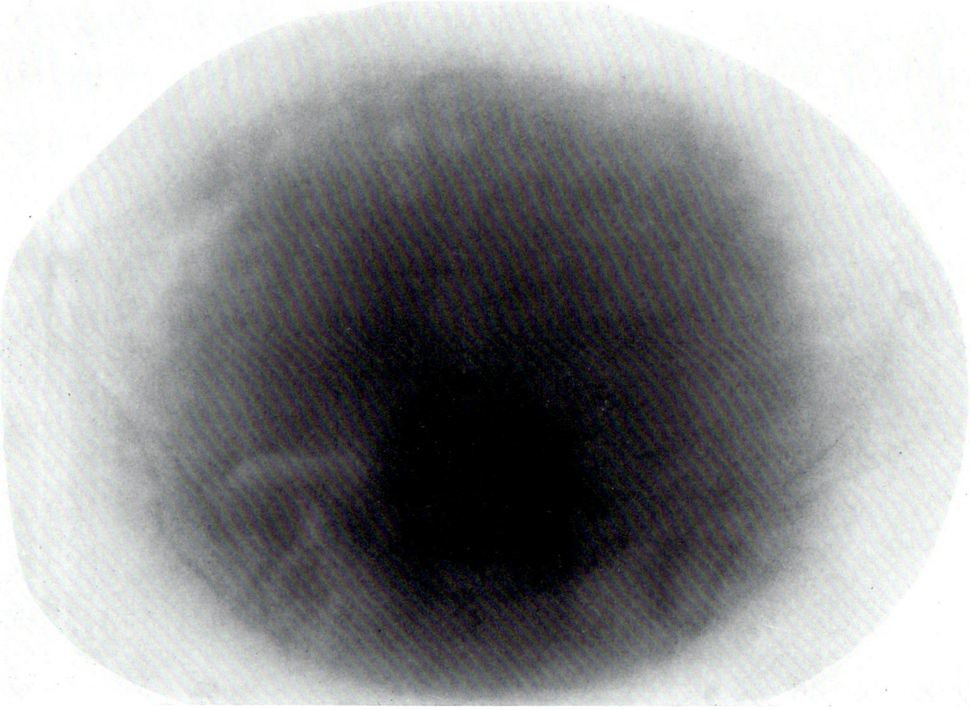

B

Fig. 567 A and B. Axial transverse tomogram of the lower abdomen of a woman at the level of the anterior superior iliac spine taken by means of the axial transverse tomograph of the erect type

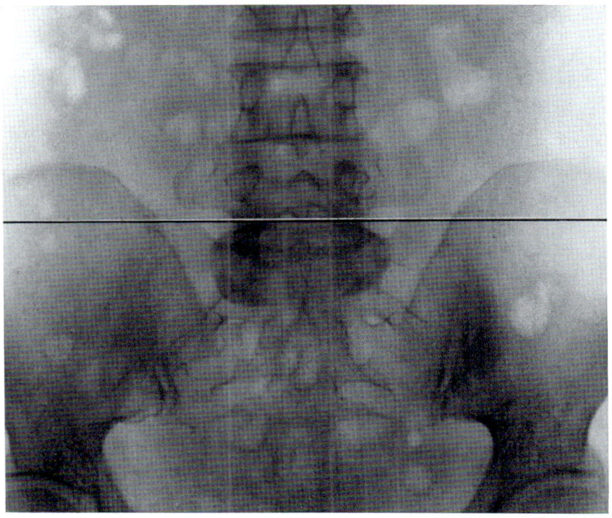

A

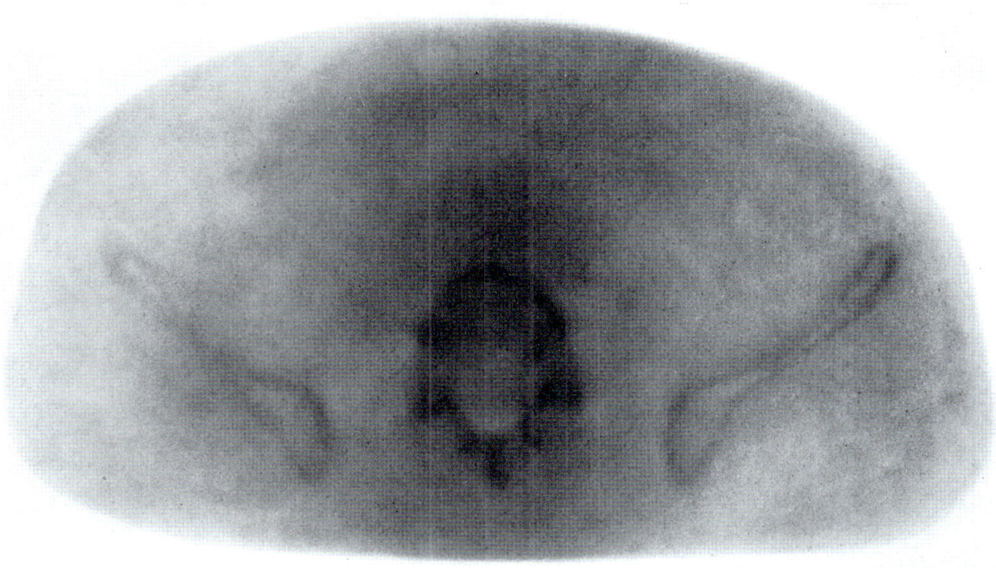

B

Fig. 568 A and B. Axial transverse tomogram at the same level of the same woman as in Fig. 567. The tomogram is taken by means of the horizontal type of unit. The difference from Fig. 567 is caused by the change in the position of the viscera.

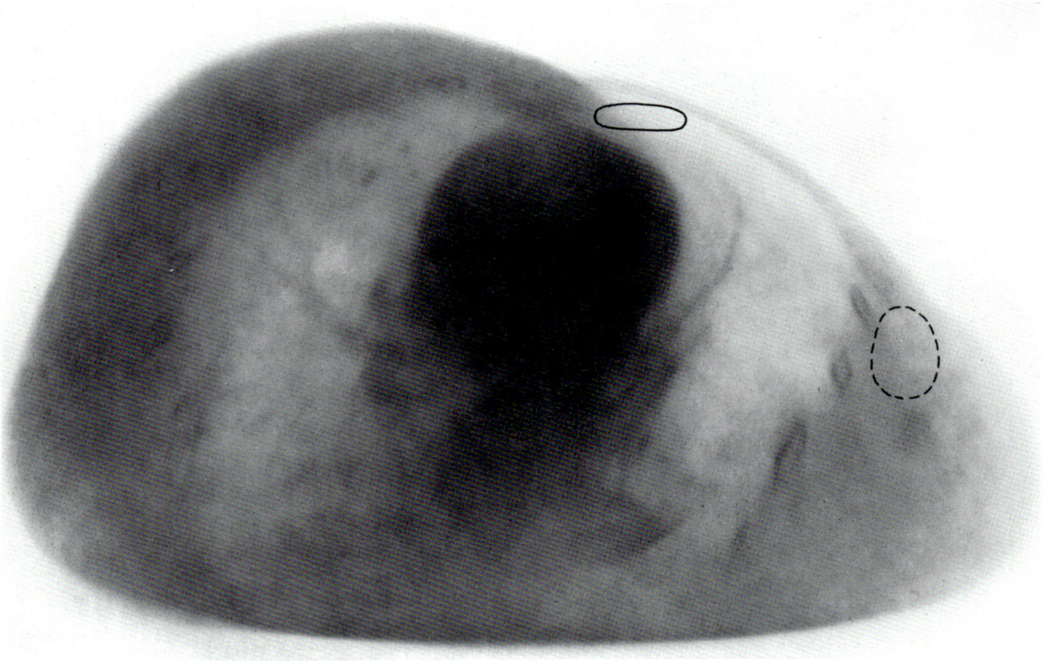

Fig. 569. Region to be treated for irradiation of postoperative breast cancer. The lymph nodes (solid line) along the internal mammary vessels and the axillary lymph nodes (broken line) are determined for irradiation. Operated breast wall is not irradiated, as the operation was radically carried out in this case

Fig. 571. Axial transverse tomogram to be applied to the positioning of a lung cancer patient. Three points on the contour of the cross section of the body represent the positioning skin marks a, b and c. Standard lines (solid lines) are drawn from the center 0 of the region to be treated so that one is parallel to the line b—c (broken line) and the other perpendicular to it. By extending these two lines to the contour of the cross section of the body, the centering skin marks A, B and C are obtained

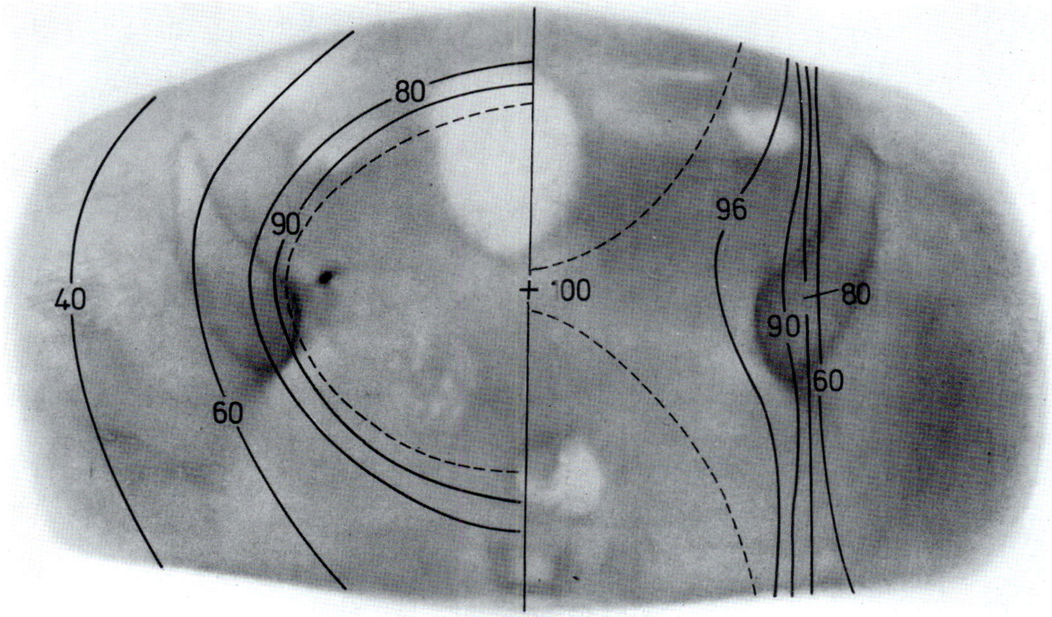

Fig. 570. Isodose curves for irradiation of cancer of the uterus by ^{60}Co conformation radiotherapy (left) and ^{60}Co radiotherapy through two portals (right). Region to be irradiated is shown by the broken line (left). The conformation radiation technique provides better dose distribution than the two-portal stationary irradiation

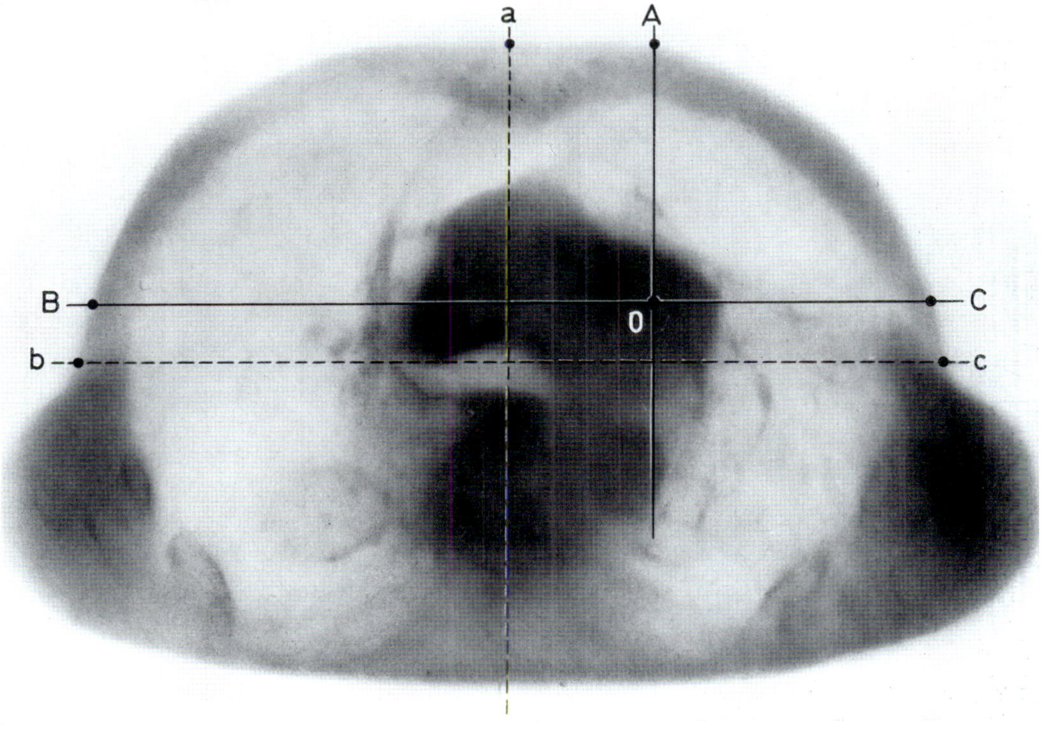

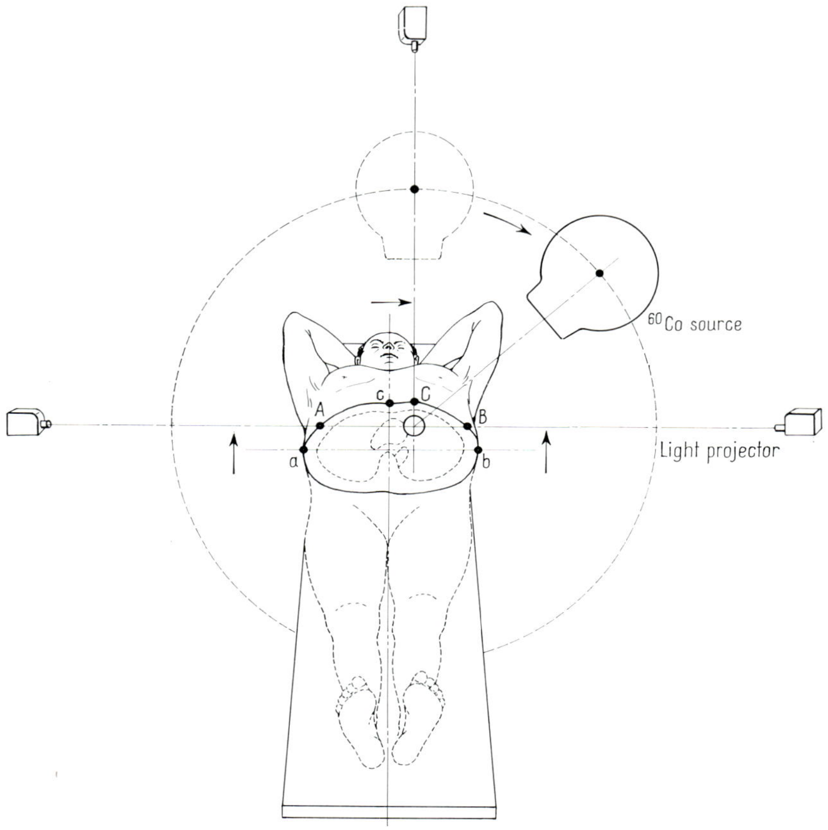

Fig. 572. Diagram illustrating adjustment of the central γ-ray of ^{60}Co to the center of the lesion by means of positioning skin marks and centering skin marks

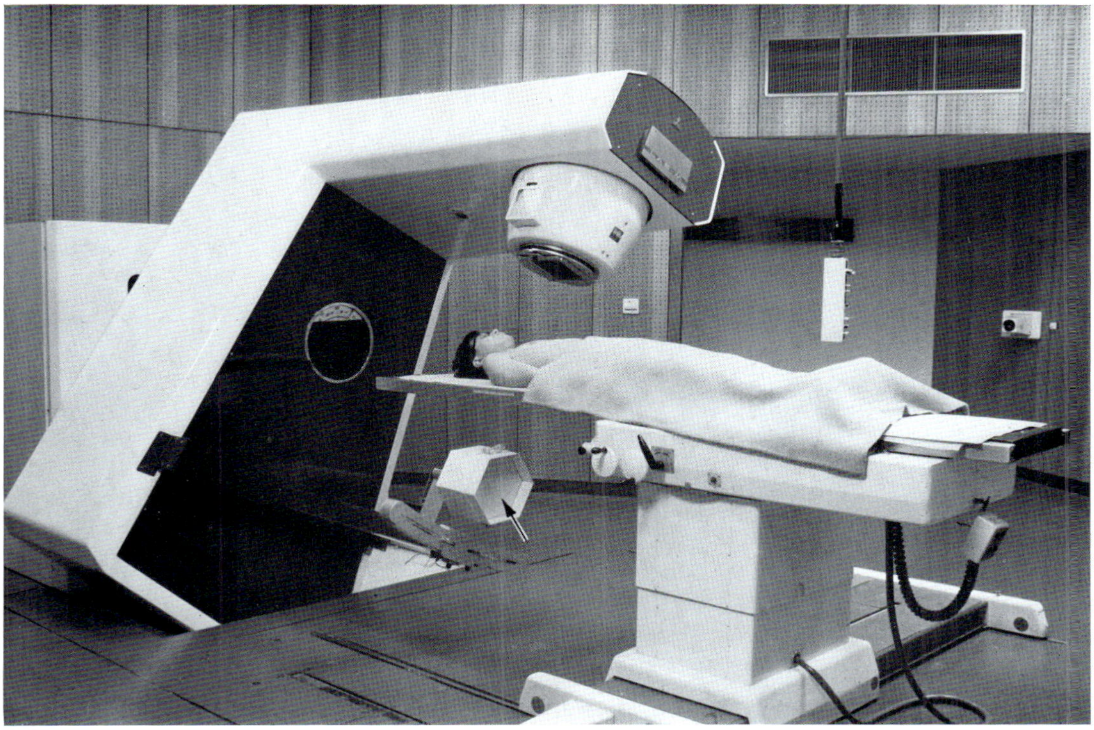

Fig. 573. Beam focus radiography in action. Beam focus radiograph (↗) is attached to the rotational accelerator therapy unit (Mitsubishi)

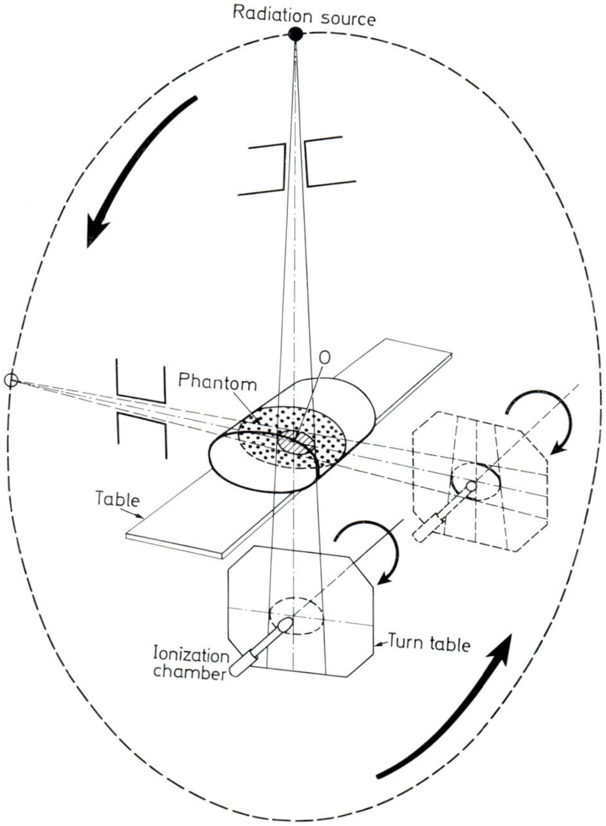

Fig. 574. Diagram illustrating the principle of beam focus radiography. The center of rotation of the film is arranged on the line joining the radiation source with the rotation center of the unit (0). With counter-clockwise rotation of the radiation source, the cassette keeping definite direction by clockwise rotation rotates around the patient

Fig. 576. Axial transverse tomogram applied to needle puncture for biopsy. a, b and c: positioning skin marks. P: point to be punctured

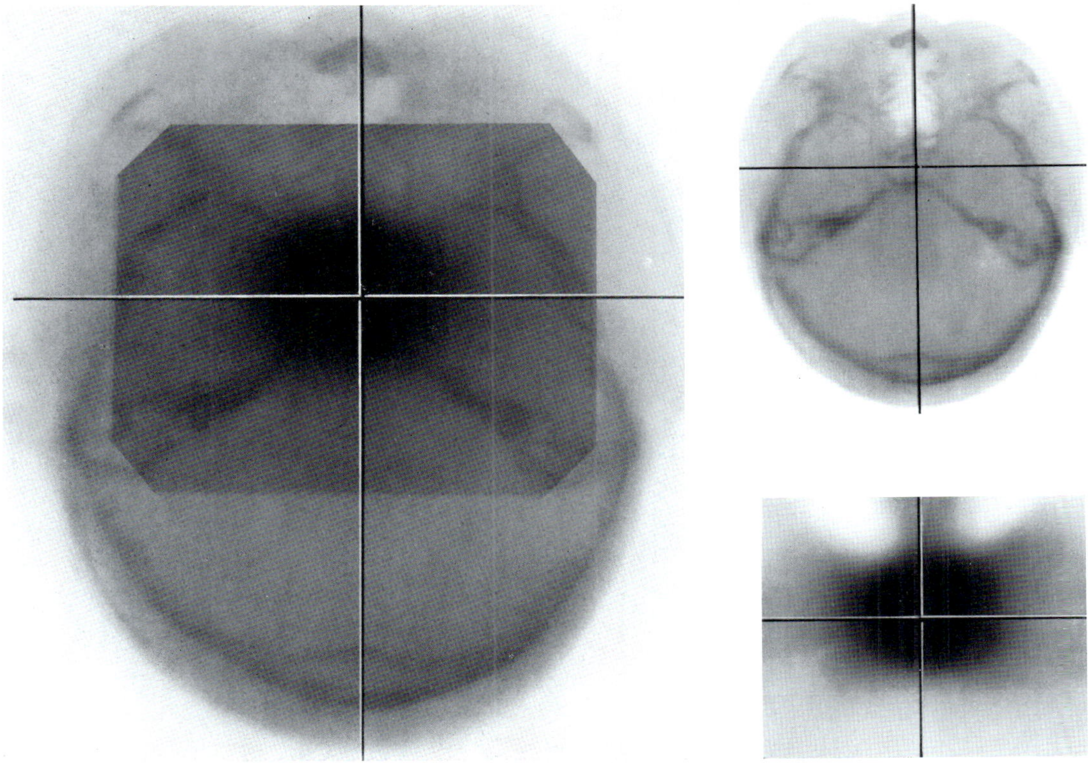

Fig. 575. Confirmation of coverage of the correct beam focus in radiation therapy. Beam focus in axial transverse cross section of the head at the level of the pituitary tumor. The large image on the left shows the overlapping of the axial transverse tomogram (top right) and the beam focus radiogram (bottom right)

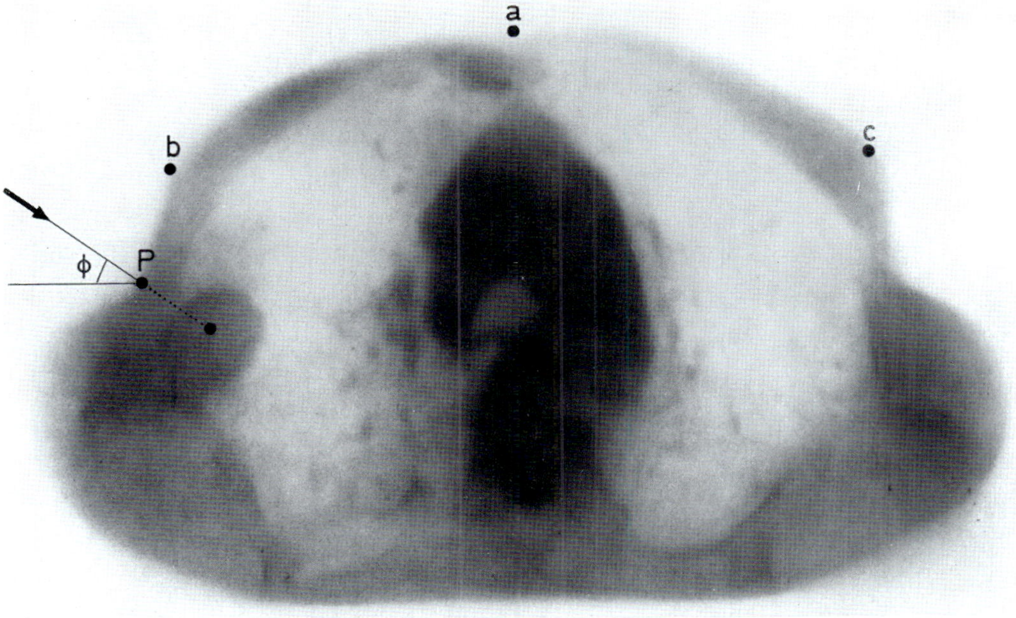

radiotherapy of a lying patient as, in the human body, the reciprocal relationship of the viscera changes very much with the change of posture (Figs. 567, 568).

Thus it is desirable to use the axial transverse tomograph of horizontal type for radiation therapy of the lying patient.

Roentgen images on the axial transverse tomogram are essentially not distorted as compared with the original figure, but enlarged with a definite magnification ratio. In accordance with this, the actual size of the cross-section is obtained by multiplying the image of the tomogram by the inverse enlargement ratio.

A. Planning for Irradiation

1. Determination of Region to be Treated. First of all the extent, shape, size and location of the region to be treated are determined as exactly as possible before radiation therapy. This procedure is simple if axial transverse tomography is used. Indeed, though the disease is varied in appearance, the treated region usually takes the common size and shape according to the stage of cancer, as, for instance, not only the original tumor with its infiltration but also the primary lymph nodes of the lesion are included in the region to be treated.

In order to obtain three-dimensional knowledge of the region there arises the need for comparative examination of normal roentgenograms with axial transverse tomograms.

For skin cancer, the treated region is simply decided by inspection of its two-dimensional extent on the skin surface. The state under the skin is not observed by the naked eye. But it can be known directly if axial transverse tomography is applied. In irradiation for postoperative breast cancer, the area from the skin to the inner wall of the thorax may at times be subject to irradiation. Moreover, the lymph nodes along the internal mammary vessels would be the target of metastasis and are irradiated in the case where the original tumor was seated upper median or median of the nipple of the affected breast. Thus the region to be treated is considered to be as shown in Fig. 569.

For the deep-seated tumor, the hypophyseal tumor, for instance, the region to be treated will be a cylinder, with the height containing the full turkish saddle imaged on the normal roentgenograms and with the circle in the axial transverse cross-section imaged on the axial transverse tomogram. However, the eye, especially the lens, should be irradiated with as small a dose as possible (Fig. 575). At any rate, by means of the tomogram the location of the eye or the distance between the tumor and the skin becomes clear.

2. *Selection of Irradiation Technique.* It is the purpose of irradiation planning to select the appropriate technique of irradiation on the basis of the axial transverse tomogram.

The actual procedure is to place an axial transverse tomogram on the viewing box. The isodose chart, in which the isodose curves are drawn on the translucent film with the same magnification ratio as that of the axial transverse tomogram, is placed over the axial transverse tomogram (Fig. 57C). If the tumor is considered to be localized in the superficial part of the body, electron beam therapy of adequate MeV would be suitable. If stationary radiation technique is considered appropriate, the number of the radiation fields, and the direction and size of the cross-section of the beam are determined to meet effective radiation planning. When the number of portals of the radiation field is increased, that will be regarded as the irradiation technique of moving field therapy. The dose distribution in the lesion as well as in the normal region is given on the isodose chart prepared by previous measurement of the dose by phantom experiment.

Indeed, there are various types of irradiation technique such as rotational, arc or conformation therapy. If moving field therapy is considered adequate for the case, the merits and defects of the rotational, arc or conformation radiation techniques are compared with each other and the most suitable one is adopted. In our opinion, the conformation irradiation technique, though not yet widely used, generally provides the ideal dose distribution.

Without axial transverse tomography, such precise determination of the region and planning of irradiation could not be realized.

B. Positioning of Patient

The next problem is to conduct irradiation with the correct positioning of the patient. With inadequate or wrong positioning, the radiation beam will stray away from the region to be treated, resulting in partial coverage of the beam focus to the treated region, which will cause recurrence. The effort to make the correct irradiation planning to produce the minimum beam focus is more likely to be harmful.

The positioning of the patient in connection with the correct planning is carried out by means of axial transverse tomography as follows:

The patient is laid supine or in a relaxed posture on the tomographic table. The body level where the region to be treated exists on the normal roentgenogram is adjusted to the plane g of the unit. The light spots are projected on to the plane g of the patient from the light projectors attached to the walls and ceilings of the tomography room (see p. 12). The light beams are contained in a vertical plane of the isocenter of the axial transverse tomograph.

The light spot projected on the anterior part of the skin of the patient is termed point a, that on the right b and that on the left c. These points marked in ink on the skin are termed positioning skin marks a, b and c (Fig. 571).

Lead wires 0.5 mm in diameter of the cross section and 1 cm long are placed at the points a, b and c respectively with the arrangement parallel to the axis of the body.

The axial transverse tomogram is taken. On the tomogram there are imaged three points on the contour of the body, corresponding to positioning skin marks a, b and c.

The line joining the points b and c is termed the horizontal line and the line which forms a perpendicular from a to this line is termed the vertical line.

By interpreting the axial transverse tomogram, the region to be treated is determined and the center 0 of this region is selected.

From this center 0 lines are drawn parallel and perpendicular to the horizontal line bc.

These new lines are termed the horizontal and vertical standard lines of the axial transverse tomogram. The crossing points of these lines and the contour of the skin on the tomogram are termed centering skin marks B, C and A.

In the rotational therapy unit three light projectors are also attached to the walls and ceiling, their light spots being adjusted to cross at the isocenter of the rotational therapy unit (Fig. 572). The patient is laid on the therapy table in the same posture as on the tomographic table. By shifting the therapy table to and fro, or right or left, the light spots are made to coincide with each of the positioning skin marks a, b and c which are drawn in ink on the skin.

Then the distances between the horizontal and vertical lines of the positioning skin marks and those of the centering skin marks on the axial transverse tomogram are measured and their values divided by the magnification ratio of the axial transverse tomogram. The therapy table is then shifted exactly up or down, right or left in accordance with the value of the distance thus obtained.

The light projectors in the radiation therapy room thus serve for the correct positioning of the patient on the therapy table.

The final position of the light spots on the skin is on the centering skin marks of the patient which correspond to the points A, B and C of the axial transverse tomogram.

After this procedure the isocenter of the rotational unit is located at the center of the region to be treated. This means that the central radiation ray will hit the center of the region to be treated irrespective of the direction of the radiation beam. If the cross-section of the radiation beam is selected by reference to the size of the lesion, the region to be treated will be covered correctly whatever the direction of the beam. Thus, both stationary radiation therapy and moving field therapy can be performed by a simple but exact procedure, with the centering skin marks contributing to the correct conduct of radiation therapy. For conducting either multiportal or moving field therapy, the rotational teleradiation therapy unit is thus recommended.

Even when the stationary teleradiation unit is used with multiportal irradiation, the procedure of planning and positioning of patients is similar to the above. The patient is laid on the therapy table in the same posture as on the tomographic table and the same procedure is followed as in the case of the rotational therapy unit. The size of the radiation beam is adjusted to that of the radiation field, and the central ray is focused with the same direction as the planning on the axial transverse tomogram.

These processes will be carried out by means of the usual light beam localizer.

C. Confirmation of Correct Positioning

Where axial transverse tomography is applied to radiation therapy, it is possible to confirm whether the radiation has been correctly planned during the actual procedure of the radiation therapy. This is the device of beam focus radiography (Fig. 573).

Under the therapy table a rotating disc having a cassette holder is attached, the center of which is located on the extension of the straight line joining the radiation source and the center of the rotational radiation therapy unit. Although the disc rotates around the patient on the therapy table simultaneously with the rotation of the radiation source, the disc itself rotates in inverse direction to the rotation of the radiation source (Fig. 574). As a result, the disc maintains its position relative to the radiation source as it rotates. Thus, the side of the cassette attached to the disc holder stays at right angles to the direction of the radiation beam. 10×12 inch industrial film, is used.

Inside the front cover of the cassette there are horizontal and vertical lines of 0.5 mm lead wire in place of the intensifying screens. The crossing point is adjusted so as to be located at the rotation center of the disc. The image of the lead wire is recorded on the film with the electron rays emitted during exposure of supervoltage rays.

The crossing lines imaged on the film are termed horizontal and vertical standard lines (Fig. 575c).

In conducting multiportal radiation therapy or moving field therapy, the radiation beam passes through the body and images dense radiation figure of beam focus on the center of this film. This image represents the figure of the treated region. The radiographic method is thus termed beam focus radiography.

The beam focus radiogram is enlarged with the magnification ratio of β.

$$\beta = \frac{A' + B'}{A'}$$

where A' is the distance between the radiation source and the rotation center of the therapy unit and B' is that between the rotation center of the unit and that of the disc.

The axial transverse tomography is not actual size but enlarged with a certain magnification ratio, say α. To get the actual size of the tomogram (Fig. 575b) and the beam focus radiogram (Fig. 575c), the radiograms are reduced by multiplying the reciprocal value of the magnification ratio.

When the figures in actual size are obtained, the two radiograms are overlapped by placing the centering vertical and horizontal standard lines of the axial transverse tomogram over those of the beam focus radiogram (Fig. 575a). The actual location, size and shape of the beam focus within the body is obtained. This procedure enables the confirmation to be made, whether the beam focus correctly covers the region to be treated or not.

In practice, it is troublesome and time-consuming to reduce the tomogram and beam focus radiogram to actual size. Thus the overlapping viewing box is used instead.

The construction of the viewing box is such that there is the following relation between the position of the eye, the axial transverse tomogram and the beam focus radiogram:

$$b = a\left(\frac{\beta}{\alpha} - 1\right)$$

where b is the distance between the beam focus radiogram and the axial transverse tomogram, a is that between the eye and the axial transverse tomogram, α the magnification ratio of the axial transverse tomogram, and β that of the beam focus radiogram.

Taking 50 cm as the distance between the eye and the axial transverse tomogram, the adequate value of b will be given, as α and β are constant in accordance with the distances between the radiation source the rotation center of the unit and that of the films for the axial transverse tomography or for the beam focus radiography.

By arranging the distances between these three points accordingly, the magnification ratio of the beam focus radiogram to the eye becomes the same as that of the axial transverse tomogram. When this viewing box technique is used, the result is effectively similar to reduction of the two radiograms to the actual size.

When the radiation technique is proved to be correct by means of beam focus radiography, the centering skin marks are tattooed intracutaneously with sterilized Indian ink.

After this procedure the positioning of the patient on the therapy table becomes simple, as the centering skin marks are merely made to coincide with the light spots of the projectors.

Usually, in order to confirm the correct coverage of the radiation beam on the treated region, radiograms are taken with the direct beam, such as ^{60}Co γ-ray, and examined. However, the radiogram taken for cancer of the esophagus, for instance, reveals the image of the esophagus with difficulty, due to lack of contrast between the bone, barium and soft tissue and so this method is of limited application.

The method of applying the beam focus radiogram to confirm the correct coverage of the tumor by the radiation beam is considered superior to the method of ^{60}Co γ-ray radiography in that the confirmation is achieved directly and it is known how the beam focus covers the lesion and whether the planning was carried out correctly or not.

The simulator on the other hand is also considered useful for correct positioning and its confirmation. Nevertheless, the whole task of determing the region to be treated, planning by using the isodose chart, positioning and confirmation may be limited when conducted only by means of the simulator.

2. Surgical Operation

According to *Iglauer* (42), *Monod* et al. (79) or *Piazza* (91) axial transverse tomography has contributed to the determination of operability. *Benedetti* (10) studied the chest after operation. *Imaoka* (43) applied rotation radiography to the removal of a foreign body in the thigh.

From the practical point of view, it is not always necessary to know thoroughly the state of lesion before the surgical operation, as more information about the lesion is usually obtainable in the course of the operation than by means of radiological examination. Moreover, trouble arises from the easy change of the relation between the tissue and organs during the operation. Nevertheless, for the puncture or the small incision of a lesion located deep in the body, it will be better to establish the size, location and shape of the lesion before operation. In order to remove a foreign body, determination of its location is also most essential.

Axial transverse tomography will contribute much to the surgical planning of the operation.

Normal radiography will, of course, inform us whether or not the lesion exists, and in what level of the body it is located.

If this lesion cannot be inspected or palpated because of its deep seated location and is considered suitable for treatment by puncture or small excision, the patient is laid on the tomographic table in the position convenient for surgical operation. The level of the lesion on the axial transverse cross section is made to coincide with plane g. For this, fluoroscopic examination or roentgenography with small-sized film will be sometimes useful.

The skin of the patient is illuminated by the three light projectors and the positioning skin marks are determined in the way described on p. 300.

The axial transverse tomogram is made and examined. The tomogram reveals the location, size and shape of the lesion. After that procedure the surgical technique is selected. The patient is laid on the table of the surgical room where the light projectors are set in the walls and ceiling in the same way as in the tomography room.

When performing a biopsy puncture, the location of the point for puncture is selected and called point P (Fig. 576). Next, the angle of the needle of the syringe to the horizontal level and the distance from the tip of the needle of the syringe to the lesion are measured by examining the axial transverse tomogram, bearing in mind what procedure will avoid injury to the critical tissue.

The distance between the point P and the lesion is deduced by multiplying the magnification ratio of the tomogram. The point P which is obtained as the point with the above distance nearest one of the positioning skin marks is marked in ink on the skin of the patient From this point P the needle is introduced into the skin at the definite angle Φ and depth planned with the axial transverse tomogram.

References

1. Papers on Axial Transverse Tomography

1. *Abreau, de:* Tomografia horizontal do torax. Radiologia (B. Aires) **7**, 223 (1944). Reported by title only in J. Radiol. Électrol. **28**, 10 (1947).
2. *Albertis, P. de:* Contributo della stratigrafia assiale trasversa associata al retropneumoperitoneo e alla insufflazione gastrica nello studio della masse abdominali. Minerva med. **50**, 3 (1959).
3. *Alè, G.*, e *L. Macchi:* Studio morfologico e topografico degli aneurismi dell'aorta toracica mediante la tomografia assiale trasversa. Ann. Radiol. diagn. (Bologna) **36**, 303 (1963).
4. *Amisano, P.:* La stratigrafia toracica a strato trasverso. Radiol. med. (Torino) **32**, 418 (1946).
5. — La stratigrafia assiale trasversa nell'età pediatrica. Policlin. infant., Suppl. al fascicolo di Gennaio, 1947.
6. — Three dimensional stratigraphic examination; axial transverse stratigraphy. Part II. Amer. J. Roentgenol. **74**, 777 (1955).
7. *Balestra, Passeri* et *Macarini:* La stratigraphie axiale transversale dans la pathologie de l'appareil pulmonaire. J. Radiol. Électrol. **31**, 462 (1950).
8. *Barenbojm, A. M.:* Die Transversaltomographie als Ergänzungsmethode für die topographische Erfassung hilusnaher Kavernen. Rozhl. Tuberk. **18**, 735 (1958).
9. *Benedetti, G.:* Studio stratigrafico assiale della regione cervicale. Radiol. sperimentale **2**, 110 (1948).
10. — Studio stratigrafico del pneumotorace extrapleurico chirurgico. Minerva med. **2**, 543 (1951).
11. *Bulgarelli, R.*, e *L. Oliva:* Su di un caso di doppio arco aortico associato a probabile morbo di Roger e su due casi accertati di morbo di Roger studiati mediante la stratigrafia assiale trasversa e la stratigrafia frontale. Minerva pediat. **3**, 1 (1951).
12. — — Prime ricerche sulla stratigrafia assiale trasversa associata alla stratigrafia frontale con o senza pneumomediastino anteriore nella tetralogia di Fallot prima e dopo intervento alla Blalock-Taussig e nella sindrome di Eisenmenger. Minerva pediat. **3**, 275 (1951).
13. *Bulgarelli, R.*, e *L. Oliva:* Prime ricerche sulla stratigrafia assiale trasversa associata alla stratigrafia frontale nelle cardiopatie acquisite reumatiche. Minerva pediat. **3**, 311 (1951).
14. — — Prime ricerche sulla stratigrafia assiale trasversa associata alla stratigrafia frontale nella pervietà del dotto di Botallo. Minerva pediat. **3**, 259 (1951).
15. *Buzzi, G.:* La stratigraphie axiale transversale dans la pathologie du médiastin. J. Radiol. Électrol. **31**, 146 (1950).
16. *Chiro, G. di:* Axial transverse encephalography. Amer. J. Roentgenol. **92**, 441 (1964).
17. — Axial transverse encephalography with the radiotome. Medica Mundi **10**, 92 (1965).
18. *Clément, J. P.:* Contribution à l'exploration radiologique de la région pancréatique par la stratigraphie axiale transverse. J. belge Radiol. **48**, 151 (1965).
19. *Duhamel, J.*, e *P. L. Martin:* Considerazioni sulla esatta determinazione del piano dei punti fissi in stratigrafia assiale trasversa. Radiol. med. (Torino) **39**, 1014 (1953).
20. — —, et *J.-C. Roques:* Théorie élémentaire des images induites thoraciques en tomographie axiale transversale. J. Radiol. Électrol. **42**, 470 (1961).
21. *Egan, R.*, and *G. C. Johnson:* Multisection transverse tomography in radium implant calculations. Radiology **74**, 407 (1960).
22. *Farinet, G., G. L. Sannazzari* e *A. Torretta:* La stratigrafia assiale trasversa quale esame complementare della radioisotopografia nello studio degli strumi benigni e maligni. Minerva fisioter radiobiol. **4**, 291 (1959).
23. *Fleischer, H., A. Gebauer* u. *F. Wachsmann:* Verwendung transversaler Schichtaufnahmen bei der Festlegung des Bestrahlungsplanes intrathorakaler Tumoren. Fortschr. Röntgenstr. **76**, 52 (1952).

24. *Frain, C.*, et *F. Lacroix:* Effet stratigraphique et coupes horizontales. C. R. Acad. Sci. (Paris) **224**, 973 (1947).
25. — — Étude expérimentale sur l'obtention de coupes horizontales. Paris méd. **37**, 94 (1947).
26. — — Courbe-enveloppe et coupes horizontales. J. Radiol. Électrol. **28**, 142 (1947).
27. — — De l'obtention de coupes horizontales. J. Radiol. Électrol. **29**, 256 (1948).
28. —, *J. Surmont, M. Tubiana, B. Pierquin, R. Marlois, J. Abbatucci* et *A. Dutreix:* Intéret de la tomographie transversale (coupes horizontales) dans le repérage, le centrage et al dosimétrie des tumeurs thoraciques traitées par radiothérapie transcutanée. J. Radiol. Électrol. **38**, 792 (1955).
29. *Frik, W., C. E. Buchheim* u. *H. Jupitz:* Der Einfluß von Rotationswinkel, Strahleneinfallswinkel und Objektlage auf die Qualität transversaler Schichtaufnahmen. Fortschr. Röntgenstr. **97**, 94 (1962).
30. *Fumagalli, G., A. Passeri* e *D. Vallebona:* Stratigrafia assiale trasversa e spirometria nella valutazione delle alterazioni ventilatorie. Contributo del singolo polmone. Minerva med. **52**, 2731 (1961).
31. *Gardella, G.:* La stratigrafia assiale dell'ilo polmonare. La stratigrafia assiale trasversa, Genova, p. 20 (1947).
32. *Gebauer, A.*, u. *F. Wachsmann:* Geometrische Betrachtungen und technische Fragen zur Herstellung transversaler (horizontaler) Körperschichtaufnahmen. Röntgen-Bl. **2**, 215 (1949).
33. — Körperschichtaufnahmen in transversalen (horizontalen) Ebenen. Fortschr. Röntgenstr. **71**, 669 (1949).
34. — Das transversale Schichtbild des normalen Thorax, ein Beitrag zur topographischen Anatomie am lebenden Menschen. Fortschr. Röntgenstr. **74**, 14 (1951).
35. — Diagnostische Vorteile und Indikationsstellung der Körperschichtaufnahmen in transversalen Ebenen gegenüber denen in vertikalen. Fortschr. Röntgenstr. **75**, 9 (1951).
36. *Giraud, M., Ch. Gros, J. P. Walter, P. Bloch* et *Y. Grumbach:* Exploration du pancréas par la tomographie axiale transverse. J. Radiol. Électrol. **46**, 863 (1965).
37. *Giraud, M., P. Bret, M. Levrat, M. Croisille* et *G. Bousquet:* Exploration radiologique du pancréas par stratigraphie axiale transverse. Bilan de dix années d'expérience.Ann. Radiol. **9**, 563 (1966).
38. *Gremmel, H.:* Die Transversalschichtuntersuchung des Herzens und der großen Gefäße. Fortschr. Röntgenstr. **96**, 3 (1962).
39. *Hachiya, H.*, and *H. Ito:* The rotatory cross-section radiography of hip joint, especially of measuring antetorsion. Centr. Jap. J. orthop. traum. Surg. **2**, 51 (1958) [Japanese].
40. *Hammer, G.:* Quere Schichtaufnahmen mit dem „Transversotom". Wien. med. Wschr. **103**, 464 (1953).
41. *Hartley, J. B.:* Localization by transverse tomography. Brit. J. Radiol. **34**, 550 (1961).
42. *Iglauer, E.:* Das transversale Schichtverfahren und das Pneumomediastinum in der Thoraxchirurgie. Kongreßber. 2. Tagg Med.-Wiss. Ges. Röntgenol. DDR, p. 208 (1958).
43. *Imaoka, M.:* Application of the discontinuous rotatography to the removal of the foreign body. Nippon Acta radiol. **10** (7), 5 (1950) [Japanese].
44. — Rotatory cross section radiography of the gall bladder. Nippon Acta radiol. **12** (8), 32 (1952) [Japanese].
45. *Janker, R.:* Ein Universal-Schichtaufnahmegerät. Fortschr. Röntgenstr. **73**, 253 (1950).
46. *Jucker, C.*, e *B. Pierquin:* Utilità della stratigrafia assiale trasversa nella radioterapia delle neoplasie endotoraciche. Radiol. med. (Torino) **48**, 740 (1962).
47. *Jusztusz, Gy.:* Transversalis rétegfelvételekről. Magy. Radiol. **3**, 84 (1951).
48. *Kitabatake, T.:* Frequency of tuberculous lesions in the mediastinal lung field. Nagoya J. med. Sci. **18**, 35 (1955).
49. *Kobayashi, T., S. Nitta, S. Kaii*, and *H. Takamura:* Rotatory cross section radiography of chest. J. Juzen med. Soc. **57**, 759 (1955) [Japanese].
50. *Kubota, Y., Y. Sato*, and *M. Yoshida:* Rotatory crossgraphy of pelvis. Hirosaki med. J. **4**, 11 (1953) [Japanese].

51. *Lacroix, F.:* I. Tomographie axiale transverse du membre inférieur. II. De l'importance du role joué en tomographie axiale par le couvercle de la cassette. J. Radiol. Électrol. **40**, 91 (1959).
52. *Levrat, M., P. Mallet-Guy, P. Bret, P. Grandmottet* et *J. Michoulier:* Le diagnostic radiologique des tumeurs endocriniennes du pancréas par la stratigraphie axiale transverse. A propos de deux observations: volumineux épithélioma, petit adénome langheransien kystique. Presse méd. **70**, 679 (1962).
53. *Lodin, H.:* Mediastinal herniation and displacement studied by transversal tomography. Acta radiol. (Stockh.) **48**, 337 (1957).
54. — Transversal tomography of the descending aorta. Acta radiol. (Stockh.) **56**, 251 (1961).
55. — Transversal tomography in the examination of thoracic deformities (Funnel chest and kyphoscoliosis). Acta radiol. (Stockh.) **57**, 49 (1962).
56. *Macarini, N.*: La stratigrafia nello studio dell'ascesso pulmonare, delle cisti da echinococco e delle pneumopatie cistiche. Lezioni del Primo Corse Internaz. Teorico-Pratico di Aggiornamento e Perfezionamento sulla Stratigrafia, 431 (1950).
57. —, e *L. Oliva:* La dimostrazione radiologica diretta del pancreas. Radiol. med. (Torino) **37** (12), 1 (1951).
58. — — Sur l'insufflation retroperitoneale associée a la stratigraphie tridimensionelle. J. belge Radiol. **34**, 281 (1951).
59. *Maestri, A. de:* Metodo di riconoscimento dello strato fisso nella stratigrafia assiale trasversa. Radiol. sperimentale **2**, 118 (1948).
60. — La stratigraphie transversale du thorax en pédiatrie. J. Radiol. Électrol. **31**, 464 (1950).
61. —, e *C. Lombroso:* Studio stratigrafico trasverso nelle iperplasie timiche. Minerva pediat. **3**, 255 (1951).
62. *Martin-Lalande, J.,* et *Y. T. Jean Lo:* Radiotomographie transverse de la trachée dans le médiastin supérieur: Quelques aspects et rapports normaux et pathologiques. Bronches **11**, 209 (1961).
63. *Matsuda, T.:* Rotatory cross section radiography of the chest. Nippon Acta radiol. **12** (2), 14 (1952) [Japanese].
64. — Evaluation of the rotatory cross section radiography applied to chest diseases. Nippon Acta radiol. **12** (10), 31 (1953) [Japanese].
65. — Position of the tuberculous cavity in the thoracs. Nippon Acta radiol. **13**, 485 (1953) [Japanese].
66. —, and *H. Yaguchi:* Rotatory cross section radiography of the upper abdomen insufflated air extraperitoneally. Jap. J. Urol. **45**, 673 (1954) [Japanese].
67. —, and *Y. Sato:* Tomography and rotatory cross section radiography of pulmonary tuberculous cavity. Nippon Acta radiol. **13**, 674 (1954) [Japanese].
68. — Rotatory cross section radiography of the stomach and the duodenum. Nippon Acta radiol. **14**, 197 (1954) [Japanese].
69. — Rotatory cross section radiography of the chest disease. Curr. Med. **5**, 121 (1957) [Japanese].
70. —, *Y. Kubota,* and *M. Yoshida:* High voltage radiographic technique applied to rotatory cross section radiography. Nippon Acta radiol. **16**, 1104 (1957) [Japanese].
71. —, and *T. Watanabe:* Rotatory cross section radiography applied to coverage of radiation beam to malignant tumor. Nippon Acta radiol. **18**, 1584 (1959) [Japanese].
72. —, *K. Ban,* and *S. Endo:* The compensating filter applied to rotatory cross section radiography. Nippon Acta radiol. **26**, 273 (1966) [Japanese].
73. — Moving filter applied to axial transverse tomography. Tohoku J. exp. Med. **94**, 163 (1968).
74. — Adjustment of axial transverse tomograph. Tohoku J. exp. Med. **95**, 331 (1968).
75. — Wedge grid applied to axial transverse tomography. Tohoku J. exp. Med. (in press).
76. *Mattina, M., G. Curiale* e *A. Cricchio:* La tomografia trasversale nello studio del mediastino. Radiol. prat. **14**, 93 (1964).
77. *Moldenhauer, W.:* Indikationen zur Transversaltomographie der Thoraxorgane. Radiol. diagn. (Berl.) **3**, 151 (1962).

78. *Monod, R., Ch. Frain* et *P. Court:* L'association tomographie transversale et pneumomédiastin. J. franç. Méd. Chir. thor. **9**, 389 (1955).
79. —, *Roche* et *Parent:* De l'intérêt des tomographies transversales en chirurgie thoracique. Lyon chir. **48**, 897 (1953).
80. *Ode, R.,* and *I. Miura:* Axial transverse tomography of the heart diseases. Therapeutics (Tokyo) **11**, 472 (1957) [Japanese].
81. *Oliva, L.:* Lo studio stratigrafico assiale trasverso dell'aorta toracica patologica. Radiologia (Roma) **6**, 649 (1950).
82. — La stratigrafia assiale trasversa nello studio delle caverne polmonari. Arch. Tisiol. **5**, 292 (1950).
83. — Le possibilità della stratigrafia assiale trasversa a giro parziale. Radiol. med. (Torino) **37**, 433 (1951).
84. *Ono, T.:* The application of the rotatory cross-section radiographing to obstetrics. Nippon Acta radiol. **13**, 141 (1953) [Japanese].
85. — The application of the rotatory cross section radiography to the diagnosis of chest diseases. Nippon Acta radiol. **13**, 469 (1953) [Japanese].
86. — An application to artificial pneumothorax of the rotatory cross-section radiography. Nippon Acta radiol. **13**, 568 (1953) [Japanese].
87. — On the rotatory cross section radiography of lower abdomen. Nippon Acta radiol. **14**, 711 (1955) [Japanese].
88. —, and *T. Sotani:* On the rotatory cross section radiogram of extrapleural thoracoplastic chest. Nippon Acta radiol. **19**, 655 (1959) [Japanese].
89. *Onuma, I.:* Conformation radiotherapy by means of stereosynthesis obtained by the axial transverse multisection radiography. Nippon Acta radiol. **26**, 201 (1966) [Japanese].
90. *Passeri, A.:* La stratigrafia assiale trasversa nella patologia polmonare. Radiol. sperimentale **2**, 122 (1948).
91. *Piazza, A.:* La stratigrafia nello studio delle indicazioni e degli esiti degli interventi chirurgici polmonari collasso-terapici. Lezioni del Primo Corso Internaz. Teorico-Pratico di Aggiornamento e Perfezionamento sulla Stratigrafia, 365—390 (1950).
92. *Pierquin, B., D. Chassagne* et *M. Gasiorowski:* Technique de dosimetrie en curietherapie interstitielle par tomographie transversale. Acta radiol. (Stockh.) **53**, 314 (1960).
93. — La tomographie transversale: Technique de routine en radiothérapie. J. Radiol. Électrol. **42**, 131 (1961).
94. *Pompili, G.,* e *G. Alè:* Molfologia degli strumi tiroidei cervico-toracici ed endotoracici in stratigrafia assiale trasversa. Ann. Radiol. diagn. (Bologna) **34**, 191 (1961).
95. *Retzepis, G.:* La tomographie transversale combinée avec bronchographie zonaire dans l'étude anatomo-radiologique de certaines zônes pulmonaires (Etude expérimentale sur des pièces anatomiques des poumons humains). Rev. Tuberc. (Paris) **17**, 1080 (1953).
96. *Rollandi, A.,* e *G. Reggiani:* Ilo del pulmone e stratigrafia assiale trasversa. Radiol. med. (Torino) **41**, 1087 (1955).
97. *Roswit, B., S. M. Unger, J. Stein, S. J. Malsky,* and *C. B. Reid:* Transverse laminagraphy: the third dimension in body section roentgenography: applications in radiation therapy. Amer. J. Roentgenol. **81**, 130 (1959).
98. — — Tumor localization with transverse tomography: diagnostic and therapeutic applications. Radiology **74**, 705 (1960).
99. *Roussel, J., P. Schoumacher, Pernot, A. Gaucher* et *R. Poire:* Intérêt de la tomographie axiale transversale dans l'étude des tumeurs bronchopulmonaires. Rev. méd. Nancy **83**, 55 (1958).
100. *Sakuma, S.,* and *S. Takahashi:* Beam focus radiography for taking the radiogram of the axial transverse cross section of the treated region in high density of dose. Tohoku J. exp. Med. **87**, 244 (1965).
101. *Sannazzari, G. L.,* e *A. Torretta:* La stratigrafia assiale trasversa nella preparazione die piani di cura radioterapici della neoplasie endotoraciche. Radiol. med. (Torino) **45**, 1 (1959).

102. *Sanquirico, G., R. Cignolini* et *F. Perassi:* La stratigraphie axiale transversale dans l'étude des organes médiastinaux. J. Radiol. Électrol. **31**, 463 (1950).

103. *Sansone, G.,* e *A. de Maestri:* Visualizzazione simultanea del mediastino posteriore ed anteriore dopo insufflazione per vis peridurale. Studio stratigrafico tridimensionale. Minerva pediat. **3**, 332 (1951).

104. — — Ulteriori ricerche sulla visualizzazione degli organi addominali dopo insufflazione retroperitoneale e stratigrafia assiale e trasversa. Minerva pediat. **3**, 328 (1951).

105. — —, *P. Durand* e *N. Macarini:* Pneumoencefalografia e stratigrafia assiale trasversa nel bambino. Minerva pediat. **3**, 358 (1951).

106. —, *N. Macarini* e *G. Corradi:* Studio stratigrafico tridimensionale della vascica dopo insufflazione extraperitoneale. Minerva pediat. **3**, 365 (1951).

107. —, e *A. de Maestri:* Stratigrafia assiale trasversa per lo studio degli organi addominali dopo insufflazione retroperitoneale nel bambino. Minerva med. **137** (1951).

108. —, *N. Macarini* e *L. Oliva:* La visualizzazione del pancreas nel bambino per mezzo della stratigrafia e della insufflazione retroperitoneale. Minerva pediat. **3**, 343 (1951).

109. — — — Nouvelle méthode d'exploration radiologique du pancréas chez l'enfant. J. Radiol. Électrol. **32**, 726 (1951).

110. *Sasaki, T.:* Rotatory cross section radiographic examination of stomach and duodenum of healthy adults in erect and supine position. Nippon Acta radiol. **19**, 1402 (1959) [Japanese].

111. — Axial transverse tomography applied to pancreas. Clin. All-round (Osaka) **14**, 1757 (1965) [Japanese].

112. *Sato, Y.:* Study on deformity of thorax and displacement of mediastinum after thoracoplasty. Observed by the rotatory cross section radiography. Therapeutics (Tokyo) **7** (11), 9 (1953) [Japanese].

113. *Sato, Y.:* Rotatory cross section radiography and artificial pneumoperitoneum. Therapeutics (Tokyo) **8**, 395 (1954) [Japanese].

114. *Schaudig, E.,* u. *J. Kirst:* Das Transversalschichtbild des Mediastinum beim Bronchialkarzinom. Radiol. diagn. (Berl.) **1**, 404 (1960).

115. *Sharma, S. R.,* and *N. G. Gadekar:* Transverse tomography in diagnosis of intrathoracic lesions. Indian. J. Radiol. **16**, 83 (1962).

116. *Shimazaki, T.:* On rotary cross-section radiography. 2. report. Nippon Acta radiol. **12** (5), 29 (1952) [Japanese].

117. — Rotatory cross section radiography. J. med. Soc. Communic. (Tokyo) **5**, 389 (1953) [Japanese].

118. — Rotatory cross section radiography. Kekkaku-Shinryo **9**, 553 (1955) [Japanese].

119. *Stevenson, J. J.:* Horizontal body section radiography. Brit. J. Radiol. **23**, 319 (1950).

120. *Suchánˇ, M.:* Transversal tomography in the diagnosis of pulmonary tuberculosis. Bratisl. lek. Listy **37**, 346 (1963).

121. *Takahashi, S.:* Study on rotation radiography. Aomori-ken Gakuzyutsu-Shinko Kenkyu-Happyo Hokokusho No. **1** (1948) [Japanese].

122. — Rotation radiography. Jap. med. J. **1313**, 3 (1949) [Japanese].

123. —, *M. Imaoka,* and *T. Shinozaki:* Rotatory cross section radiography. Nippon Acta radiol. **10**, 1 (1950) [Japanese].

124. — — — Rotatory cross-section radiography of the living human body. Nippon Acta radiol. **10** (8), 29 (1950) [Japanese].

125. — Rotatory cross section radiography of the pulmonary tuberculosis. Jap. J. clin. Tuberc. **9**, 587 (1950) [Japanese].

126. — A method to take radiograms of the transsection of the body at any inclination and curvature. Prel. report. Tohoku J. exp. Med. **52**, 138 (1950).

127. —, and *T. Nikaido:* A method to take a radiogram of the body in three dimensions. Prel. report. Tohoku J. exp. Med. **52**, 144 (1950).

128. *Takahashi, S.:* Study on rotatography. Hirosaki med. J. **2**, 1 (1951) [Japanese].

129. —, *M. Imaoka,* and *T. Shinozaki:* Rotatory cross-section radiography. Study on the rotatography, 4. report. Tohoku J. exp. Med. **54**, 59 (1951).

130. —, *T. Matsuda,* and *T. Nikaido:* Obstructive shadow superimposed to the pulmonary field of the rotatory cross section radiogram of the chest. Nippon Acta radiol. **12** (7), 10 (1952) [Japanese].

131. — *S. Anzai,* and *J. Obara:* Rotatory crossgraphy (rotatory cross section radiography) of ventricles and subarachnoid cisterns. Tohoku J. exp. Med. **56**, 161 (1952).

132. —, and *J. Obara:* Rotatory crossgraphy (rotatory cross section radiography) of the head. Tohoku J. exp. Med. **56**, 311 (1952).

133. — — Rotatory crossgraphy (rotatory cross section radiography) of the neck. Tohoku J. exp. Med. **57**, 17 (1952).

134. — Theory of blurring of X-ray images and occurrence of obstructive shadows in rotatory cross section radiography. Tohoku J. exp. Med. **58**, 63 (1953).

135. —, and *T. Matsuda:* Clinical evaluation of rotatory cross section radiography (rotatory crossgraphy) applied to chest diseases. Tohoku J. exp. Med. **58**, 179 (1953).

136. —, and *T. Shinozaki:* Solidography of the heart. Acta radiol. (Stockh.) **41**, 435 (1954).

137. —, u. *T. Kitabatake:* Über einen Versuch zum ständigen Kontrollieren des Krankheitsherdes bei der Rotationsbestrahlung, mit Hilfe des Prinzips der transversalen Schichtaufnahme. Nagoya J. med. Sci. **17**, 461 (1954).

138. — High voltage macroradiography and high voltage rotation radiography. Recent Advanc. Tuberc. Res. (Tokyo) **15**, 44 (1956) [Japanese].

139. —, and *T. Matsuda:* Simultaneous multisection radiography by means of rotatory cross section radiography. Nippon Acta radiol. **18**, 191 (1958) [Japanese].

140. *Takahashi, S., and T. Matsuda:* Axial transverse laminagraphy applied to rotational therapy. Radiology **74**, 61 (1960).

141. — Axial transverse tomography and beam focus radiography applied to conformation radiotherapy. Jap. J. Cancer Clin. (Tokyo) **10**, 364 (1964) [Japanese].

142. *Takamatsu, I.,* and *Y. Imai:* Axial transverse tomogram of the mediastinal hernia. Hirosaki med. J. **3**, 349 (1952) [Japanese].

143. *Takeuchi, A.:* Experimental study on obstructive shadow formation in axial transverse tomography applied to chest. Nippon Acta radiol. **27**, 134 (1967) [Japanese].

144. — Obstructive shadow of ribs imaged on the axial transverse tomogram of the chest. Nagoya J. med. Sci. **31**, 509 (1969)

145. *Thomas, G.,* u. *A. Stecken:* Transversaltomographie normaler und pathologischer Befunde der Lungengefäße und der Aorta. Radiol. diagn. (Berl.) **2**, 375 (1961).

146. — Transversaltomographie normaler und pathologischer Befunde der Lungengefäße und der Aorta. II. Erweiterung der Diagnostik pathologischer Aortenbefunde durch das Schichtverfahren unter besonderer Berücksichtigung der Transversaltomographie. Radiol. diagn. (Berl.) **3**, 447 (1962).

147. *Vallebona, A.:* Nouvelle méthode roentgenstratigraphique. Radiol. clin. (Basel) **16**, 279 (1947).

148. — Vecchi e nuovi methodi stratigrafici. Radiol. med. (Torino) **33**, 601 (1947).

149. — L'esplorazione stratigrafica tridimensionale. Radiol. sperimentale **2**, 95 (1948).

150. — I nuovi orizzonti della stratigrafia nei verî campi della medicina. Inform. med. (Genova) **2** (4), 1—159 (1948).

151. — Prime ricerche su di un nuovo metodo radiografico: Stratigrafia assiale con radiazioni perpendicolari all'asse. Ann. Radiol. diagn. (Bologna) **20**, 57 (1948).

152. — Transversal Axial Stratography. Sci. med. ital. **1**, 152 (1950).

153. — Axial transverse laminagraphy. Radiology **55**, 271 (1950).

154. *Vallebona, A.:* La stratigrafia nelle sue origini e nei suoi attuali sviluppi. Minerva med. **2** (35), 1 (1950).
155. — Demonstration von transversalen Schichtbildern des Herzens. Fortschr. Röntgenstr. **76**, 508 (1952).
156. — Récents progrès dans le domaine de la stratigraphie. Seventh Internat. Congr. of Radiology (The invited papers). Acta radiol. (Stockh.), Suppl. **116**, 175—183 (1954).
157. — Three dimensional stratigraphic examination; axial transverse stratigraphy. I. Amer. J. Roentgenol. **74**, 769 (1955).
158. — Les récents développements de la stratigraphie et particulièrement de la stratigraphie axiale transversale. Gaz. Hôp. (Paris) **127**, 449 (1955).
159. — Methoden und Hilfsmittel zur Lokalisation tiefliegender Tumoren mit besonderer Berücksichtigung der Bewegungsbestrahlung. Strahlentherapie **97**, 489 (1955).
160. *Vallebona, D.:* La tomografia assiale trasversa nella preparazione del piano di trattamento dei tumori del polmone. Nunt. radiol. (Roma) **31**, 562 (1965).
161. *Vieten, H.:* Grundlagen und Möglichkeiten der Röntgendarstellung von Querschnitten (Transversalschichten) langgestreckter Körper mittels kreisförmiger Verwischung der nicht abzubildenden Objektteile. Fortschr. Röntgenstr. **73**, 226 (1950).
162. *Vignolini, R.:* Studio stratigrafico assiale dei seni costomediastinali. Radiol. med. (Torino) **36**, 36 (1950).
163. *Voigt, O.,* u. *M. Thümmler:* Zur Anwendung des transversalen Schichtverfahrens in der Lungenklinik unter Einsatz eines selbstkonstruierten Gerätes. Z. Tuberk. **118**, 274 (1962).
164. *Vulpian, P. de:* Tomographie transversale thoracique. J. Radiol. Électrol. **33**, 280 (1952).
165. *Wangermez, Ch., A. Rigaud, P. Boujean* et *J. P. Meyruis:* La stratigraphie axiale transverse dans l'examen de la partie supérieure de l'abdomen. (Confrontations anatomo-radiologiques). J. Radiol. Électrol. **40**, 109 (1959).
166. *Watanabe, T., N. Ono,* and *K. Nagai:* Telecobaltradiation therapy which composed of rotatory cross section radiograph and rotatory conformation therapy unit. Nippon Acta radiol. **23**, 841 (1963) [Japanese].
167. *Watson, W.:* Differential radiography. Radiography **9** (1939).
168. *Wilk, S. P.:* Axial transverse tomography of the chest. Radiology **72**, 42 (1959)

2. Books on Axial Transverse Tomography

169. *Bonte, G., M. Brenot* et *G. Trinez:* La tomographie axiale transversale. Paris: Doin 1955.
170. *Farr, R. F., A. C. H. Scott, R. Ollerenshaw* and *G. J. H. Everard:* Transverse axial tomography. Oxford: Blackwell Sci Publ. 1964.
171. *Gebauer, A.,* u. *A. Schanen:* Das transversale Schichtverfahren. Stuttgart: Georg Thieme 1955.
172. —, *E. Muntean, E. Stutz* u. *H. Vieten:* Das Röntgenschichtbild. Stuttgart: Georg Thieme 1959.
173. *Takahashi, S.:* Tomography and axial transverse tomography. Tokyo: Igakushoin 1954 [Japanese].
174. *Takahashi, S.:* Rotation radiography Japan Society for the Promotion of Science. Tokyo: Maruzen 1957.
175. — Conformation radiotherapy. Rotation technique as applied to radiography and radiotherapy of cancer. Stockholm: Acta Radiologica Suppl. 242. 1965.
176. *Vallebona, A.* (by edited): La stratigrafia assiale trasversa. Genova: G. Sambolino e Figli 1947.
177. — Trattato di stratigrafia. Milano: Casa Editrice Dottore F. Vallardi 1952 [Excerpta Medica, Sect. 14, Vol. 7, p. 97 (383), 1953].

3. Books on Anatomy of Axial Transverse Cross Section

178. *Doyen, E., J. P. Bouchon* et *R. Doyen:* Atlas d'anatomie topographique. Paris: A. Maloine 1911.
179. *Hovelacque, A., O. Monod* et *H. Evrard:* Treize coupes horizontales du thorax. Paris: Librairie Maloine 1938.
180. *Nishi, S., H. Oka, T. Sasa, K. Otsuki,* and *T. Hasegawa:* Clinical demonstration of axial transverse cross section of adult. Tokyo: Kanehara 1949.
181. *Nishi, S.* (by edited): Atlas of human anatomy. Tokyo: Kanehara 1956.
182. *Pernkopf, E.:* Topographische Anatomie des Menschen. München: Urban & Schwarzenberg 1943.
183. *Roy-Camille, R.:* Coupes horizontales du tronc. Paris: Masson & Cie. 1959.
184. *Eycleshymer, A. C.,* and *D. M. Schoemaker:* A cross-section anatomy. New York: D. Appleton-Century Co. 1938.

Author Index

The numbers in *italics* shown in paranteses are the numbers of the references in the bibliography.

Page numbers in *italics* refer to the bibliography.

Abbatucci, J., see Frain, C. (*28*), 1, 289, *308*
Abreau, de (*1*), 1, *307*
Albertis, P. de (*2*), 13, *307*
Alè, G., and L. Macchi (*3*), 235, *307*
— see Pompili, G. (*94*), 235, *310*
Amisano, P. (*4*), (*5*), (*6*), 1, 235, *307*
Anzai, S., see Takahashi, S. (*131*), 13, *312*

Balestra, Passeri, and Macarini (*7*), 235, *307*
Ban, K., see Matsuda, T. (*72*), 6, *309*
Barenbojm, A. M. (*8*), 235, *307*
Benedetti, G. (*9*), (*10*), 235, 304, *307*
Bloch, P., see Giraud, M. (*36*), 235, *308*
Bonjean, P., see Wangermez, Ch. (*165*), 235, *313*
Bonte, G., M. Brenot, and G. Trinez (*169*), 1, 5, *313*
Bouchon, J. P., see Doyen, E. (*178*), 2, *314*
Bousquet, G., see Giraud, M. (*37*), 235, *308*
Brenot, M., see Bonte, G. (*169*), 1, 5, *313*
Bret, P., see Giraud, M. (*37*), 235, *308*
— see Levrat, M. (*52*), 235, *309*
Buchheim, C. E., see Frik, W. (*29*), 5, *308*
Bulgarelli, R., and L. Oliva (*11*), (*12*), (*13*), (*14*), 235, *307*
Buzzi, G. (*15*), 235, *307*

Chassagne, D., see Pierquin, B. (*92*), 289, *310*
Chiro, G. di (*16*), (*17*), 13, 235, *307*
Cignolini, R., see Sanquirico, G. (*102*), 235, *311*
Clément, J. P. (*18*), 235, *307*
Corradi, G., see Sansone, G. (*106*), 236, *311*
Court, P., see Monod, R. (*78*), 235, *310*
Cricchio, A., see Mattina, M. (*76*), 235, *309*
Croisille, M., see Giraud, M. (*37*), 235, *308*
Curiale, G., see Mattina, M. (*76*), 235, *309*

Doyen, E., J. P. Bouchon, and R. Doyen (*178*), 2, *314*
Doyen, R., see Doyen, E. (*178*), 2, *314*
Duhamel, J., and P. L. Martin (*19*), 1, *307*
— — and J.-C. Roques (*20*), 13, *307*
Durand, P., see Sansone, G. (*105*), 235, *311*
Dutreix, A., see Frain, C. (*28*), 1, 289, *308*

Egan, R., and G. C. Johnson (*21*), 289, *307*
Endo, S., see Matsuda, T. (*72*), 6, *309*
Everard, G. J. H., see Farr, R. F. (*170*), 1, *313*
Evrard, H., see Hovelacque, A. (*179*), 2, *314*
Eycleshymer, A. C., and D. M. Schoemaker (*184*), 2, *314*

Farinet, G., G. L. Sannazzari, and A. Torretta (*22*), 235, *307*
Farr, R. F., A. C. H. Scott, R. Ollerenshaw, and G. J. H. Everard (*170*), 1, *313*
Fleischer, H., A. Gebauer, and F. Wachsmann (*23*), 289, *307*
Frain, C., and F. Lacroix (*24*), (*25*), (*26*), (*27*), 1, *308*
— J. Surmont, M. Tubiana, B. Pierquin, R. Marlois, J. Abbatucci, and A. Dutreix (*28*), 1, 289, *308*
Frain, Ch., see Monod, R. (*78*), 235, *310*
Frik, W., C. E. Buchheim, and H. Jupitz (*29*), 5, *308*
Fumagalli, G., A. Passeri, and D. Vallebona (*30*), 235, *308*

Gadekar, N. G., see Sharma, S. R. (*115*), 235, *311*
Gardella, G. (*31*), 13, *308*
Gasiorowski, M., see Pierquin, B. (*92*), 289, *310*
Gaucher, A., see Roussel, J. (*99*), 235, *310*
Gebauer, A. (*33*), (*34*), (*35*), 1, 13, 235, *308*
— E. Muntean, E. Stutz, and H. Vieten (*172*), 1, 235, *313*
— and F. Wachsmann (*32*), 1, *308*
— and A. Schanen (*171*), 1, 235, *313*
— see Fleischer, H. (*23*), 289, *307*
Giraud, M., P. Bret, M. Levrat, M. Croisille, and G. Bousquet (*37*), 235, *308*
— Ch. Gros, J. P. Walter, P. Bloch, and Y. Grumbach (*36*), 235, *308*
Grandmottet, P., see Levrat, M. (*52*), 235, *309*
Gremmel, H. (*38*), 235, *308*
Gros, Ch., see Giraud, M. (*36*), 235, *308*
Grumbach, Y., see Giraud, M. (*36*), 235, *308*

Hachiya, H., and H. Ito (*39*), 236, *308*
Hammer, G. (*40*), 235, *308*
Hartley, J. B. (*41*), 304, *308*
Hasegawa, T., see Nishi, S. (*180*), 2, *314*
Hovelacque, A., O. Monod, and H. Evrard (*179*), 2, *314*

Iglauer, E. (*42*), 304, *308*
Imai, Y., see Takamatsu, I. (*142*), 235, *312*
Imaoka, M. (*43*), (*44*), 13, 304, *308*
— see Takahashi, S. (*123*), (*124*), (*129*), 1, 5, 8, *311*, *312*
Ito, H., see Hachiya, H. (*39*), 236, *308*

Janker, R. (45), 5, *308*
Jean Lo, Y. T., see Martin-Lalande, J. (*62*), 235, *309*
Johnson, G. C., see Egan, R. (*21*), 289, *307*
Jucker, C., and B. Pierquin (*46*), 289, *308*
Jupitz, H., see Frik, W. (*29*), 5, *308*
Jusztusz, Gy. (*47*), 1, *308*

Kaii, S., see Kobayashi, T. (*49*), 235, *308*
Kirst, J., see Schaudig, E. (*114*), 235, *311*
Kitabatake, T. (*48*), 235, *308*
— see Takahashi, S. (*137*), 289, *312*
Kobayashi, T., S. Nitta, S. Kaii, and H. Takamura (*49*), 235, *308*
Kubota, Y., Y. Sato, and M. Yoshida (*50*), 13, *308*
— see Matsuda, T. (*70*), 8, *309*

Lacroix, F. (*51*), 6, *309*
— see Frain, C. (*24*), (*25*), (*26*), (*27*), 1, *308*
Levrat, M., P. Mallet-Guy, P. Bret, P. Grandmottet, and J. Michoulier (*52*), 235, *309*
— see Giraud, M. (*37*), 235, *308*
Lodin, H. (*53*), (*54*), (*55*), 235, *309*
Lombroso, C., see Maestri, A. de (*61*), 235, *309*

Macarini, see Balestra (*7*), 235, *307*
Macarini, N. (*56*), 235, *309*
— and L. Oliva (*57*), (*58*), 235, *309*
— see Sansone, G. (*105*), (*106*), (*108*), (*109*), 235, 236, *311*
Macchi, L., see Alè, G. (*3*), 235, *307*
Maestri, A. de (*59*), (*60*), 1, 235, *309*
— and C. Lombroso (*61*), 235, *309*
— see Sansone, G. (*103*), (*104*), (*105*), (*107*), 235, 236, *311*

Mallet-Guy, P., see Levrat, M. (*52*), 235, *309*
Malsky, S. J., see Roswit, B. (*97*), 289, *310*
Marlois, R., see Frain, C. (*28*), 1, 289, *308*
Martin-Lalande, J., and Y. T. Jean Lo (*62*), 235, *309*
Martin, P. L., see Duhamel, J. (*19*), (*20*), 1, 13, *307*
Matsuda, T. (*63*), (*64*), (*65*), (*68*), (*69*), (*73*), (*74*), (*75*), 6, 8, 13, 235, *309*
— K. Ban, and S. Endo (*72*), 6, *309*
— Y. Kubota, and M. Yoshida (*70*), 8, *309*
— and Y. Sato (*67*), 235, *309*
— and T. Watanabe (*71*), 289, *309*
— and H. Yaguchi (*66*), 13, *309*
—, see Takahashi, S. (*130*), (*135*), (*139*), (*140*), 8, 235, 240, 289, *312*
Mattina, M., G. Curiale, and A. Cricchio (*76*), 235, *309*
Meyruis, J. P., see Wangermez, Ch. (*165*), 235, *313*
Michoulier, J., see Levrat, M. (*52*), 235, *309*
Miura, I., see Ode, R. (*80*), 235, *310*
Moldenhauer, W. (*77*), 235, *309*
Monod, O., see Hovelaque, A. (*179*), 2, *314*
Monod, R., Ch. Frain, and P. Court (*78*), 235, *310*
— Roche and Parent (*79*), 304, *310*
Muntean, E., see Gebauer, A. (*172*), 1, 235, *313*

Nagai, K., see Watanabe, T. (*166*), 289, *313*
Nikaido, T., see Takahashi, S. (*127*), (*130*), 8, 240, *311*, *312*
Nishi, S. (*181*), 2, *314*
— H. Oka, T. Sasa, K. Otsuki, and T. Hasegawa (*180*), 2, *314*
Nitta, S., see Kobayashi, T. (*49*), 235, *308*

Obara, J., see Takahashi, S. (*131*), (*132*), (*133*), 13, *312*
Ode, R., and I. Miura (*80*), 235, *310*
Oka, H., see Nishi, S. (*180*), 2, *314*
Oliva, L. (*81*), (*82*), (*83*), 5, 235, *310*
— see Bulgarelli, R. (*11*), (*12*), (*13*), (*14*), 235, *307*
— see Macarini, N. (*57*), (*58*), 235, *309*
— see Sansone, G. (*108*), (*109*), 235, *311*
Ollerenshaw, R., see Farr, R. F. (*170*), 1, *313*
Ono, N., see Watanabe, T. (*166*), 289, *313*
Ono, T. (*84*), (*85*), (*86*), (*87*), 13, 235, 236, *310*

Ono, T., and T. Sotani (*88*), 235, *310*
Onuma, I. (*89*), 289, *310*
Otsuki, K., see Nishi, S. (*180*), 2, *314*

Passeri see Balestra (*7*), 235, *307*
Passeri, A. (*90*), 235, *310*
— see Fumagalli, G. (*30*), 235, *308*
Parent see Monod, R. (*79*), 304, *310*
Perassi, F., see Sanquirico, G. (*102*), 235, *311*
Pernkopf, E. (*182*), 2, *314*
Pernot, see Roussel, J. (*99*), 235, *310*
Piazza, A. (*91*), 304, *310*
Pierquin, B. (*93*), 289, *310*
— D. Chassagne, and M. Gasiorowski (*92*), 286, *310*
— see Frain, C. (*28*), 1, 289, *308*
— see Jucker, C. (*46*), 289, *308*
Poire, R., see Roussel, J. (*99*), 235, *310*
Pompili, G., and G. Alé (*94*), 235, *310*

Reggiani, G., see Rollandi, A. (*96*), 235, *310*
Reid, C. B., see Roswit, B. (*97*), 289, *310*
Retzepis, G. (*95*), 13, *310*
Rigaud, A., see Wangermez, Ch. (*165*), 235, *313*
Roche, see Monod, R. (*79*), 304, *310*
Rollandi, A., and G. Reggiani (*96*), 235, *310*
Roques, J.-C., see Duhamel, J. (*20*), 13, *307*
Roswit, B., and S. M. Unger (*98*), 289, *310*
— — J. Stein, S. J. Malsky, and C. B. Reid (*97*), 289, *310*
Roussel, J., P. Schoumacher, Pernot, A. Gaucher, and R. Poire (*99*), 235, *310*
Roy-Camille, R. (*183*), 2, *314*

Sakuma, S., and S. Takahashi (*100*), 289, *310*
Sannazzari, G. L., and A. Torretta (*101*), 289, *310*
— see Farinat, G. (*22*), 235, *307*
Sanquirico, G., R. Cignolini, and F. Perassi (*102*), 235, *311*
Sansone, G., N. Macarini, and G. Corradi (*106*), 236, *311*
— — and L. Oliva (*108*), (*109*), 235, *311*
— and A. de Maestri (*103*), (*104*), (*107*), 235, 236, *311*
— — P. Durand, and N. Macarini (*105*), 235, *311*
Sasa, T., see Nishi, S. (*180*), 2, *314*
Sasaki, T. (*110*), (*111*), 13, *311*
Sato, Y. (*112*), (*113*), 13, 235, *311*
— see Kubota, Y. (*50*), 13, *308*
— see Matsuda, T. (*67*), 235, *309*
Schanen, A., see Gebauer, A. (*171*), 1, 235, *313*
Schaudig, E., and J. Kirst (*114*), 235, *311*
Schoemaker, D. M., see Eycleshymer, A. C. (*184*), 2, *314*
Schoumacher, P., see Roussel, J. (*99*), 235, *310*
Scott, A. C. H., see Farr, R. F. (*170*), 1, *313*
Sharma, S. R., and N. G. Gadekar (*115*), 235, *311*
Shimazaki, T. (*116*), (*117*), (*118*), 1, 235, *311*
Shinozaki, T., see Takahashi, S. (*123*), (*124*), (*129*), (*136*), 1, 5, 8, 240, *311*, *312*
Sotani, T., see Ono, T. (*88*), 235, *310*
Stecken, A., see Thomas, G. (*145*), 235, *312*
Stein, J., see Roswit, B. (*97*), 289, *310*
Stevenson, J. J. (*119*), 1, *311*
Stutz, E., see Gebauer, A. (*172*), 1, 235, *313*
Sucháñ, M. (*120*), 235, *311*
Surmont, J., see Frain, C. (*28*), 289, *308*

Takahashi, S. (*121*), (*122*), (*125*), (*126*), (*128*), (*134*), (*138*), (*141*), (*173*), (*174*), (*175*), 1, 5, 8, 14, 235, 289, *311*, *312*, *313*
— S. Anzai, and J. Obara (*131*), 13, *312*
— M. Imaoka, and T. Shinozaki (*123*), (*124*), (*129*), 1, 5, 8, *311*, *312*
— and T. Kitabatake (*137*), 289, *312*
— and T. Matsuda (*135*), (*139*), (*140*), 235, 240, 289, *312*
— — and T. Nikaido (*130*), 8, *312*
— and T. Nikaido (*127*), 240, *311*
— and J. Obara (*132*), (*133*), 13, *312*
— and T. Shinozaki (*136*), 240, *312*
— see Sakuma, S. (*100*), 289, *310*
Takamura, H., see Kobayashi, T. (*49*), 235, *308*
Takamatsu, I., and Y. Imai (*142*), 235, *312*
Takeuchi, A. (*143*), (*144*), 10, *312*
Thomas, G. (*146*), 235, *312*
— and A. Stecken (*145*), 235, *312*
Thümmler, M., see Voigt, O. (*163*), 235, *313*
Torretta, A., see Farinat, G. (*22*), 235, *307*
— see Sannazzari, G. L. (*101*), 289, *310*
Trinez, G., see Bonte, G. (*169*), 1, 5, *313*
Tubiana, M., see Frain, C. (*28*), 1, 289, *308*

Unger, S. M., see Roswit, B. (*97*), (*98*), 289, *310*

Vallebona, A. (*147*), (*148*), (*149*), (*150*), (*151*), (*152*), (*153*), (*154*), (*155*), (*156*), (*157*), (*158*), (*159*), (*176*), (*177*), 1, 13, 235, 289, *312*, *313*
Vallebona, D. (*160*), 289, *313*
— see Fumagalli, G. (*30*), 235, *308*
Vieten, H. (*161*), 1, *313*
— see Gebauer, A. (*172*), 1, 235, *313*
Vignolini, R. (*162*), 235, *313*
Voigt, O., and M. Thümmler (*163*), 235, *313*
Vulpian, P. de (*164*), 235, *313*

Wachsmann, F., see Fleischer, H. (*23*), 289, *307*
Wachsmann, F., see Gebauer, A. (*32*), 1, *308*
Walter, J. P., see Giraud, M. (*36*), 235, *308*
Wangermez, Ch., A. Rigaud, P. Bonjean, and J. P. Meyruis (*165*), 235, *313*
Watanabe, T., N. Ono, and K. Nagai (*166*), 289, *313*
— see Matsuda, T. (*71*), 289, *309*
Watson W,. (*167*), 1, *313*
Wilk, S. P. (*168*), 235, *313*

Yaguchi, H., see Matsuda, T. (*66*), 13, *309*
Yoshida, M., see Kubota, Y. (*50*), 13, *308*
— see Matsuda, T. (*70*), 8, *309*

Subject Index

Normal type refers to figure numbers and *italics* refer to page numbers.

Acanthiomeatal line *15, 33, 35, 37, 39, 41, 43, 45, 47, 49, 51, 241*
Acetabulum 406, 436, 438
Acromion 150
Adjustment of tomograph *8*
Ala ossis ilii 378, 381, 383, 386, 388, 391, 393, 396
Aneurysm 538, 539, 540
Anus 426
Aorta abdominalis 302, 305, 307, 310, 312, 315, 317, 320, 322, 325, 327, 330, 332, 335, 337, 340, 342, 345, 347, 350, 352, 355, 357, 360, 362, 365, 367, 370
Aorta ascendens 192, 197, 207, 212, 217, 222, 227
Aorta descendens 192
Aorta thoracica 194, 197, 204, 207, 209, 212, 214, 217, 219, 222, 224, 227, 229, 232, 234, 237, 239, 242, 244, 247, 249, 252, 254, 257, 259, 262, 264, 267, 269, 272, 287, 290, 292, 295, 297, 300, 302, 305
Aponeurosis palmaris 483
Aquaeductus cerebri 35, 40, 65, *70*
Arachnoidea encephali 10
Arcus aortae 184, 187, 189, 192, 199, 202
Arcus vertebrae (C_2) 102, 105
Arcus vertebrae (C_3) 112, 115
Arcus vertebrae (C_4) 117, 120, 122, 125
Arcus vertebrae (C_5) 127, 130, 132, 135
Arcus vertebrae (C_6) 137, 140, 142, 145
Arcus vertebrae (C_7) 147, 150
Arcus vertebrae (Th_1) 162
Arcus vertebrae (Th_2) 172
A. axillaris 167, 172, 177, 182, 187, 192, 197
A. basilaris 40, 65, 70, 75
A. brachialis 471, 473, 475
A. carotis communis 137, 140, 142, 145, 147, 150, 162, 167, 172, 177
A. carotis externa 85, 90, 100, 105, 110, 112, 115, 120, 122, 125, 127, 130, 132, 135
A. carotis interna 40, 45, 65, 70, 85, 90, 95, 100, 105, 110, 112, 115, 120, 122, 125, 127, 130, 132, 135
A. cerebelli inferior anterior 75
A. cerebri anterior 35, 50, 55
A. cerebri media 30, 60
A. cerebri posterior 35, 65
A. V. circumflexa femoris lateralis 451
A. V. N. dorsalis clitoridis 426
A. dorsalis pedis 501
A. V. facialis 100, 105, 120
A. femoralis 416, 421, 426, 431, 441, 446, 451, 456, 487, 489
A. fibularis 497, 499
A. gastrica sinistra 295, 300
A. glutaea inferior 406, 411, 416, 436, 441, 446, 451, 456
A. hepatica 300
A. hepatica communis 310
A. iliaca communis 381, 386
A. iliaca externa 391, 396, 401, 406, 411, 436, 462, 463, 464, 465
A. iliaca interna 391, 396, 401, 406, 411, 436
A. intercostalis 172, 177, 182, 192, 197, 202, 207, 212, 222, 227, 232, 237, 242, 247, 252, 257, 262, 267, 272, 290, 295, 300, 305, 310, 315, 320, 330, 335, 345
A. lienalis 300, 305
A. lingualis 125
A. lumbalis 335, 340, 345
A. mesenterica inferior 355, 360, 365
A. mesenterica superior 325, 330, 335, 340, 345
A. obturatorius 416, 436, 441
A. pancreaticoduodenalis 315
A. poplitea 492
A. profunda femoris 487
A. pudenda interna 416, 421, 426, 441, 446, 451, 456
A. pulmonalis 212, 214, 217, 219, 222, 224, 227
A. radialis 479
A. rectalis superior 401, 406
A. renalis 320, 325, 327, 330
A. sacralis lateralis 386, 391, 396
A. sacralis mediana 401
A. subclavia 162, 167, 172, 177, 182
A. thoracica interna 172, 177, 182, 187, 192, 197, 202, 207, 212, 217, 222, 227, 232, 237, 242, 247, 252, 257
A. tibialis anterior 497, 499
A. tibialis posterior 494, 497, 499, 501
A. ulnaris 479, 481
A. uterina 401
A. vertebralis 45, 80, 85, 90, 95, 100, 105, 110, 115, 120, 125, 130, 135, 140, 145, 150
Articulatio coxae 403, 406, 408, 411, 433, 436, 438, 441
Articulatio humeri 164, 169
Articulatio sacroiliaca 383, 386, 388, 391, 393, 396
Atlas 92, 95

Subject Index

Atrium dextrum 232, 237, 242, 247, 252, 257
Atrium sinistrum 232, 237, 242, 247
Auricula 32, 35, 37, 40, 42, 45, 67, 70, 72, 75, 77, 80, 82, 87, 90, 92, 95
Axial transverse tomograph of erect type *5, 289,* 567
Axial transverse tomograph of horizontal type *5, 7,* 568, *298*
Axial transverse tomography (ICRU) *1*

Beam focus *289,* 575
Beam focus radiography 573, 574, *301, 302, 303*
Bifurcatio tracheae 204, 207
Bronchus 209, 212, 214, 217, 219, 222, 224, 227
Bulbus oculi 35, 40, 45, 60, 65, 70
Bulbus penis 451
Bulbus vestibuli 426
Bursa subcutanea olecrani 475
Bursa subcutanea prepatellaris 492

Caecum 378, 381, 386, 388, 391, 393, 396
Canalis vertebrae 287, 290, 292, 295, 297, 300, 302, 305, 307, 310, 312, 315, 317, 320, 322, 325, 332, 335, 337, 340, 342, 345, 347, 352, 355, 357, 360, 362, 365, 367, 370
Cancer of the mandible 507, 508, 509
Cancer of the maxillary sinus *241,* 504, 505, 506
Capsula articularis coxae 406
Capsula interna 20
Caput femoris 403, 406, 408, 411, 433, 436, 438, 441
Caput humeri 159, 162, 169, 172
Cartilago costalis 252, 262, 267, 272
Cartilago costalis I 174, 177
Cartilago thyreoidea 132, 135, 137, 140
Cassette for axial transverse tomography *6*
Cauda equina 335, 340, 345, 350, 355, 360, 365, 370, 381, 386, 391, 396
Caudalocranial direction of central X-ray *10*
Cavitas glenoidalis 172
Cavum articulare genus 492
Cavum laryngis 140
Cavum nasi 75
Cavum oris 82, 85, 87, 90, 92, 95, 97, 100
Cavum pericardii 232, 262, 267
Cavum pharyngis 82, 85, 87, 90, 95, 97, 100, 102, 105, 107, 110, 112, 115, 117, 120, 122, 125, 127, 130, 132, 135, 137
Cavum pleurae 232, 237, 242
Cavum subarachnoidale 10, 70
Cellulae ethmoidales anteriores 37, 40, 42, 48, 62, 65, 67, 70
Cellulae ethmoidales posteriores 37, 40, 42, 45, 62, 65, 67, 70
Cellulae mastoideae 42, 45, 72, 75, 77
Cerebellum 35, 40, 75, 80
Cisterna cerebellomedullaris 95
Cisterna chyli 330
Clavicula 147, 150, 159, 162, 164, 167, 169, 172, 174, 177
^{60}Co γ-ray radiography *303*
Cold abscess 544, 545, 546
Collum femoris 413, 416, 438, 441, 443, 446
Collum scapulae 159, 162
Colon ascendens 327, 330, 332, 335, 337, 340, 342, 345, 347, 350, 352, 355, 357, 360, 362, 365, 367, 370
Colon descendens 320, 322, 325, 327, 330, 332, 335, 337, 340, 342, 345, 347, 350, 352, 355, 357, 360, 362, 365, 367, 370, 381, 386, 388, 391, 393, 396, 398, 401
Colon sigmoideum 459
Colon transversum 312, 315, 317, 320, 322, 325, 327, 330, 332, 335, 337, 340, 357, 360, 378, 381, 383, 386, 463, 464
Concha nasalis 67, 70
Concha nasalis inferior 77, 80
Concha nasalis media 72, 75, 80
Condylus lateralis femoris 492
Condylus medialis femoris 492
Confluens sinuum 40, 45, 80
Conformation therapy *299,* 570, 575
Cor 224, 229, 234, 239, 244, 249, 254, 259, 264, 267
Corpus adiposum retrosternale (= Thymus rest) 177, 182, 187, 192, 197, 202, 207, 212
Corpus callosum 20, 25, 50, 55, 60
Corpus cavernosum penis 451, 456
Corpus femoris 418, 421, 423, 426, 428, 431, 448, 451, 453, 456, 487, 489
Corpus fibulae 494, 497, 499
Corpus humeri 469, 471, 473
Corpus penis 451, 453, 456
Corpus spongiosum penis 451, 456
Corpus sterni 194, 197, 199, 202, 204, 207, 209, 212, 214, 217, 219, 222, 224, 227, 229, 232, 234, 237, 239, 242, 244, 247, 257
Corpus striatum 50, 60
Corpus tibiae 494, 497, 499
Corpus uteri 406
Corpus ventriculi 292, 295, 297
Corpus vertebrae (C_2) 97, 100, 102, 105
Corpus vertebrae (C_3) 107, 110, 112, 115
Corpus vertebrae (C_4) 117, 120, 122, 125
Corpus vertebrae (C_5) 127, 130, 132, 135

Corpus vertebrae (C_6) 137, 140, 142, 145
Corpus vertebrae (C_7) 147, 150
Corpus vertebrae (Th_1) 159, 162
Corpus vertebrae (Th_2) 164, 167, 169, 172
Corpus vertebrae (Th_3) 174, 177, 179, 182, 184, 187
Corpus vertebrae (Th_4) 189, 192, 204, 207
Corpus vertebrae (Th_5) 194, 197, 214, 217, 219, 222
Corpus vertebrae (Th_6) 224, 227
Corpus vertebrae (Th_9) 229, 232, 249, 252, 254, 257
Corpus vertebrae (Th_{10}) 239, 242, 244, 247, 259, 262, 264, 267, 287, 290
Corpus vertebrae (Th_{11}) 269, 272, 292, 295, 297, 300
Corpus vertebrae (Th_{11-12}) 302, 305
Corpus vertebrae (Th_{12}) 307, 310, 312, 315
Corpus vertebrae (L_1) 317, 320, 322, 325
Corpus vertebrae (L_{1-2}) 327, 330
Corpus vertebrae (L_2) 332, 335, 337, 340
Corpus vertebrae (L_{2-3}) 342, 345
Corpus vertebrae (L_3) 347, 350, 352, 355
Corpus vertebrae (L_{3-4}) 357, 360
Corpus vertebrae (L_4) 362, 365, 367, 370
Corpus vertebrae (L_5) 381
Costa 287, 290, 292, 295, 297, 300, 302, 305, 307, 310, 312, 315, 317, 320, 322, 325, 327, 330, 335
Costa I 147, 150, 159, 164, 167, 169, 172, 187
Costa II 159, 162, 164, 167, 169, 172, 174, 177, 179, 182, 184, 187, 189, 192, 194, 197, 199, 202, 204, 207
Costa III 172, 174, 177, 179, 182, 184, 187, 189, 192, 194, 197, 199, 202, 204, 207, 209, 212, 214, 217, 219, 222, 224, 227
Costa IV 179, 182, 184, 187, 189, 192, 194, 197, 199, 202, 204, 207, 209, 212, 214, 217, 219, 222, 224, 227,
Costa V 189, 192, 197, 209, 214, 217, 219, 222, 224, 227, 229
Costa VI 219, 222, 224, 227, 229, 232, 234, 237, 239, 244, 249, 252, 254, 257
Costa VII 229, 232, 234, 237, 239, 242, 244, 247, 249, 252, 254, 257, 259, 262, 264, 267, 269, 272
Costa VIII 229, 232, 234, 237, 239, 242, 244, 247, 249, 252, 254, 257, 259, 262, 264, 267, 269, 272
Costa IX 229, 232, 234, 237, 239, 242, 244, 247, 249, 252, 254, 257, 259, 262, 264, 267, 269, 272
Costa X 239, 242, 244, 247, 249, 252, 254, 257, 259, 262, 264, 267, 269, 272
Costa XI 269, 272
Craniocaudal direction of central X-ray *10*
Crena ani 428, 431, 453
Crista galli 32, 35, 52, 55
Crista sacralis intermedia 388, 391, 393, 396
Crista sacralis lateralis 388, 391, 393, 396
Crista sacralis mediana 383, 386, 388, 391, 393, 396

Dentes 87, 90, 92, 95, 97, 100
Dens artificialis 97, 100
Dens axis 92, 95
Diaphragma 244, 247, 249, 252, 254, 257, 259, 262, 264, 267, 269, 272, 287, 290, 292, 295, 300, 305, 310, 312, 315, 320, 325, 330
Diaphragma: Pars costalis 272
Diaphragma: Pars lumbalis 272
Diaphragma pelvis 426, 436, 446, 451
Diaphragma urogenitale 411
Discus intercostalis (Th_{3-4}) 199
Discus intercostalis (Th_{4-5}) 209
Discus intercostalis (Th_{9-10}) 234, 237
Discus intervertebralis (Th_{3-4}) 202
Discus intervertebralis (Th_{4-5}) 212
Dorsum sellae 67, 70
Ductus choledochus 310, 315
Ductus hepaticus 300
Ductus thoracicus 172, 177, 182, 187, 192, 197, 202, 207, 212, 217, 222, 227, 232, 237, 242, 247, 252, 257, 262, 267, 272, 287, 290, 295, 300, 305, 310, 315, 320, 325
Duodenum 312, 317, 322, 327, 332
Duodenum: Flexura duodenojejunalis 315
Duodenum: Pars ascendens 320, 322, 325
Duodenum: Pars descendens 315, 320, 325, 330, 335, 340
Duodenum: Pars horizontalis 330, 337
Duodenum: Pars superior 310
Dura mater encephali 10, 15, 25, 30, 40, 50, 55, 60, 65

Epiglottis 115, 120, 125, 127, 130
Excavatio rectouterina 405, 411, 416
Excavatio rectovesicalis 446
Excavatio vesicouterina 406, 411, 416

Faeces 398, 401, 433
Falx cerebri 10, 15, 20, 25, 30, 50, 55
Fascia antebrachii 479, 481
Fascia brachii 469, 471, 473
Fascia cervicalis 110, 120, 125

Fascia iliotibialis 487
Fascia lata 411, 421, 426, 431, 451, 456, 487, 489
Fascia nuchae 100, 105, 110, 115, 117, 120, 125, 130, 135, 140, 150
Fascia prevertebralis 102, 107, 110
Fascia temporalis 15, 20, 45
Fibrosarcoma 564, 565, 566
Filum metallicum 97, 100
Fissura longitudinalis cerebri 10, 52, 60
Fissura orbitalis superior 62
Flexura coli dextra 317, 320
Flexura coli sinistra 287, 290, 292, 295, 297, 300, 302, 305, 307, 310, 315
Foramen jugulare 77, 80, 82
Foramen lacerum 42, 77
Foramen rotundum 42
Foramina sacralia 383, 388, 393
Foreign body (nail) 521, 522, 523
Fornix 25
Fossa interpeduncularis 35
Fossa lateralis cerebri 20, 27, 30, 32, 35
Fossa supraspinata 207
Fracture of the iliac bone 558, 559
Funiculus spermaticus 441, 446, 451

Galea aponeurotica 15, 20, 25, 35
Ganglion coeliacum 305, 310
Glandula lacrimalis 40, 60, 65
Glandula parathyreoidea 150
Glandula parotis 85, 90, 95, 100
Glandula sublingualis 110
Glandula submandibularis 105, 107, 110, 112, 115, 117, 120, 122, 125
Glandula suprarenalis 302, 305, 307, 310, 312, 315
Glandula thyreoidea 142, 145, 147, 150

Hemisphaerium cerebelli 45, 85, 90
Hemisphaerium cerebri 10, 15
Hepar 259, 262, 264, 267, 269, 272, 287, 290, 292, 295, 297, 300, 302, 305, 307, 310, 312, 315, 317, 320, 322, 325, 327, 330
Humerus 174, 177, 182, 184, 187, 192, 194
Hypophysis 70

Ileum 378, 381, 383, 386, 388, 391, 393, 396, 398, 401, 436
Inclination angle *8*, ***10***
Insula 20, 25, 30, 55
Intestinum tenue 292, 295, 297, 300, 302, 305, 307, 310, 312, 317, 322, 325, 327, 330, 332, 335, 337, 340, 342, 345, 347, 350, 352, 355, 357, 360, 362, 365, 367, 370

Jejunum 315

Labium inferius 92, 95, 100
Labium majus pudendi 428, 431
Labium superius 82
Lien 272, 287, 290, 292, 295, 297, 300, 302, 305, 307, 310, 312, 315
Ligamentum falciforme hepatis 290, 295, 300
Ligamentum inguinale 406, 411, 416
Ligamentum ischiofemorale 416
Ligamentum latum uteri 406
Ligamentum nuchae 80, 85, 90, 95
Ligamentum teres uteri 406, 411
Linea alba 290, 295, 300, 305, 310, 315, 320, 325, 330, 335, 340, 345, 350, 355, 360, 365, 370, 381, 386, 391, 396, 401, 406, 411, 416
Lingua 87, 95, 100
Lobus frontalis cerebri 17, 20, 22, 25, 27, 30, 35, 50
Lobus frontalis cerebri: Gyrus rectus 60
Lobus occipitalis cerebri 20, 30, 35, 40, 55, 60, 65, 75, 80, 85
Lobus temporalis cerebri 20, 30, 35, 40, 42, 45, 65, 70
Lymphonodi aortici 300, 305, 310, 315, 320, 325, 330, 335
Lymphonodi axillares 192, 197
Lymphonodi bronchopulmonales 227
Lymphonodi cervicales profundi 115, 130, 140, 145, 150
Lymphonodi cervicales superficiales 120, 150
Lymphonodi gastrici sinistri 295
Lymphonodi hepati 300
Lymphonodi iliaci aggregati 378, 383, 386
Lymphonodi iliaci externi 388, 391, 393, 396, 398, 401, 403, 406, 408, 411, 436
Lymphonodi iliaci interni 391, 396, 401, 406, 411
Lymphonodi infraclaviculares 282
Lymphonodi inguinales 416, 421, 423, 426, 428, 431, 441, 446, 451, 456
Lymphonodi lienales 300, 305
Lymphonodi lumbales 340, 345, 350, 355, 360, 365, 370
Lymphonodi mediastinales anteriores 197
Lymphonodi mediastinales posteriores 290, 295
Lymphonodi obturatorius 416, 436
Lymphonodi pancreaticoduodenalis 315, 320
Lymphonodi pancreaticolienales 300, 305
Lymphonodus popliteus 492
Lymphonodi sacrales 396

Lymphonodi submandibulares 115, 120
Lymphonodi sympathicus 355
Lymphonodi tracheales 162, 167, 172, 177, 182, 187, 192, 202, 207, 283, 284
Lymphonodi tracheobronchiales inferiores 217, 222
Lymphonodi tracheobronchiales superiores 212, 285

Magnification rate *8, 298, 299, 302, 303, 305*
Malignant lymphoma 524, 525, 526, 527, 528
Malleolus lateralis 501
Malleolus medialis 501
Mandibula: Corpus mandibulae 102, 105, 107, 110, 112, 115, 117, 120
Mandibula: Ramus mandibulae 82, 85, 87, 90, 92, 95, 97, 100
Manubrium sterni 174, 177, 179, 182, 184, 187, 189, 192
Maxilla 85, 90
Maxilla: Facies infratemporalis 72, 75, 77, 80
Maxilla: Processus frontalis 57, 62, 65, 67, 70, 72, 77
Maxilla: Processus palatinus 82, 87
Meatus nasi 72
Mediastinal tumor 529, 530, 531
Medulla oblongata 75, 80, 85, 90
Medulla spinalis 95, 100, 105, 110, 115, 120, 125, 130, 135, 140, 145, 150, 232, 237, 247, 290, 295, 300, 305, 310, 315, 320, 325, 330
Mesencephalon 35
Metastatic cancer of the pleura 541, 542, 543
Mons pubis 416, 418, 421, 423, 426
Moving filter *6*
Multisection radiography *240*
M. abductor pollicis 481
M. abductor pollicis longus 479, 483
M. adductor brevis 421, 426, 431, 451, 456
M. adductor longus 421, 426, 431, 451, 456, 487
M. adductor magnus 421, 426, 431, 451, 456, 487, 489
M. adductor minimus 456
M. anconeus 475, 477
M. biceps brachii 187, 469, 471, 473
M. biceps brachii: Caput breve 177
M. biceps femoris 492
M. biceps femoris: Caput breve 487, 489
M. biceps femoris: Caput longum 431, 456, 487, 489
M. brachialis 471, 473, 475, 477
M. brachioradialis 475, 477, 479, 481
M. buccinator 85, 90, 95, 100, 105
Mm. constrictores pharyngis 100, 105, 110, 115, 120, 125, 130, 135, 140
M. coracobrachialis 172, 469
M. corrugator supericlii 40
M. deltoideus 145, 150, 162, 167, 172, 177, 182, 187, 192, 197, 469
M. depressor anguli oris 105, 110, 115
M. depressor labii inferioris 105, 110, 115
M. digastricus: Venter anterior 115, 120, 125
M. digastricus: Venter posterior 90, 95, 115
Mm. profundi dorsi 162, 167, 172, 177, 182, 187, 192, 197, 202, 207, 212, 217, 222, 227, 232, 237, 242, 247, 252, 257, 262, 267, 272
M. erector trunci 290, 295, 300, 305, 310, 315, 320, 325, 330, 335, 340, 345, 350, 355, 360, 365, 370, 381, 386, 391, 396
M. extensor carpi radialis 475, 477, 479, 481, 483
M. extensor carpi ulnaris 477, 479, 481, 483
M. extensor digitorum 479, 481, 483
M. extensor digitorum brevis: Tendo 501
M. extensor digitorum longus 494, 497, 499, 501
M. extensor hallucis brevis: Tendo 501
M. extensor hallucis longus 497, 499
M. extensor hallucis longus: Tendo 501
M. extensor pollicis brevis 479
M. extensor pollicis longus 481
Mm. extensores pollicis: Tendines 483
Mm. faciei 75
Mm. fibulares 499, 501
M. fibularis longus 494, 497
M. flexor carpi radialis 475, 477, 479, 481
M. flexor carpi ulnaris 475, 479, 481
M. flexor digitorum longus 497, 499, 501
M. flexor digitorum profundus 477, 479, 481, 483
M. flexor digitorum superficialis 475, 477, 479, 481, 483
M. flexor hallucis longus 497, 499, 501
M. flexor pollicis longus 481
M. gastrocnemius 494, 497
M. gastrocnemius: Caput laterale 492
M. gastrocnemius: Caput mediale 492
M. genioglossus 105, 110
M. geniohyoideus 120
M. glutaeus maximus 381, 386, 391, 396, 401, 406, 411, 416, 421, 426, 431, 436, 441, 446, 451, 456
M. glutaeus medius 381, 386, 391, 396, 401, 406, 411, 416, 436, 441, 446
M. glutaeus minimus 386, 391, 396, 401, 406, 411, 436

M. gracilis 426, 431, 451, 456, 487, 489
M. hyoglossus 110, 120
Mm. hypothenaris 483
M. iliacus 381, 386, 391, 396, 401, 436
M. iliopsoas 406, 411, 416, 421, 426, 441, 446, 451
M. infraspinatus 150, 162, 167, 172, 177, 182, 187, 192, 197, 202, 207, 212, 217, 222, 227
Mm. intercostales 162, 167, 172, 177, 182, 187, 192, 202, 207, 212, 222, 227, 232, 237, 242, 247, 252, 257, 262, 267, 272, 290, 295, 300, 305, 310, 315, 320, 325, 330
M. latissimus dorsi 202, 207, 212, 217, 222, 227, 232, 237, 242, 247, 252, 257, 262, 267, 272, 290, 295, 300, 305, 310, 315, 320, 325, 330, 335, 340, 345, 350, 355, 360, 365
M. levator ani 416, 421, 426, 446, 451
M. levator scapulae 105, 110, 115, 120, 125, 130, 135, 140, 145, 150
M. levator labii superioris etc. 85, 90
M. levator veli paratini 85
M. longissimus capitis 95
M. longus capitis 90, 95
M. longus colli 90, 95, 162, 167, 172, 177, 187
M. masseter 80, 85, 90, 95, 100, 105, 110, 115
M. mentalis 110, 115
M. mylohyoideus 110, 112, 115, 120, 125
Mm. nuchae 100, 105, 110, 115, 120, 125, 130, 135, 140, 145, 150
M. obliquus capitis superior 95
M. obliquus abdominis externus 290, 295, 300, 305, 310, 315, 320, 325, 330, 335, 340, 345, 350, 355, 360, 365, 370, 381, 386, 391, 396, 401
M. obliquus abdominis internus 315, 320, 325, 330, 335, 340, 345, 350, 355, 360, 365, 370, 381, 386, 391, 396, 401
M. obturatorius externus 416, 421, 426, 446, 451
M. obturatorius internus 411, 416, 421, 426, 436, 441, 446, 451
M. occipitofrontalis: Venter frontalis 35, 50
M. occipitofrontalis: Venter occipitalis 20, 25, 35, 40, 55, 60, 65, 70
M. omohyoideus 130, 135, 140, 145, 150
M. orbicularis oculi 40, 45, 60, 65, 70
M. orbicularis oris 85, 90, 95, 105, 110
M. palmaris brevis 483
M. palmaris longus 477, 479
M. pectineus 416, 421, 426, 441, 446, 451
M. pectoralis major 162, 167, 172, 177, 182, 187, 192, 197, 202, 207, 212, 217, 222, 227, 232, 237, 242, 247, 252, 257
M. pectoralis minor 167, 172, 177, 182, 187, 192, 197, 202, 207, 212, 217, 222, 227
M. phrenicus 150
M. piriformis 401, 406, 411, 436
M. plantaris 492
M. popliteus 494
Mm. praevertebrales 100, 105, 110, 115, 120, 125, 130, 135, 140, 145, 150
M. pronator teres 475, 479
M. pronator teres: Caput humerale 477
M. pronator teres: Caput ulnare 477
M. psoas major 320, 325, 330, 332, 335, 337, 340, 342, 345, 347, 350, 352, 355, 357, 360, 362, 365, 367, 370, 381, 386, 391, 396, 401, 436
M. pterygoideus lateralis 80
M. pterygoideus medialis 85, 90, 95, 100, 105
M. pyramidalis 436
M. quadratus femoris 421, 426, 446, 451
M. quadratus lumborum 330, 335, 340, 345, 350, 355, 360, 365, 370
M. rectus abdominis 272, 290, 295, 300, 305, 310, 315, 320, 325, 330, 335, 340, 345, 350, 355, 365, 370, 381, 386, 391, 396, 401, 406, 411, 416, 421, 436, 441
M. rectus capitis anterior 95
M. rectus capitis lateralis 95
M. rectus capitis posterior major 95
M. rectus capitis posterior minor 95
M. rectus femoris 416, 421, 426, 431, 441, 446, 451, 456, 487, 489
M. rectus inferior 70
M. rectus lateralis 40, 45, 65
M. rectus medialis 40, 45
M. rectus superior 40
M. rhomboideus 145, 150
M. rhomboideus major 162, 167, 172, 177, 182, 187, 192, 197, 202, 212, 217, 222, 227
M. sartorius 406, 411, 416, 421, 426, 441, 446, 451, 456, 487, 489, 492
Mm. scaleni 100, 105, 110, 115, 120, 125, 130, 135, 140, 145, 150
M. semimembranosus 456, 487, 489, 492
M. semispinalis capitis 45, 80, 85, 90, 95
M. semitendinosus 456, 487, 489, 492
M. serratus anterior 162, 167, 172, 177, 182, 187, 192, 197, 202, 207, 212, 217, 222, 227, 232, 237, 242, 247, 252, 257, 262, 267, 272, 290, 295, 300, 305
M. soleus 494, 497, 499
M. sphincter ani externus 426, 451, 456
M. sphincter ani internus 416, 426, 451, 456
M. splenius capitis 75, 90

M. sternocleidomastoideus 95, 100, 105, 107, 110, 112, 115, 117, 120, 122, 125, 127, 130, 132, 135, 137, 140, 142, 145, 147, 150, 162, 167, 172
M. sternohyoideus 125, 130, 135, 140, 142, 145, 147, 150, 177
M. sternothyreoideus 140, 145, 150
M. styloglossus 90
M. stylohyoideus 90, 110, 115
M. stylopharyngeus 90
M. subclavius 162, 172
M. subscapularis 162, 167, 172, 177, 182, 187, 192, 197, 202, 207, 217, 222, 227
M. supinator 477, 479
M. suprascapularis 145
M. supraspinatus 150, 162, 167, 172, 202, 207, 212
M. temporalis 10, 15, 20, 25, 30, 35, 40, 45, 50, 55, 60, 65, 70, 75
M. tensor 85
M. tensor fasciae latae 401, 406, 411, 416, 421, 426, 431, 436, 441, 446, 451, 456, 487
M. teres major 192
M. teres minor 177, 187, 192, 197, 202, 207, 212, 217, 227
M. thenaris 483
M. thyreohyoideus 125, 130, 135
M. tibialis anterior 494, 497, 499, 501
M. tibialis posterior 494, 497, 499, 501
M. transversus abdominis 320, 325, 330, 335, 340, 345, 350, 355, 360, 365, 370, 381, 386, 391, 396, 436
M. trapezius 95, 100, 105, 110, 115, 120, 125, 130, 135, 140, 145, 150, 162, 167, 172, 177, 182, 187, 192, 197, 202, 207, 212, 217, 222, 227, 232, 237, 242, 247, 257, 262, 267, 272
M. triceps brachii 187, 192, 197
M. triceps brachii: Caput laterale 469, 471, 473
M. triceps brachii: Caput longum 177, 469, 471, 473
M. triceps brachii: Caput mediale 469, 471, 473
M. vastus intermedius 421, 426, 431, 487, 489
M. vastus lateralis 421, 426, 431, 451, 456, 487, 489
M. vastus medialis 431, 456, 487, 489, 492
Myoma uteri 555, 556, 557
Myositis ossificans 510, 511, 512

Nasus 67, 70
N. accessorius 95, 100, 105, 110, 115, 120, 125
N. cutaneus antebrachii medialis 471, 473
N. dorsalis clitoridis 426
N. facialis 85, 90
N. femoralis 381, 386, 391, 396, 401, 406, 411, 416, 421, 426, 431, 436, 441, 446, 451, 456
N. fibularis superficialis 494, 497, 499, 501
N. glossopharyngeus 85, 95, 105, 120
N. hypoglossus 85, 90, 95, 100, 105, 110, 115, 120, 125
N. intercostalis 172, 177, 182, 192, 197, 202, 207, 212, 222, 227, 232, 237, 242, 247, 252, 257, 262, 267, 272, 290, 295, 300, 305, 310, 315, 320, 330, 335, 345
N. ischiadicus 401, 406, 411, 416, 421, 426, 431, 436, 441, 446, 451, 456, 487, 489
N. laryngeus recurrens 135, 140, 145, 150, 162, 167, 172, 177, 182, 192
N. lumbalis 345, 350, 355, 360, 365, 370
N. maxillaris 45
N. medianus 469, 471, 473, 475, 477, 479, 481, 483
N. obturatorius 386, 391, 396, 401, 406, 411, 416, 436, 441
N. phrenicus 130, 135, 140, 145, 172, 177, 182, 187, 192, 197, 202, 207, 212, 217, 222, 227, 232, 237, 242, 247, 252
N. radialis 469, 471, 473, 475, 477, 479
N. sacralis 386, 391, 396
N. saphenus 487, 489
N. splanchnicus major 290, 295, 300, 305, 310, 315, 320, 325, 330, 335
N. thoracicus longus 290, 300
N. tibialis 492, 494, 497, 499, 501
N. ulnaris 469, 471, 473, 475, 477, 479, 481, 483, 495
N. vagus 85, 95, 100, 105, 110, 115, 120, 125, 130, 135, 140, 145, 150, 167, 172, 177, 182, 187, 192, 197, 202, 207, 212, 222, 227, 232, 237, 247, 252, 257, 262, 267, 272
Nucleus caudatus 20, 25, 50, 55
Nucleus lentiformis 20, 25, 50, 55

Obstructive shadow *8*
Oesophagus 140, 145, 150, 162, 167, 172, 174, 177, 179, 182, 187, 192, 197, 202, 207, 212, 217, 219, 222, 227, 232, 237, 242, 247, 252, 257, 262, 267, 272, 273, 274, 275, 276, 277, 278
Olecranon 475
Omentum majus 320, 325, 330, 335, 340, 345
Orbita 32, 35, 37, 42, 52, 57, 62, 67, 70
Orbitomeatal line *15, 17, 19, 21, 23, 25, 27, 29, 31, 241*
Os capitatum 483
Os coccygis 403, 406, 408, 411, 433, 436

Os coxae 403, 406, 408, 411, 433, 436
Os ethmoidale 57, 60
Os frontale: Pars nasalis 37, 40, 42, 45, 57, 60, 62, 65
Os frontale: Pars orbitalis 52, 55, 57, 60
Os frontale: Processus zygomaticus 37, 40, 42, 45, 55, 57, 60
Os frontale: Sinus frontalis 50
Os frontale: Squama frontalis 7, 10, 12, 15, 17, 20, 22, 25, 27, 30, 32, 47, 50, 52, 55
Os hamatum 483
Os hyoideum 122, 125
Os ilium 383, 388, 398, 401,
Os ilium: Crista iliaca 367, 370
Os ischii 413, 416, 418, 421, 423, 426, 438, 441, 443, 446, 448, 451
Os occipitale: Pars basilaris 40, 77, 80, 82, 85, 87
Os occipitale: Squama occipitalis 7, 10, 12, 15, 17, 20, 22, 25, 27, 30, 32, 35, 37, 40, 42, 45, 47, 50, 52, 55, 57, 60, 62, 65, 67, 70, 72, 75, 77, 80, 82, 85, 87, 90, 92, 95
Os parietale 7, 10, 12, 17, 22, 25, 27, 30, 47
Os parietale: Angulus sphenoidalis 32, 35
Os pubis 413, 416, 418, 421, 438, 441, 443, 446.
Os sacrum 378, 381, 383, 386, 388, 391, 393, 396, 398, 401
Os sphenoidale 72
Os sphenoidale: Ala major 32, 42, 45, 57
Os sphenoidale: Corpus 42, 45
Os sphenoidale: Processus pterygoideus 77
Os temporale 15
Os temporale: Pars petrosa 72, 75, 80, 82, 85
Os temporale: Pars squamosa 32, 35, 37, 40, 50, 52, 55, 57, 60, 62, 65, 67, 70
Os temporale: Processus mastoideus 80, 82, 85
Os trapezium 483
Os trapezoideum 483
Os triquetrum 483
Os zygomaticum 72, 75, 77
Os zygomaticum: Processus frontalis 62, 67, 70
Ostium cardiacum 290
Ostium pyloricum 310
Ovarium 401
Overlapping viewing box *302*

Palatum durum 85, 90
Palatum osseum 82
Pancreas cancer 547, 548
Pancreas: Caput pancreatis 312, 315, 322, 325
Pancreas: Corpus pancreatis 297, 300, 302, 305, 307, 310, 317, 320
Paracystium 416
Paraproctium 416, 436
Patella 492
Pedunculus cerebri 40, 65
Pericardium 217, 222, 227
Peritonaeum 381, 406, 411, 436
Peritonaeum parietale 305, 310, 315, 320, 325, 330, 335, 340, 345, 350, 355, 360, 365, 370, 386, 391, 396, 401
Plane g *5, 6, 300, 304*
Platysma 85, 95, 100, 105, 110, 115, 120, 125, 130, 135, 140, 145, 150
Plexus brachialis 120, 130, 135, 140, 145, 150, 162, 167, 172, 177, 182, 187, 192
Plexus cervicalis 100, 105, 110, 115, 125
Plexus chorioideus 20, 25, 30, 35, 50, 80
Plexus chorioideus ventriculi lateralis 65
Plexus chorioideus ventriculi quarti 75
Plexus ischiadicus 391
Plexus prostaticus 446
Plexus venosus prostaticus 441
Plexus venosus rectalis 421
Plexus venosus vaginalis 416, 421, 426
Plexus venosus vesicalis 416, 421, 426
Pons 45, 70, 80
Positioning skin mark 571, 572, 576, *300, 301, 303, 304, 305*
Processus articularis inferior (Th_2) 172
Processus articularis superior (Th_2) 162
Processus articularis superior (Th_3) 172
Processus clinoideus anterior 62, 67
Processus condylaris 77, 80
Processus coronoideus 77, 80
Processus mastoideus 87, 90
Processus pterygoideus 82, 85
Processus spinosus (C_3) 107, 110
Processus spinosus (C_6) 142, 145
Processus spinosus 164, 197, 287, 290, 292, 295, 297, 300, 302, 305, 307, 310, 312, 315, 322, 325, 327, 330, 337, 340, 342, 345, 347, 350, 352, 355, 357, 360, 362, 365, 367, 370, 378, 381
Processus styloideus 87, 90
Processus transversus (C_2) 97, 105
Processus transversus (C_7) 142, 145
Processus transversus (Th_1) 147, 150
Processus transversus (Th_2) 167
Processus transversus (Th_3) 172
Processus transversus 159, 287, 307, 310, 317, 322, 332, 347, 357, 362, 365, 367, 370
Processus xiphoideus 262

Promontorium 378, 381
Prostata 441, 446
Protuberantia occipitalis externa 87, 90
Protuberantia occipitalis interna 42, 72, 75, 77, 80, 85, 87
Pulmo dexter 164, 169, 174, 179, 184, 189, 194, 199, 204, 209, 214, 219, 224, 229, 234, 239, 244, 249, 254, 259, 264, 269, 290
Pulmo dexter: Apex pulmonis 159, 162
Pulmo dexter: Lobus inferior 187, 192, 197, 202, 207, 212, 217, 222, 227, 232, 237, 242, 252, 257, 262, 267, 272
Pulmo dexter: Lobus medius 227, 232, 237, 242, 252, 257, 262
Pulmo dexter: Lobus superior 167, 172, 177, 182, 187, 192, 197, 202, 207, 212, 217, 222, 227
Pulmo sinister 164, 169, 174, 179, 184, 189, 194, 199, 204, 209, 214, 219, 224, 229, 234, 239, 244, 249, 254, 259, 264, 269, 290
Pulmo sinister: Apex pulmonis 159, 162
Pulmo sinister: Lobus inferior 187, 192, 197, 202, 207, 212, 217, 222, 227, 232, 237, 242, 247, 252, 257, 262, 267, 272
Pulmo sinister: Lobus superior 167, 172, 177, 182, 187, 192, 197, 202, 207, 212, 217, 222, 227, 232, 237, 242, 252, 257, 262

Radius 477, 479, 481
Radix linguae 100, 105
R. profundus n. radialis 477
R. superficialis n. radialis 477
Rectum 398, 401, 403, 406, 408, 411, 416, 421, 433, 436, 438, 441, 443, 446, 451, 459, 460
Ren dexter 312, 315, 317, 320, 322, 325, 327, 330, 332, 335, 337, 340, 342, 345, 347, 350, 352, 355
Ren sinister 302, 305, 307, 310, 312, 315, 317, 320, 322, 325, 327, 330, 332, 335, 337, 340, 342, 345, 347, 350
Retinaculum patellae laterale 492
Retinaculum patellae mediale 492
Rima pudendi 428, 431
Rotation center: Axial transverse tomograph *8*
Rotation center: Radiation therapy unit 574, *301, 302*
Rotation radiography *1*

Sarcoidosis 532, 533, 534
Scapula 137, 140, 142, 145
Scapula: Acromion 147, 150
Scapula: Angulus inferior 229, 232
Scapula: Angulus superior 159, 162
Scapula: Facies costalis 172, 182, 202, 207, 212, 217, 222, 227
Scapula: Fossa infraspinata 172, 202, 207, 212, 217, 222, 227
Scapula: Margo lateralis 169, 174, 177, 179, 182, 184, 187, 189, 192, 194, 197, 199, 202, 204, 207, 209, 212, 214, 217, 219, 222, 224, 227
Scapula: Margo medialis 147, 150, 169, 174, 177, 179, 182, 184, 187, 189, 192, 194, 197, 199, 202, 204, 207, 209, 212, 214, 217, 219, 222, 224, 227
Scapula: Margo superior 150
Scapula: Spina scapulae 147, 150
Scrotum 453, 456
Septum nasi 70, 75, 77, 80
Simulator *303, 304*
Sinus costomediastinalis 232, 237, 242, 247
Sinus frontalis 27, 30, 32, 35, 45, 47, 52, 55,
Sinus maxillaris 72, 75, 77, 80
Sinus occipitalis 85
Sinus petrosus superior 45
Sinus rectus 75
Sinus sagittalis inferior 50
Sinus sagittalis superior 10, 15, 20, 25, 30, 35, 50, 55, 60, 65, 75
Sinus sigmoideus 75, 80, 85, 90
Sinus sphenoidalis 37, 40, 42, 45, 62, 65, 70, 72, 75
Spatium retrooesophageum 140
Spatium retropharyngeum 90, 97, 100, 102, 105, 107, 110, 112, 115, 117, 120, 122, 125, 130
Spina scapulae 164, 167, 199, 202, 204, 207, 209, 212
Sulcus lateralis 50
Sulcus parietooccipitalis 25
Suprarenal cyst 549, 550
Symphysis pubica 418, 421, 438, 441, 443, 446

Talus 501
Tendo calcaneus (Achillis) 501
Tendo musculi bicipitis brachii 475, 477
Tentorium cerebelli 70, 80, 85
Thalamus 20, 30, 55, 60
Thickening of the periosteum 560, 561, 562, 563
Thorotrast liver 551, 552
Tonsilla palatina 85, 90
Tonsilla pharyngea 102, 105

Trachea 142, 145, 147, 150, 159, 162, 164, 167, 169, 172, 174, 177, 179, 182, 184, 187, 189, 192, 194, 197, 199, 202
Tractus iliotibialis 489, 492
Trochlea humeri 475
Truncus brachiocephalicus 177, 182
Truncus coeliacus 310, 315, 320
Truncus lumbosacralis 381
Truncus pulmonalis 217, 222, 227
Truncus sympathicus 95, 100, 105, 110, 115, 120, 125, 130, 135, 140, 145, 150, 162, 167, 172, 177, 182, 187, 192, 197, 202, 207, 212, 217, 222, 227, 232, 237, 242, 247, 252, 257, 262, 267, 272, 290, 295, 340, 345, 350, 355, 360, 365, 370
Tuba uterina 401
Tuberculous calcification of the mesenteric lymph nodes 553, 554
Tuberculous cavity of the lung 516, 517, 518, 519, 520
Tumor of the thyroid 513, 514, 515

Ulna 477, 479, 481
Umbilicus 352, 355, 357, 360
Ureter 335, 340, 345, 350, 355, 360, 365, 370, 381, 386, 391, 396, 401, 406, 411, 436, 458, 459, 460, 463
Urethra 421, 426, 441, 446, 451, 456

Vagina 408, 411, 413, 416, 418, 421, 423, 426
Vallecula cerebri lateralis 55
Vanishing tumor 535, 536, 537
Vas lymphaticum 471, 475, 477, 497, 501
Vasa brachialia 469
Vasa interossea anteriora 479
Vasa lymphatica 473, 479, 481, 483, 487, 497, 499
Vasa radialia 477
Vasa tibialis anteriora 494
Vasa ulnaria 477
V. axillaris 167, 172, 177, 182, 187, 192, 197
V. azygos 207, 212, 217, 222, 227, 232, 237, 242, 247, 252, 257, 262, 267, 272, 290, 295, 300, 305, 310, 315, 320
V. basilica 469, 471, 473, 475, 477, 479, 481
V. brachialis 473, 475
V. brachiocephalica 172, 177, 182
V. cava inferior 237, 242, 247, 249, 252, 254, 257, 259, 262, 267, 272, 287, 290, 292, 295, 297, 300, 302, 305, 307, 310, 312, 315, 317, 320, 322, 325, 327, 330, 332, 335, 337, 340, 342, 345, 347, 350, 352, 355, 357, 360, 362, 365, 367, 370, 381
V. cava superior 184, 187, 189, 192, 194, 197, 199, 202, 204, 207, 212, 217, 222, 227
V. cephalica 469, 471, 473, 475, 477, 479, 481
V. cerebri interna 30, 60
V. cerebri magna 65
V. circumflexa femoris lateralis 451
V. dorsalis clitoridis 426
V. dorsalis pedis 501
V. facialis 100, 105, 120
V. femoralis 416, 421, 426, 431, 441, 446, 451, 456, 487, 489
V. gastrica sinistra 300
V. glutea inferior 406, 411, 416, 436, 441, 446, 451, 456
V. hemiazygos 232, 237, 242, 247, 252, 257, 262, 267, 272
V. iliaca communis 381, 386
V. iliaca externa 391, 396, 401, 406, 411, 436
V. iliaca interna 391, 396, 401, 406, 411, 436
V. intercostalis 172, 177, 182, 192, 197, 202, 207, 212, 222, 227, 232, 237, 242, 247, 252, 257, 262, 267, 272, 290, 295, 300, 305, 310, 315, 320, 330, 335, 345
V. jugularis externa 105, 110, 115, 120, 125, 130, 135, 140, 145, 150
V. jugularis interna 85, 90, 95, 100, 105, 110, 112, 115, 120, 122, 125, 127, 130, 132, 135, 140, 145, 147, 150, 162, 167,
V. lienalis 300, 305
V. lingualis 125
V. lumbalis 335, 340, 345
V. lumbalis ascendens 325, 330
V. mesenterica superior 325, 330, 335, 345
V. obturatorius 416, 436, 441
V. peronea 497, 499
V. poplitea 492
V. portae 300, 310
V. profunda femoris 487
V. pudenda interna 416, 421, 426, 441, 446, 451, 456
V. pulmonalis 229, 232
V. radialis 479
V. rectalis superior 401, 406
V. renalis 320, 322, 325, 327, 330
V. retromandibularis 85, 90, 95, 100, 105, 110, 115
V. sacralis lateralis 386, 391, 396
V. sacralis mediana 401
V. saphena magna 487, 489, 492, 494, 497, 499
V. saphena parva 494, 497, 499

V. subclavia 162
V. thoracica interna 172, 177, 182, 187, 192, 197, 202, 207, 212, 217, 222, 227, 232, 237, 242, 247, 252, 257
V. tibialis anterior 497, 499
V. tibialis posterior 494, 499, 501
V. ulnaris 479, 481
V. uterina 401
V. vertebralis 100, 105, 110, 115, 120, 125, 130, 135, 140, 145, 150
Ventriculus 267, 307, 310
Ventriculus: Corpus ventriculi 292, 295, 297, 300
Ventriculus dexter 232, 237, 242, 247, 252, 257, 262
Ventriculus: Pars cardiaca 287, 290
Ventriculus: Pars pylorica 302, 305
Ventriculus lateralis 30, 35
Ventriculus lateralis: Cornu anterius 17, 20, 22, 25, 47, 50, 55
Ventriculus lateralis: Cornu posterius 20, 25, 50, 55, 60
Ventriculus lateralis: Pars centralis 12, 15
Ventriculus quartus 75, 80, 85
Ventriculus sinister 232, 237, 242, 247, 252, 257, 262
Ventriculus tertius 17, 20, 27, 57
Vermis cerebelli 45, 70, 85, 90
Vertebra lumbalis (L_5) 378
Vesica fellea 302, 305
Vesica urinaria 398, 401, 403, 406, 408, 411, 413, 416, 433, 436, 459, 460, 464, 465
Vestibulum laryngis 132, 135

Wedge grid *6*

Universitätsdruckerei H. Stürtz AG Würzburg